Family Nursing as Relational Inquiry

Developing Health-Promoting Practice

Family Nursing as Relational Inquiry

Developing Health-Promoting Practice

Gweneth Hartrick Doane, RN, PhD

Associate Professor
School of Nursing
University of Victoria
Victoria, British Columbia,
Canada

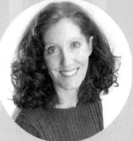

Colleen Varcoe, RN, PhD

Associate Professor
School of Nursing
University of Victoria,
Lower Mainland Campus
Vancouver, British Columbia,
Canada

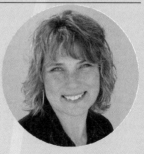

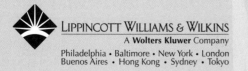

LIPPINCOTT WILLIAMS & WILKINS
A **Wolters Kluwer** Company
Philadelphia • Baltimore • New York • London
Buenos Aires • Hong Kong • Sydney • Tokyo

Acquisitions Editor: Margaret Zuccarini
Managing Editor: Helen Kogut
Editorial Assistant: Delema Caldwell-Jordan
Project Management: TechBooks
Director of Nursing Production: Helen Ewan
Art Director: Carolyn O'Brien
Design: BJ Crim
Cover Design: BJ Crim
Senior Manufacturing Manager: William Alberti
Compositor: TechBooks
Printer: Data Reproductions Corporation

9 8 7 6

ISBN 13: 978-0-7817-4841-4
ISBN 10: 0-7817-4841-0

Library of Congress Cataloging-in-Publication Data

Doane, Gweneth Hartrick, 1954–
  Family nursing as relational inquiry : developing health-promoting
practice / Gweneth Hartrick Doane, Colleen Varcoe.
      p.   cm.
  Includes bibliographical references and index.
  ISBN 0-7817-4841-0
  1. Family nursing.   2. Family nursing—Philosophy.   I. Varcoe, Colleen, 1952–   II. Title.
RT120.F34D63 2004
610.73—dc22

                                                        2004021490

LWW.com

To my children, Adrian, Taylor, and Teresa, with whom I share love, life, and laughter—and the joy of family.

And to my Aunt, Lucille Meaney, RN (1954), who lived the nursing ideals I aspire toward and who, through example, was the one to teach me what nursing was 'really' all about.

Gweneth

To my grandmother, Elizabeth Mosher (1885–1986), for lending me the courage, faith, and strength to survive the hard spots of family.

To my children, Alex, Megan, and Aaron, and my partner, Jim, who make the idea of family surpass my greatest hopes.

Colleen

Reviewers

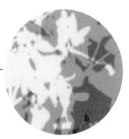

Jan Andrews, RNC, PhD
Associate Professor, Nursing
    International Liaison
School of Health Sciences
Georgia College & State University
Milledgeville, Georgia

Sharon Jackson Barton,
    RN, PhD
Professor
University of Kentucky
Lexington, Kentucky

Elizabeth Bethune
Senior Lecturer, Associate Head School
    of Nursing
Deakin University
Burwood, Victoria, Australia

Terry Buford, RN, PhD, CPNP
Assistant Professor
University of Missouri School of
    Nursing
Kansas City, Missouri

Martha M. Colvin, PhD, RN
Professor & Chair, Dept of Family
    Health
Georgia College & State University
Milledgeville, Georgia

Gail Diachuk, RN, MN
Professor
Athabasca University
Athabasca, Alberta, Canada

Kathleen Gates, RN, BScN, MHSc,
    EdD
Professor
Ryerson University
Toronto, Ontario, Canada

Norma Goldie, RN, BSN, MA
Instructor
Douglas College Nursing Department
New Westminster, British Columbia,
    Canada

Kristen A. Gulbransen, BScN, MN
Faculty of Nursing
Red Deer College
Alberta, Canada

Deborah K. Hartman, MSN, RN, CS
Professor
Millersville University
Millersville, Pennsylvania

Lynn Van Hofwegen, RN, MS, ARNP-C
Assistant Professor of Nursing
Trinity Western University
Langley, British Columbia, Canada

Joanne Kaakinen, PhD, RN
Associate Professor
University of Portland
Portland, Oregon

Judith C. Kulig, RN, DNSc
Professor
School of Health Sciences University of
    Lethbridge
Lethbridge, Alberta, Canada

Anne Marie Levac, RN, MN
Lecturer, Faculty of Nursing
University of Toronto
Toronto, Ontario, Canada

Heather Meyerhoff, MSN, RN
Assistant Professor of Nursing
Trinity Western University
Langley, British Columbia, Canada

Dianne Cooney Miner, PhD, RN, CNS
Associate Dean Undergraduate
    Programs
Decker School of Nursing
Binghamton University
Binghamton, New York

Yvonne Moore, RNBN, MSc (MFT)
Associate Professor, Faculty of Nursing
Okanagan University College
Kelowna, British Columbia, Canada

Verna C. Pangman, RN, MEd, MN
Lecturer, Faculty of Nursing
University of Manitoba
Winnipeg, Manitoba, Canada

Maureen Parkes, RN, BScN, MEd
Nurse Educator
Malaspina University College
Nanaimo, British Columbia, Canada

Cindy Peternelj-Taylor, RN, MSc
Professor
College of Nursing
University of Saskatchewan
Saskatoon, Saskatchewan, Canada

Marcia Van Riper, RN, PhD
Associate Professor, Joint Position-
    School of Nursing & Center for
    Home Science
University of North Carolina
Chapel Hill, North Carolina

Sylvia Streitberger, RN, MN, RMFT
Instructor of Nursing, Calgary Health
    Region Family Therapy Training
    Program Adjunct
Faculty Member
Red Deer College
Red Deer, Alberta, Canada

Judy Yarwood, RGON, MA (Hons), Dip Tchg (Tertiary), MCNA (NZ)
Principal Lecturer
Christchurch Polytechnic Institute
    of Technology
Christchurch, New Zealand

FOREWORD

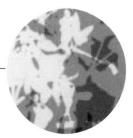

Nurses have always worried about which aspects of our work were reproducing the social injustices implicated in health disparities. Because many of us are women, we've worried a great deal about sexism; because too many of us are white, we've worried too little about racism. Because the bulk of the scholarship has come from the United States, where almost any meaningful criticism of a class system is impossible, nursing's participation in class-based inequities is hardly mentioned. Widespread homophobia has dampened debate about heteronormativity. The intersection of all of these with various forms of Western imperialism and colonialism has entered the conversation relatively recently.

Yet each of these generalizations are patently false because they assume a 'center' from which the extent of the discussion is appraised. People who have been denied entry into our field, who are denied access to health care, who have suffered our arrogance, blindness and selfishness have not been "quiet," not "without voice." But they have often been without an audience in nursing and in academic nursing.

Even those of us in academic nursing who have struggled to get clearer about these issues, to understand our participation in them, to be an audience for those criticisms, have been carrying on a fairly quiet conversation. Few of us expected it to erupt in basic nursing textbooks and perhaps next-to-last (after 'medical-surgical') in textbooks about "the family," that mythical, ideological formation with which we have often aligned our professionalist agendas.

Doane and Varcoe have made an intelligent, courageous and gentle effort to achieving just that: a "family nursing" textbook through which student nurses are invited to be that audience, to understand the inseparability of their own lives, the illness care system and enduring historical and structural injustices. At the same time, they are coached into seeing their practice as a form of inquiry into these relationships, not a pulpit of righteousness nor a confessional of guilt and despair.

"The family" is just a phrase, nine letters on a page. In modern parlance, a "floating signifier" that is mobilized in service of myriad conflicting values and political commitments. As I write these words today, in the U.S., the paroxysms over "gay marriage" are just the most recent site of struggle over who gets to define "the family" and whose interests that definition will serve. In my own nursing education, some thirty years ago, a favorite book that helped balance the pablum fed to us as "nursing theory" about "the family" was The Anti-Social Family by Barrett and McIntosh. One of their arguments is that if "the family" were such a "natural" and positive site of human relationships that it's often made out to be, capitalism and the state wouldn't have to work so hard to undermine every other form of collective life and enact everything from tax laws to mortgage qualifications that compel people to remain in them. The same argument has been made about women and heterosexual marriage.

Given my own personal and social awareness of "families"—that most violence happened there, that they were sites of meanness and stunted development as much as they were nurturance, that they made (white middle class) men seem "independent" and autonomous while we stood on the backs of women, and that they were fundamentally anti-democratic in terms of character development—I found nursing's untroubled alliance with "the family" alarming and alienating. As I learned more about the historical and colonialist imposition of that social unit on other cultures (such as American Indians), I grew ever more wary.

At the same time, most of my clients (and, of course, many parts of myself) were deeply committed to keeping families "whole," and health care increasing shifted expensive labor for chronic care onto "families." In many ways, you were in deep trouble if you didn't have one.

That's what I most appreciate about this textbook: that it sustains a very complex and historical understanding about how this form of social organization became omnipresent *and* remains compassionate and open-minded about those who embrace it—as students, as nurses, as patients. But students who are fortunate to be assigned this text—in contrast to the vast genre of "family" textbooks—will be equipped to think complexly about their role in supporting or resisting any configuration of affiliation and shared labor. And no doubt will have their understandings of their own social histories made more rich and dynamic.

I just wish I'd had it in my "family nursing" courses.

David G Allen, PhD
Professor, Psychosocial & Community Health
University of Washington
Seattle, Washington
(August, 2004)

Preface

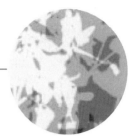

● Notes to Teachers

A Note of Invitation

Thank you for picking up this book. . . . We want to invite you to join us in making this book useful to nursing students at a wide range of places in their learning. For that reason, we thought it might be helpful if we highlighted and/or explained a few things about the book and how we have approached the presentation of family nursing content.

A Note on Pedagogy

As educators we have approached the book through a constructive-developmental pedagogy (Magolda, 1999). Constructive-developmental pedagogy seeks to create opportunities for students to learn not only content but also the process of knowledge construction and to practice that knowledge construction process within their everyday practice. We believe that for nursing students to become safe and competent practitioners they must develop the ability to be self-initiating, self-correcting, and self-evaluating in each practice moment. They must, as Kegan (1994) describes, be able to take responsibility for what happens, to be guided by their own visions and make informed decisions in conjunction with families and coworkers and within the complexities of health care situations.

    As a result of these underlying assumptions and educational goals, we believe that nursing and nursing knowledge must be presented in all of its complexity. As nurse educators we believe it is our responsibility to create opportunities for students of all levels (and especially undergraduate and/or beginning students) to experience the complex and messy world of nursing work with families and to learn how to navigate through it. Subsequently, rather than simplifying and/or reducing the complexity of either the theoretical ideas or practice examples we present in this book, we have purposefully written the book in such a way that invites learners into the complexity. We see ourselves in partnership with the students who might read this book and with you as their instructors. We intend the book to open up opportunities for you to be with students to explore the uncertain and complex terrain of family nursing and to help them develop the skills and confidence to navigate through such complexity.

It is important to be clear that we believe there is no theory or concept that is too difficult for a first year nursing student to grasp.[1] For that reason rather than simplifying and/or reducing the complexity of ideas or concepts we have attempted to present them in such a way that allows readers of all levels to make meaning of them and to be able to link them to their everyday nursing experiences. Pedagogical strategies we have used to help us do so include introducing the concepts and then building and further elaborating on those concepts gradually throughout the book. This strategy has implications for the way that you as a teacher use this book. Because concepts are built on throughout the book, the book makes most sense when read from the beginning. That is, a chapter later in the book will build on ideas, examples, and learning activities from earlier chapters. We suggest using the book by assigning each chapter in sequence.

A Note on Learning

Throughout the book we attempt to model and cultivate the development of 'self-authorship' (Magolda, 1999). Self-authorship is the ability to construct knowledge in the contextual moment. It involves the ability to articulate one's own perspective and to not lose one's center when coming in contact with external influences. The development of self-authorship involves learning at the cognitive level (making meaning of knowledge), at the interpersonal level (awareness of oneself in relationship to others), and at the intrapersonal level (self-consciousness) (Magolda, 1999). To that end, in contrast to many family nursing textbooks, we have not delineated a predetermined structured process of family nursing assessment or intervention for students to follow. Rather we have attempted to invite students to freely examine the theories and processes in light of their own beliefs, values, and practice. For students to become self-authoring nurses we believe it is vital that they engage in their own knowledge construction process and examine their own personal experience, their values and assumptions, and their nursing knowledge within the uncertainty of nursing situations. In our work as educators and consultants we have found that all levels of students have the capacity and ability for such work. At the same time we have found that prestructured processes often contravene such a knowledge construction process and subsequently hinders the development of self-authoring skills. Throughout the book we model self-authoring by presenting examples of our own evolving process of self-authorship.

A Note about Research, Theory, and Nursing Literature That Has Informed This Book

We feel it is important to highlight that we do not think of any literature as 'outdated'. Rather, we approach any existing knowledge and writing in

---

[1] The assumption that some theories are too abstract or difficult for beginning students to learn has been challenged by many in the field of postsecondary education (Doane, 2002; Hudspith & Jenkins, 2001; Kenny, 1998; Magolda, 1999; Palmer, 1998; Stables, 2003). We concur with these educators who contend that students of all levels have the capacity to engage with complex material if it is presented in a meaningful way and if teachers provide the needed support to help students make meaning of the concepts.

terms of its contribution. For that reason if you peruse the reference list you will notice that we have purposefully chosen to include not only very recent literature or research but literature spanning several decades. One of our central goals in this book is to invite a rethinking of family nursing. To achieve that goal we have found it necessary to turn to numerous writers in nursing and other disciplines. The literature we cite ranges from classic writings of pragmatist philosophers dating back to the early 1900s to literature in nursing and other disciplines from the past three decades, to research that is currently in process. This range of literature in many ways reflects the evolution that has occurred in the nursing world and highlights how this book is only possible because of the valuable work that has been done by many others in nursing throughout the past decades.

As we have attempted to articulate our perspective, we have drawn on rich and varied theoretical traditions, including phenomenological thought, feminist thought, critical thought, and so on. Some of the schools of thought on which we have drawn may be seen to be opposed to other schools of thought we have used, variety that is exactly suited to our purpose. Our intent is not to create a coherent whole but to present various theoretical perspectives as lenses. What we offer are the meanings that the ideas have had for our practice and how we see the ideas as relevant to family nursing. We hope that this approach will be useful to you in sharing with students various ways of seeing the world and in developing critical-thinking skills.

We have chosen to take a 'cross-sectional' approach to some of the 'traditional' areas of family nursing. That is, we have addressed the concerns that might be most salient to nurses working with particular groups (for example, childbearing families, grieving families, or families with children with chronic illnesses) *throughout the book*. We hope that this will make for a more coherent and comprehensive approach than if we had addressed such concerns in relation to particular groups.

A Note on Special Features and Learning Activities

In order to support the understanding of complex concepts we have included various learning activities that can be incorporated into activities in classrooms, in clinical settings, online, or in other teaching-learning settings.

- **Chapter Notes** At the end of each chapter, we pose three questions for the students/readers to respond to. These questions can be used by instructors for discussion purposes and/or by students to note important learning and track ideas they may want to follow up.
- **Try It Out** The Try It Out sections are learning activities that feature a range of ways of engaging with the content in the chapter. Typically we have three or four per chapter.
- **This Week In Practice** Each chapter has a learning activity, near the end of the chapter, that integrates the ideas presented in the chapter and draws on readers' past or current practice experiences.
- **An Example** This feature presents a story that illustrates a point being made in the text. Often we return to the story in the chapter in which it is presented, and in subsequent chapters.

- **To Illustrate** This feature focuses on a particular idea that illustrates some larger and more general argument. So, for example, we focus on the media as an example of how ideas are shaped by broader contexts.

Although we have written the book for the individual reader, we hope that individuals will learn together with colleagues or classmates. To that end, our Try It Out activities and suggestions for This Week In Practice often incorporate ideas for working together, with the hope that teachers will expand these creatively. We have also incorporated art into each chapter with the intention that teachers might use the art to create learning activities. For example, in the first chapter we include a picture of men, some of whom are in wheelchairs. This image of family could be used as a spring board or catalyst to envision and explore a range of alternate images of families. For example, students could be invited to offer their own images. They could take their own photos or create images or collages from various sources. The art we have offered could be used in relation to particular concepts. For example, students could be invited to write responses to particular images, using a relevant concept. Our hope is that you will use the book in conjunction with your own unique teaching skills in a way that enhances both!

A Note of Thanks

We appreciate that your use of the book will determine its relevance and so we thank you for joining us in this work.

REFERENCES

Doane, G. (2002). In the spirit of creativity: The learning and teaching of ethics in nursing. *Journal of Advanced Nursing,*

Hudspith, B., & Jenkins, H. (2001). *Teaching the art of inquiry.* Halifax, NS: Society for Teaching and Learning in Higher Education.

Kegan, R. (1994). *In over our heads: The mental demands of modern life.* Cambridge MA: Harvard University Press.

Kenny, R. W. (1998). *Reinventing undergraduate education: A blueprint for America's research universities.* The Boyer Commission on Educating Undergraduates in the Research University. Stony Brook: State University of New York at Stony Brook.

Magolda, M. (1999). Creating contexts for learning and self-authorship. *Constructive-Developmental Pedagogy.*

Palmer, P. (1998). *The courage to teach: Exploring the inner landscape of a teacher's life* (1st ed.). San Francisco: Jossey-Bass.

Stables, A. (2003). From discrimination to deconstruction: Four modulations of criticality in the humanities and social sciences. *Assessment and Evaluation in Higher Education, 28*(6), 665–672.

ACKNOWLEDGMENTS

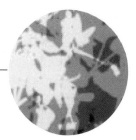

We would like to express our thanks:

To all the families who we have known and with whom we have worked—you have been instrumental in our learning.

To all of our students, from whom we continuously learn.

To all the nurses with whom we have worked over the years, you have inspired us and contributed to our understanding of family nursing.

To the people who offered their stories of health and health care experiences in this book—Gary and Lynn Fjellgaard, Helene Jospe and Dana Perlman, Helen Brown, Zoe, Lindsey, Jan and Mikaela Graham-Radford, Sheila Dick and Janet Munro.

To nursing students and colleagues who shared experiences, stories, insights, and other resources—including Mary Cleland, Susan Connolly, Maureen Murphy-Dyson, Inge Kaasteen, Robin McMillan, Nancy Moules, Valerie Olynyk, Janet Rankin, Camille Roberts, Diane Tran, Coby Tschanz, the public health nurse team members from the Northern Health Region of British Columbia, and the nurses who have worked with us in our ethics research team.

To our colleagues who have offered their encouragement, support, and critical feedback during our writing: Jinny Hayes, Rose Steele, Mary Kruger.

To the many faculty, students, and practicing nurses in New Zealand whose stories and questions convinced me (Gweneth) that it was time to write this book, and especially to Helen Nielsen, Trish Wright, and Sally Greenwood who arranged my visits and shared time, ideas, and laughter with me.

To the artists who offered their images and imagination.

About the Artists

Danaca Ackerson is a visual artist living with her family in Vancouver, Canada. She received her BFA from the Emily Carr Intitute of Art and Design in Vancouver and also studied art at the Universidad Politecnica de Valencia, Spain. Her interest in colour, pattern, and the human condition are reflected in her paintings. Danaca works with childbearing families as a registered nurse at the Children's & Women's Health Centre of British Columbia.

Fiona Raven is a book designer living in Vancouver, Canada. Photography is one of her passions. She experiments with image creation both in the darkroom and digitally. Her focus has been on black-and-white portraits, but recently she has branched out into color photography and combining images into collage and photomontage.

Jocelyne Robinson's process is to experiment with ideas, materials, and techniques that both challenge and reorder her understanding of our social environment. She creates sculptures that are influenced by her early years growing up playing in the sawdust fields in a French logging town. Jocelyne uses sawdust shapes, pulp, paper, print, and a mix of techniques as a metaphor for the layered memories and coexisting hybrids of visible/invisible boundaries that we continually negotiate among our social landscapes. The physical interplay between shapes and forms in her work evokes metaphorically the capacity we have to coexist and achieve an aesthetic of *balance* and *beauty* among the fragmented memories of our shared environment.

Gayle Allison is a registered nurse with 23 years of experience, who studied visual arts at the Emily Carr Institute of Art and Design. Gayle actively explores the idea of art in her life. The photographs seen in this book are part of a photo-documentation process Gayle engaged in while providing care for her mother during a period of convalescence at home following total hip surgery.

Connie Sabo's sculpture and mixed media work explores the connections between her Chinese ancestry and the culture of the Canadian west coast. She was born and raised in Vancouver and lives in Burnaby with her husband and two daughters.

Alex Grewal is a recent graduate of Emily Carr Institute receiving a bachelor of visual arts. Alex is a painter, sculptor, and photographer and is currently painting abstract and process-oriented paintings but goes back to figurative work.

Len Budiwski works mainly in sculptural assemblages and installations with occasional forays into photography. His work ranges in scale from the very small to entire environments involving the combining and transformation of a large diversity of materials.

CONTENTS

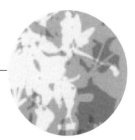

1

Rethinking
Family Nursing
Knowledge

1 The Living Experience of Family Nursing

OVERVIEW

In Chapter 1 we begin by locating ourselves philosophically, theoretically, and practically as the writers and by describing how we have located you as the reader. We outline some of the major premises and goals of this book and invite you to begin your study of family nursing by examining your current habits of knowing.

Perhaps the biggest challenge in writing a book on family nursing is to know where to start. One could begin by defining the terms—what it is we mean when we speak of family, of health, of nursing practice. Or one could begin with theory—presenting the latest theoretical perspectives that govern the domain of family nursing. In contemplating this question of where to start, it seemed to us that the way we have come to *know* family nursing is by experiencing it. As Paterson and Zderad (1988) described, nursing is an experience lived between people. In its very essence, family nursing is a relational living experience. Although definitions and theories offer knowledge that can help us in our work with families (and we will certainly get to these), they do not reveal what it is like to live family nursing—to navigate through the complexity and challenges of each new situation. Theories do not illuminate what we as nurses experience as we strive to 'do good' and 'do the right thing' within the uncertainty of any nursing moment.

As nurses who have lived this experience, we have had the opportunity, each in our own way, to try on and try out countless theories and approaches in our desire to enhance our nursing practice. Our experiences have led us to view particular perspectives as more relevant and helpful than others and we have drawn on those perspectives in the writing of this book. Because we are inviting you to join us in an examination of family nursing, it is important for us to be explicit about the values, assumptions, and theories that guide us and also about how we have gone about choosing what to include and what not to include. Therefore, we have decided to begin by articulating where we are located philosophically, theoretically, and practically and to share with you as we proceed our experience of family nursing. We also explicitly describe how we have located you as a learner/reader.

● Locating Ourselves

Examining the Cartesian View

The typical Western view of knowledge and truth is often termed the Cartesian view because the ideas of René Descartes, a French philosopher and mathematician, underpin much of Western thinking. Within this Cartesian view of knowledge, it is assumed that mind and body are distinct and separate entities (for example, we can separate 'mental illness' from 'physical' illness). Parallel to this notion of mind and body as separate is the idea that subjective knowledge can be separated from objective knowledge. For example, it is assumed that we can separate ourselves from our own feelings or interpretations and make assessments in a rational, objective way. Truth and knowledge are therefore considered to be detached and separate from human beings and contexts. And, from this Cartesian view, objective truth is considered not only possible but also desirable (for example, think of the saying 'Don't let your emotions rule your head').

'Objective truth' is also assumed to be universal (there is one truth/reality) and generalizable (between people and contexts). That is, it is assumed that people can determine 'the truth' by looking at the 'facts'—what can be seen, heard, smelled, tasted, or verified in some concrete way—and that those facts are the same regardless of who is doing the knowing. For example, from this perspective, it doesn't matter which nurse assesses a family because it is assumed that assessment is objective; therefore, any two nurses would come to the same truth and conclusions about the family. Similarly, from a Cartesian perspective, it is presumed that the facts are unchangeable from context to context, so what is known about a family is transferable to all situations. Overall, if a nurse was assessing a family through a Cartesian lens of objectivity, the nurse would be attempting to come to the one true interpretation of the family—namely one objective truth based on the facts.

In thinking critically about this view of knowledge as objective and universal, it is likely that many of you could identify times when this assumption does not hold up—times when there has seemed to be more than one truth. For example, if you have ever asked people to tell you about a movie they have seen, you will have likely heard different things from different people about the same movie—different versions regarding what the movie was about, whether it was good or not good, and so forth. Although each person has seen the same movie, each has experienced it, and come to know it, quite differently. They each offer a different truth about the movie and you are left with multiple truths to sort through when deciding whether you will see the movie or not.

We have found our nursing work to be similar. That is, rather than being able to determine one clear truth, we most often find ourselves in complex situations where there are multiple truths (interpretations, experiences, perspectives). Yet because the Cartesian view of knowledge has dominated the scientific world, including the world of nursing, knowledge and practice are often taken up as though there is one truth or certainty to find and follow. If you observe how many nurses and other health care professionals go about their work, it becomes apparent that health care knowledge and practice are often grounded in the notion of a Cartesian objective truth. For example, families are assessed by expert (objective) professionals whose job it is to come up with an accurate problem definition or diagnosis (objective truth). Similarly, in learning about family nursing, students are often taught to follow formalized models of assessment and intervention in an objective way (Hartrick, 2002).

Limitations of Objective Knowledge

Although there is no doubt that expert knowledge (such as that expressed in nursing theory, biomedical knowledge, and so on) can inform our nursing practice, what is problematic is that, based on the notion of an objective truth, expert knowledge is often taken up and used as though it represents the complete reality of families. For example, when a nurse assesses a family it is assumed that the conclusions the nurse reaches reflect the truth or reality of the family's health and healing situation. This is problematic because often objective knowledge of a family is limited. In many ways, objective knowledge is surface knowledge in that it most often reveals only what can be externally accessed. Objective knowledge is knowledge 'about' things (Thayer-Bacon, 2003) and thus does not penetrate into inner depths and/or ever-changing aspects of family health and healing. In addition, because objective knowledge arises from a detached observer (the objective nurse), it is often decontextualized and depersonalized knowledge. As James (1907) contended, the detached objective way of approaching knowing and knowledge may result in the ability to name objects but it does not allow us to come to know human experience in any depth.

The limitations of objective knowledge were exemplified by a physician during a forum on breast cancer that I (Gweneth) attended a few years ago. The physician who was speaking began his presentation by putting up a slide of a microscopic view of breast cancer cells. As he put the slide on the screen, he commented that if he were to ask the oncologists in the room about how best to treat the particular type of breast cancer represented on the slide, although there might be slight variation, a fairly standard way of approaching treatment likely would be agreed on. Next, the speaker put up a slide that pictured a woman standing in a garden of flowers. As we all looked at the woman in the slide, the

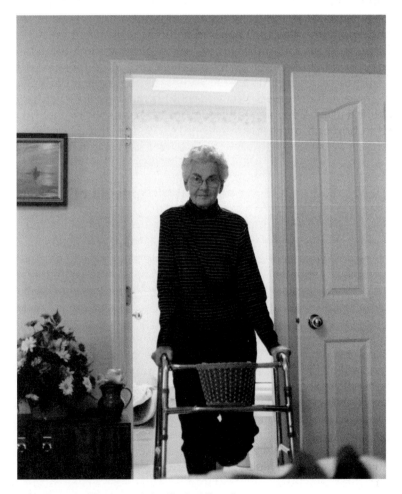

A family truth. (Photograph by Gayle Allison.)

speaker stopped and very pointedly stated, "This is the woman whose breast cancer you just saw and this is where the treatment changes." What the physician was pointing to was how vitally important it is to look beyond the surface, beyond the diagnosis and disease state and beyond the objective features of peoples' health and healing situations. The physician was illustrating that even the treatment of physical disease must be located within the personal and contextual uniqueness of people and their everyday lives.

In line with this physician, we believe that the process of health and healing is relational, contextual, and unique. Although five women may be living with breast cancer, because they are unique beings who each inhabit particular contextual and relational locations in life, those unique personal, relational, and contextual aspects must be taken into consideration if health and healing are to be promoted. Unfortunately, we have found that an objective view of knowledge severely constrains our ability to know and respond to people/families' unique health and healing processes. Therefore, in this book we have intentionally and explicitly moved beyond a Cartesian view of knowledge and in particular beyond the notion of objective truth. Specifically we present a *relational view* of family and family nursing that challenges many of the assumptions of Cartesian thought. Relational in this sense means connection in many forms. That is, we believe that we come to know family and promote health and healing through a process of being in relation personally, socially, physically, intellectually, and spiritually, as we live in relation not only to other human beings, but also to our environments. Nursing practice that is relational and responsive to the uniqueness of people/families must be informed by multiple knowledges including experiential, contextual, spiritual, theoretical, biomedical, ethical, and ideological knowledge.

What Has Guided the Writing of This Book?

We begin by identifying the beliefs and assumptions that underpin our relational approach and that have guided us in deciding what theory and literature to include and not to include in this book. We invite you to consider the following statements in light of your own knowledge and experience as people in the world. Instead of just reading the statements through, as you read each one, stop and ask yourself what you think about what we have said. Pay attention to how these statements differ from Cartesian assumptions. Also, try to identify what *you* believe about people and families. We have included some questions to help you think about your own beliefs and assumptions in relation to ours.

1. *People are contextual beings who live in relation with others and with social, cultural, political, and historical processes and communities* (Thayer-Bacon, 2003). This relational connection exists at both intimate and generalized levels. Stop for a minute and think about this statement. Do you believe that people are integrally connected to their social world or do you believe in the autonomous, independent person who is somehow self-sustaining? For example, when you made your decision to enter nursing school, although it was a personal decision

did you make it in relation to your world? Did you think about what it would mean in terms of getting a job, being able to travel, having economic security? Did you consider that nursing would enable you to work with people? Did you take into account the opinions of other important people in your life? In what ways were your own personal thoughts sparked and/or influenced by what you had heard and learned in your sociocontextual world?

2. *People are products of relational interactions. These relational interactions and practices promote us to believe certain things and not others.* Do you believe you are the product of relational interactions? For example, have you been shaped by the relational interactions you have had with your nursing instructors and other nurses in your clinical placements? Have you come to believe certain things about nursing and act in certain ways as a result of those interactions? What do *you* think about the idea that people are products of relational interactions?

3. *Sociohistorical values, knowledges, practices, attitudes, and structures are passed on through relational interactions. These sociohistorical forces become so taken for granted that people often take them as the only reality, forgetting that they can be remade.* Thus particular knowledge and practices become habituated and through a process of socialization people begin fulfilling certain roles in particular ways. Do you believe that you have been socialized into the person you are today? Have you taken up ways of thinking and practicing assuming they are 'just the way things are'? For example, can you identify how you have adhered to social expectations regarding what it means to be a man or woman? Has your socialization in nursing led you to take up the role of nurse in particular ways and not in others? Or do you see it differently?

4. *Each person has a unique context that affects and shapes that person's identity, knowing, experience, and way of being in the world.* Peoples' contextuality including their own personal experiences, social and cultural history, and location affect how they make sense of their world and how they participate in it. Do you believe that the context in which you grew up and/or the context in which you currently live has shaped you as a person? What about others you have known—can you see how their context has shaped them differently than you? Do you think it is possible not to be affected by your context?

5. *People gain insight into their contextuality—into themselves (for example, their beliefs, values, theories, way of being, cultural beliefs, and practices) through interactions with others.* Thus our relational experiences offer a site for knowledge development and transformation of practices. Have you ever learned something important about yourself through your interactions with others? Have your interactions with others helped you notice things about your own life context (for example, family, home, community, culture) that were previously less noticeable and/or taken for granted?

6. *People not only are shaped by their relational experiences and contexts, but also shape those experiences and contexts.* Subsequently, people have the potential to improve on the knowledge and practices that

have been handed down to them. This improvement is achieved by scrutinizing knowledge, developing broader understandings, and enlarging perspectives. Have you ever found yourself thinking differently from your parents? Have you made decisions that were different from what people in your world were telling you to make? Have you ever decided that you had to change the way something was done because it didn't seem right or didn't fit for you or someone for whom you cared?

7. *Because people are relational beings, their experiences of health and healing are complex and multifaceted.* To attend to this complexity, multiple forms of knowledge are required including experiential, contextual, spiritual, theoretical, biomedical, and so forth. What knowledges have you drawn on in your work as a nurse? Do you give particular types of knowledge authority over other types? Why or why not?

Overall these beliefs and assumptions highlight how you as a nurse are integral to the development of any family nursing knowledge. For example, these assumptions highlight that when you approach a family to do an assessment, what is focused on, what is noticed, and/or not noticed, and the conclusions that are reached about the family will be strongly shaped by you—the particular nurse who is doing the assessment. Moreover, this means that because all nurses are shaped by their sociohistorical location and background, if two nurses were to assess the same family, although there would be similarities in what they 'saw', there would also likely be differences. As nurses we have the capacity to interpret our own experiences and make our own decisions and choices and the interpretations and choices we make are shaped by our relational world.

Why a Relational Approach to Family Nursing?

The main reason we have taken up a relational approach to family nursing is that we have found it greatly enhances our ability to know and respond to people/families. In particular, it allows us as nurses to connect across differences. As nurses we continually experience similarities and differences between ourselves and the people/families with whom we come in contact. A guiding intent of a relational approach to family nursing is to more intentionally recognize and attend to those similarities and differences. Specifically this relational approach seeks to make similarities and differences more transparent in order to learn from them (Thayer-Bacon, 2003). As the similarities and differences are made transparent, we are better able to attend to issues of meaning, experience, race, history, culture, health, and sociopolitical systems. In addition, as we relationally honor and attend to such differences the potential for growth, change, and knowledge development is enhanced.

We have also shaped this book according to a relational approach in order to more accurately reflect the complexity of family nursing practice. We want to provide the opportunity for you as a reader/student/nurse to experience and learn to navigate through the 'messiness' (Tanner, 1988) of everyday practice. A relational approach to knowledge and theory grounds knowledge development in experiences and practices that take place in the contingent and ever-changing world of family nursing.

Finally, we believe that to meaningfully employ knowledge in practice, you as a nurse must actively take part in the knowledge development process. A relational approach to knowledge development and theory building enlists nurses as active participants. However, development of knowledge is not limited to nurses. As Thayer-Bacon (2003) contends, if we limit our knowledge development to conversations with 'scholars' or 'experts', we limit the scope of our understanding. 'For the standards we use to determine expertise are also fallible and embedded within social contexts. . . . Our standards need to be continually questioned and this can only happen at a deep level, re-examining foundational background assumptions, if we allow in outsiders' perspectives' (p. 70). Therefore, a relational approach to knowledge recognizes the value of multiple and differing forms of knowledge and enlists the 'knowing' and experience of families as well as knowledge from outside the discipline of nursing.

A Pragmatic Understanding of Knowledge and Truth

Our relational view of family nursing arises through a pragmatic understanding of knowledge and knowledge development as outlined by pragmatist philosophers such as William James, John Dewey, Richard Rorty, and Barbara Thayer-Bacon. A pragmatic view of knowledge assumes the existence of multiple truths and interpretations and considers knowing to be a relational process. Pragmatists reject the idea that the mind and body are separate and that objective knowledge is possible. From a pragmatic perspective, it is understood that we can never really separate ourselves from our experiences. This means that the knower is always central to the knowing process (the nurse assessing the family is central to the interpretations and diagnoses that are made). Pragmatists contend that all knowledge is 'socially constructed by embedded, embodied people who are in relation with each other' (Thayer-Bacon, 2003, p. 10). Said another way, pragmatists assume that what is known is always shaped by who it is that is doing the knowing, emphasizing that even facts are interpreted by people and subsequently who we are as people integrally shapes what we know and how we experience others.

There are three features of a pragmatic perspective that are important to highlight in thinking about family nursing knowledge and knowledge development. First, because it is impossible to separate human beings from human knowing, according to pragmatists there can be no such thing as objective knowledge or truth. And it is impossible to obtain knowledge that is certain and/or universal. Knowledge is never certain because, as Thayer-Bacon (2003) describes, 'the only truths we have access to are derived through our own error-prone . . . procedures' (p. 63). Similarly, because all knowers are limited by their particular location and embedded-ness, any knowledge is understood to be limited in its scope and depth. This is because as socially embedded people we each bring our 'selective interest' to any experience or situation. Thayer-Bacon (2003) describes selective interest as the bias or attitude that exists in each thought we have. It is our own attitude or selective interest that determines the questions we ask and even the way we go about answering our questions! Selective interest causes us to notice certain things and not others and to attend to certain experiences and not others.

Even scientists and theorists have been shaped by their social worlds and bring selective interests to their work. Thus, research, no matter how strong the claims to 'objectivity', always reflects selective interest. And, because family theory and assessment frameworks have been created by socially embedded people with selective interests, it is important to understand that any theory and/or assessment framework is selective. That is, any theory or framework offers a biased and selected view of family. Subsequently, from a pragmatic perspective all knowledge is understood to be limited and fallible and any theory or expert truth is considered to be in need of continual scrutiny. One must always scrutinize how any particular theory may be limiting one's view and knowing of a particular family.

The second important feature of a pragmatic approach to knowledge is the connection of knowledge, experience, and practice. In contrast to the Cartesian view that separates theoretical knowledge from practical knowledge, pragmatists do not see a deep split between theory, practice, and experience. Knowing is considered to be a relational, experiential action. According to pragmatists, all knowing occurs in relation to a range of other ideas and people, is experienced, and is an active rather than passive occurrence. Pragmatists take this link between theory and practice seriously. From a pragmatic perspective, all so-called theory is understood to arise from and be grounded in experiences and practices (Rorty, 1999). Subsequently, pragmatists share Berman's (2000) contention that truth is a verb, it *happens* to an idea. Ideas become true, are *made* true by events (James, 1907). For example, according to a pragmatic perspective, one's theory of family (what one believes a true family looks and acts like) arises through the events and experiences in one's life (which include experiences in one's family of origin, the theories one is exposed to in nursing school, the books one reads, the media, and so forth). As we live and experience family in our personal and professional lives we are (although often unconsciously) continuously theorizing and retheorizing family. And our experiences serve to change or modify our understanding of what a true family looks and acts like. In this way, knowledge development (and theory) is understood to be a living, active process.

Third, from a pragmatic perspective the value of knowledge lies in its pragmatic contribution. That is, knowledge is not valued because it offers us more theoretical understanding but rather because it pragmatically enables us to be more effective in the world. While a Cartesian way of evaluating any theory might be to try to determine how true or accurate it is, from a pragmatic perspective we can never know which theory is more true (since there is no one truth). What is important— what gives any theory its value—is not how true it is but how it fosters increased responsiveness to people. For this reason pragmatism directs us to be less confident in what we think we know and to approach our practice aware of the uncertainty of any truth. Because theories are valuable to the extent that they enhance our knowing and responsiveness, any theories guiding family nursing must be scrutinized according to how useful they are in enhancing our capacity to respond and practice in ways that promote the health and well-being of particular families in particular moments.

 ## To Illustrate

A good example of how ideas (and knowledge) of family come into being and are 'made' true relationally is the media in Western countries. If one looks closely at media representations of family, it is possible to see particular Eurocentric truths of family being promoted. For example, marketing people promoting everything from food to health to real estate promote the truth of family (usually mom, dad, and the two children) as a warm, nurturing, safe haven; similarly politicians seeking election will speak of 'getting back to family values' as though all families share the same values (Doane, 2003). Journalists wanting to incite people to listen to their news coverage will use the family truths and images (for example, smiling faces depicting closeness and safety) to emotional-ize stories with headlines that read 'family devastated by. . .'. As we are bombarded by such media and live within these strong value messages, we begin to assume certain things about family. Perhaps the most problematic thing we begin to assume is that these values and images are true. Worse yet, we begin to expect families to function according to these images and truths. Families who model themselves according to these images are seen as healthy, normal, and well-functioning. Families who do not reflect these stereotypical images are deemed 'other' and often 'less than'. Instead of seeing these images and truths as problematic and therefore revising the truths to more accurately reflect the reality of family in contemporary society, we begin to see families as lacking and in need of revision. One just has to look at the language of 'broken family', 'single-parent family', 'gay-lesbian families', and so forth to see the 'othering' that routinely takes place. These descriptions (many of which have been coined by 'experts' in academic fields and have subsequently been taken up and used by nurses and other human-service professionals) depict how families are other than the norm, which usually requires no modifiers: the dual-parent, heterosexual norm. Within this othering is the implicit message that families who do not fit the norm are somehow less than. This is an example of how taken-for-granted ways of thinking and conceptualizing families can constrain our understanding and responsiveness. Throughout this book we continually invite you to scrutinize the taken-for-granted assumptions about family that are lived out in the relational world around you.

What We Offer in This Book

Because we concur with the pragmatist view of knowledge and truth, the intent guiding this book is somewhat different from what you might have found in other textbooks. Our pragmatic underpinnings lead us to believe that the value of knowledge and theory lies in how it enhances our knowing of and response to people/families. Therefore, we have attempted to create an opportunity for you to enhance your conscious and intentional *living* knowledge. We hope to inspire you to scrutinize *how you are living your knowledge* and to *develop wider possibilities for knowing and responding to families*. To support the achievement of that goal, we are intentionally going beyond the bounds of current habits of knowing and practice that we believe constrain family nursing practice. In articulating our relational view, we have drawn on knowledge, theory, and research in nursing and from other disciplines to help us refine, strengthen, and present what we believe to be a more expansive way of approaching and knowing family. Overall, the relational view we present highlights the interconnectedness of people; families; sociopolitical contexts and cultures; past, present, and future experiences; and the natural world. We attempt to explicitly show how families, nurses, and family nursing exist and occur within webs of interrelationality that integrally connect and shape people/families' health and healing.

As a result of our pragmatic location, the truth that governs this book is a truth we hold about the most responsive (and responsible) way to live knowledge. Rather than identifying a particular theoretical framework of family nursing for you to learn and follow, we suggest that the way to foster knowledgeable and competent family nursing practice is to develop a more conscious, intentional, and responsive way of living knowledge. Subsequently, we invite you into a knowledge development process through which you will have the opportunity to consider what happens when you *live* different theories in your practice. As we examine theoretical knowledge throughout the book, we employ questions of adequacy (Rorty, 1999) to help us consider the adequacy of the theories in terms of their practical contribution to our everyday work with families. We invite you to scrutinize the theories in light of your experiences and to ask: 'Is our knowledge of things adequate to the way things really are? Are our ways of describing things, of relating them to other things so as to make them fulfill our needs more adequately, as good as possible?' (Rorty, 1999, p. 72). As James (1907) described, 'experience has ways of boiling over, and making us correct our present formulas' (James, 1907, p. 170). As you read this book, participate in the learning activities we suggest, and consider the theories in light of your family nursing experiences, our intent is to support you in developing ways of viewing and responding to families— ways of living family nursing knowledge—that enable you to know more deeply and respond more fully to the people/families with whom you work.

What Might Make Theory 'Adequate' for Family Nursing Practice?

The question of adequacy always begs the question of 'adequate for what?' Thus, adequate theory for family nursing depends on the goal of family nursing practice. Here we may depart from some nurses who hold the view that nursing can be guided by goals that are determined outside of our relations with families. Indeed, we believe that the goal of nursing is not an end, but a way of being. By this we mean that while we think that nursing practice should be ethical, health promoting, and safe for families (that is to say, practice should not harm families), the specific goals and outcomes of practice cannot be predetermined. The outcomes of family nursing are arrived at in relation with and in response to families. Thus, we are seeking theories that will enhance the nurse's way of being—to support nurses to be in-relation with people/families in ways that are more responsive, more health promoting, more ethical, more safe, and thereby increasingly more competent.

With this goal in mind, we are interested in knowledge that is 'useful and purposeful for answering our questions and solving our problems' (Thayer-Bacon, 2003, p. 40). Therefore, it is important to consider the extent to which any theory helps us do so. Because theories presuppose a certain way of defining a family or situation, questions we need to ask of any theory include:

- What is the focus of this theory?
- How does this theory define the focus of family nursing?
- To what does the theory, idea, or concept draw my attention?
- What does it take for granted or assume about family, health, and/or nursing?
- How does it expand my view and help me move beyond my own selective interests?

To consider a theory's adequacy in terms of its usefulness it would be further helpful to ask,

- How does this theory inform and/or constrain my knowing?
- What does it overlook?
- What does it lead me to question?
- What does it lead me to doubt?
- What does it lead me to take for granted?

Finally, because we are concerned with practice and knowledge as action, we think it is important to consider what direction for practice any given theory provides. Useful questions here might be:

- What would this lead me to do?
- What actions would I be compelled to take?

Such questions can be useful in assessing the adequacy of various theories, ideas, or concepts for family nursing practice.

 ## To Illustrate

The idea of 'cultural safety' is one we introduce in detail later in this book, and it serves as a possible illustration of how we might consider the adequacy of a theory. Briefly, because we see people and families as socially embedded, we believe that understanding families' contexts is necessary if we are to practice competently. In considering various ways to seek connections across similarities and differences, we have found the concept of cultural safety to be more adequate than other ways of theorizing multicultural practice (Papps &

Ramsden, 1996; Polaschek, 1998; Smye & Browne, 2002). This idea was originally introduced in New Zealand out of concern about the health care of Maori people and to assist nurses (many of whom were descended from white settlers) to work across their differences with Maori people. The idea was that any actions that demeaned, disrespected, or disempowered Maori people created 'un-safety'. As initially conceptualized, this idea drew attention, for example, to the historical oppression of Maori people. The idea helped nurses (regardless of ethnicity) to move beyond their selective interests and to question their taken-for-granted assumptions about Maori people. The idea dealt with the problems occasioned for Maori people by colonialism and racism. The theory provided direction toward actions that recognize, respect, and nurture the unique cultural identity of individuals and safely meet their needs, expectations, and rights (Smye & Browne, 2002). Within New Zealand/Aotearoa, the theory has focused on the ethnicity and culture of Maori people with the intent of promoting recognition and respect, particularly by non-Maori nurses. A number of people, in recognizing the value and importance of cultural safety for nursing practice, have considered how the ideas that underpin cultural safety as developed in New Zealand might also be useful in other contexts. For example, considering the ideas for their relevance within their own contextual location, nursing authors writing within the Canadian context have considered how cultural safety might be useful in providing safe nursing care with Aboriginal people (Browne & Fiske, 2001; Smye & Browne, 2002) and immigrant groups in Canada (Reimer Kirkham et al., 2002). Informed by existing work in cultural safety, these authors have argued that the distinct histories and experiences of both immigrant groups and Aboriginal people in Canada have implications for how the theory might be taken up in the Canadian context. This is an example of how, to be helpful and informative, any theory needs to be scrutinized within particular contexts and within the everyday experience of particular families and how such scrutiny can enhance theoretical adequacy for nursing practice.

What Is the Goal of This Book?

It is our hope that through the knowledge development process this book provides, you will develop a more conscious, intentional, and responsive family nursing practice. We hope that you will engage in continuously questioning and redeveloping your own knowledge. Given our pragmatic approach to knowledge, it is our intent to challenge the normative truths that currently govern understandings of family and thus family nursing. James (1907) argued that our theories and beliefs 'pass so long as nothing challenges them, just as bank notes pass so long as nobody refuses them' (p. 163). We believe that many truths and theories currently dominating understanding of family and family nursing are no longer passable. They do not do justice to the diverse, living experience of families nor adequately support nurses to promote the health and well-being of families in their diverse everyday lives. Our pragmatic view has led us to believe that it is not families that are problematic or other than. Rather, the problem lies with the theories, truths, and norms that limit what family might be. It is the truths and theories of family that need 'unstifling' and 'limbering up' (James, 1907, p. 145). Thus, we have purposefully brought our pragmatic attitude to explorations of family nursing. We have carefully chosen theoretical perspectives and research that we feel have the potential to expand the understanding of family and family nursing. At the same time, we have included narrative examples of real experiences of people/families, other nurses, and ourselves. The theories, research, and stories we include are ones that we have found helpful in limbering up our thinking and in providing direction for everyday practice with families. It is important to emphasize that the theories and processes we include in this book have not been chosen because of their truth value but rather because we believe they offer views of family and family nursing more adequate to the purpose of expanding understanding and enhancing responsiveness toward health promotion. In offering these perspectives, we have attempted to refrain from giving authority to any particular idea or theory. Rather we hope to set theory to work within your everyday nursing experiences.

Locating Ourselves Theoretically

Drawing on James' (1907) contention that theories are *'instruments, not answers to enigmas, in which we can rest'* (our emphasis, p. 147), we employ critical and experiential theories, nursing theories from the human science tradition, and contemporary ethical theories to invite a new view *into* family and family nursing. Our intent is to present and use the theories as instruments to aid us in articulating understandings of family and family nursing that have yet to be made explicit. Most importantly, we do not offer the ideas as yet another prescription for practice. Rather, it is our hope that this book allows readers to engage in a very thoughtful inquiry into their own experiences of family and family nursing that enables them to intentionally and consciously develop their own theory and truth of family nursing practice.

Locating Ourselves Practically

Although we do not intend to present our ideas as solidified truths or prescriptions for practice, we do offer what we think are possibilities for relationally responsive practice with families. We present theories and processes that offer and support a relational approach to family nursing. This relational approach is guided by an *ethic of social justice*—where decisions and actions are not only health promoting and/or economically viable but are *socially just*. Practice guided by an ethic of social justice continually asks 'so what?' If I do or do not do this, so what may the impact be? Such practice is not idealistic in the sense of 'being able to fix things' or in overlooking the limitations of the 'real world', but it is practice that is *inspired by ideals*. As nurses we strive toward the ideals of compassion, respect, equitable relations, and the honoring of human life. Regardless of whether we are able to change a particular situation or fix what is wrong in the world, striving toward these ideals supports us to act in ways that are respectful, compassionate, and equitable and that leave us feeling that we have somehow 'done good'.

The practice processes we offer stand in contrast to most family nursing textbooks that provide structured models of assessment and intervention. We view practice as a way of being as much as a form of action. Subsequently, we view relationships, ethics, health promotion, culture, safety, diversity, power, communication, and economics (ideas we explore in detail later in this book) as integral to any nursing moment. We do *not* consider these elements to be domains of assessment or areas of content that can be grafted onto existing theories or assessment frameworks. Rather, in a relational approach to family nursing these elements fundamentally shape and determine the how, what, and why of practice. They are integrally related living processes that support each other. For example, practicing ethically and practicing in a way that ensures the emotional and cultural safety of families are inseparable; to do both, nurses must have the opportunity to learn and become relational practitioners. They must approach knowledge in a way that fosters such practice. This relational way of being and approach is lived and evident in all moments of practice regardless of whether it is an emergency room nurse helping a person in a 1-minute transfer to a stretcher or a community health nurse working with a family with high priority needs over a 2-year period. It is the *way* a nurse works with people/families; *what* the nurse sees, thinks, and takes note of when assessing families; and *how* he or she goes about promoting health that makes practice relational.

● Locating You As a Learner/Reader

In addition to the pragmatic approach to theory that underpins this book, our writing has also been guided by experiential and critical-learning theories. As learners and teachers, we have come to understand learning as not merely an intellectual activity but a deeply embodied and personal process that requires active and substantial engagement at the experiential level. To become an intentional, competent nurse the learning process must bring intellectual understanding (for example, theory) together with embodied, emotional experience (for example, personal experience, nursing practice experience). As a result of our pragmatic understanding of knowledge, and our concern for connections and context, we see you the learner/reader in much the same way as we see ourselves. That is, to follow Thayer-Bacon (2003), as people we each have the potential to learn to be more critical, creative, and constructive. As you read what we have written from your own location, you may actually find yourself identifying limitations in our thinking. Rather than being concerned about this, we welcome your differing perspectives and insights. As writers we see ourselves as being in-relation with you the reader and assume that we will continue to expand our knowing and understanding of family nursing. In that spirit we have chosen to take up a conversational style of writing. As we present ideas throughout the book, we at times speak about our own locations and experiences, about how our thinking has changed over time, and about questions we are currently exploring. And we invite you to consider your own experiences and ideas in-relation to ours. At the same time we are aware that you are also in-relation with many others who will influence and inform your knowing of family. We hope that as you work your way through this book, you will use the numerous other relational connections you have to further your knowledge development process.

Given our belief that learning is a deeply embodied process, we have presented the ideas in this book in such a way that you as a reader will require certain learning skills and attitudes in order to reap the most benefit. First, as a reader you will need to be willing to take a *stance of unknowing*. As learners and teachers we have found that when people think they know something they are less likely to see what they do not know and thereby less likely to learn. We invite you to step out of a stance of knowing and explore an infinite number of previously un-thought-of possibilities. For example, we will be asking you to step out of what you already 'know' about family from your life experience and/or prior study and consider other ideas and conceptualizations. Second, to get the most from this book, you will need to *risk trying new ways* and looking through new lenses. Learning is risky business. It is far less risky to carry on with the status quo and do things according to the dominant norms that exist in family nursing and in health care practice. Throughout the book, however, we ask you to look through new lenses to see families and nursing practice from angles and vantage points from which you may not have looked before. Third, you will need the skill of *self-observation* and *critical self-reflection* (what we will call reflexivity) to honestly look at who you are, discover what you believe and value, and determine how you are living those values and beliefs in practice, and you will need the willingness to challenge your taken-for-granted beliefs and practices. Finally, you will need to *be open to discomfort*—to be willing to be perturbed and discover things about yourself or your practice that you may not like. Discomfort is a catalyst for learning. When your solid foundations of knowledge and practice are called into question, it may feel uncomfortable, yet this discomfort sparks questions and exploration that have the potential to foster your ongoing development as a relational, ethical, and culturally safe practitioner.

● Questioning Our Habitual Knowing-in-Action

We begin the exploration of family nursing with a discussion about *habits*. In particular we want to begin by exploring the habits that currently dominate the knowing and understanding of family. As human beings we have all developed habits. Habits do not merely shape our thinking but they also shape the way we act in the world. Habits can be thought of as the taken-for-granted truths that shape our practice. Taken up in a nonreflective way, these truths become ingrained in our bodily responses and flow through us unconsciously. For example, the dominant truths governing our views of good nutrition lead us to take up certain nutritional habits and also potentially confine how we think, feel, and go about ensuring adequate nutrition. The dairy industry has done such a good job of promoting the truth that four glasses of milk is a daily nutritional requirement that even though I (Gweneth) found that milk was actually problematic for two of my children, I would find myself habitually pouring milk into their glasses at dinner (children need four glasses of milk a day for strong bones—don't they?). I would suddenly realize what I was doing and replace it with water or something else, yet as I watched my children drink from their glasses during the meal I would actually find myself lamenting over them not being able to get the milk they needed. This habit of thought and action not only set limits on my views of what was necessary nutrition but also confined the paths for action I saw available to me for meeting my children's nutritional needs. Elias (1978, 1982) has clearly described how habitual ways of acting are so deeply integrated that they extend to how we conduct ourselves bodily. People learn to discipline and control their own bodies according to the social groups within which they live and work. The 'busy gait' of nurses (Tomlinson, 1988) is an example of embodied habits of conduct. This busy gait conveys messages to patients and other staff about how efficient and organized a nurse is and the extent to which a nurse has time, is available, or can be interrupted or asked for help.

It is important to emphasize that these patterns of activity—these habits—are constantly reproduced by us in a nonreflective way. As we learn to think and act in particular ways, those ways become ingrained in our bodily responses and flow through us unconsciously. As habits, they become conditions of intellectual and bodily efficiency (Dewey, 1922). However, this efficiency comes with a price. The habits operate to set boundaries and restrictions on our reach. They serve as blinders that confine what we see in families as well as the paths for action we see open to us.

Habits Are Helpful

Dewey (1922) contended that part of the reason habits are so powerful is that they start out as helpful. They provide an expertise and efficiency that is necessary for daily living. They offer comfort in particular areas of our lives (as a mother who gave her children, milk I could rest assured that they were getting what they needed to develop strong bones). As Dewey described, a sailor can be at home on the sea, a hunter in the forest, a scientist in the laboratory. Concrete habits do all the perceiving, recognizing, imagining, recalling, judging, conceiving, and reasoning in such an efficient way, that energy and attention can be freed up for other activities and possibilities (Dewey, 1922). Therefore, the mechanism of habit is indispensable. The constant interruption of consciously searching for and intentionally performing each act would make daily life impossible.

Driving is a good example of how one develops and integrates habits. If you drive a car, think back to when you first learned and how everything felt so strange—how each time you got in the car you had to think about starting the car, putting it in gear, releasing the parking brake, and so forth. For those of you who have driven for a while, however, it is likely that the action of starting the car and driving off has became so ingrained that when you now hop in the car you no longer need to think about what you are doing and you are busy thinking about the class you are heading to or what you have to do during the day. Your mind is freed up to think of other things. In this way, habits are very helpful.

Habits Are Problematic

Nevertheless, habits alone are problematic. 'With habit alone there is a machine-like repetition, a duplicating recurrence of old acts' (Dewey, 1922, p. 180). By themselves, habits are too organized, too insistent, and too determinate. Because they are so adapted to the environment, they no longer need to be analyzed and if left unchecked habits end in thoughtless action (Dewey, 1922). The power of habit was brought home to me (Gweneth) during a recent trip to New Zealand. Having learned to drive in Canada where the passenger seat is on the right-hand side of the car, as a passenger I found it amazingly difficult to move beyond the habit of walking to the right-hand side of the car to get in. Although I knew that in New Zealand the passenger seat is on the left-hand side of the car and would of course intend to walk to the correct side of the car, unless I paid very close attention I would inadvertently walk to the wrong side. Because I was usually in conversation with people as we walked to the car, my habit of going to the right-hand side of the car would kick in and it would take one of the nurses I was with to jokingly ask me if I preferred to drive to make me realize I had done it again!

Throughout the book we present narratives, learning activities, and theoretical understandings in a way that might help you to see into your practice—to see what habits you have developed and how you are habitually living knowledge in your everyday actions as a nurse. We begin that process by offering the story below.

 An Example: A Family Experience

The following is a story of a family experience; however, it is not typical of those told in the family nursing literature or in family nursing practice. Moreover, the way family is depicted in the story is not how most people usually think of family. We have purposefully chosen to begin with this story because we are hoping it will help you begin to identify some of the taken-for-granted knowledge (and habits) of family that you already bring with you and at the same time perhaps challenge the truth of this knowing.

A few years ago I (Gweneth) was asked to be a parent-driver for a trip my daughter's grade six class took to a drop-in center for people who were homeless and living on the street. During our time at the center, one of the staff members, named John, told the children about his experience of 'living on the street' for 20 years. As John told his story, he invited the children to ask questions. Because it was close to Christmas one child asked him how he spent Christmas when he lived on the street. This idea of Christmas suddenly sparked a flurry of questions about family. Didn't he have a family? Where was his family all those years he was living on the street? What was it like to live on the street without your family? In response, John began talking about how very lonely he had felt during that time. He described how people would walk by him as though he didn't exist and that he gradually began to feel invisible. At first it did not really seem like John was addressing the children's family questions. However, as I listened I realized that he was in fact talking about his 'family experience.' In being asked about family he had begun to describe his experience of 'not mattering to people' of being 'invisible' to others. The reason that I had difficulty at first connecting his response to the children's questions was that his experience in no way resembled what *I* expected in a response to questions about family. John did not talk about his parents or his brothers and sisters. He did not talk about people at all. Rather he talked about *how family was meaningful to him*. Living in a society in which the family unit is the main organizing social structure and being treated as nonexistent, the family questions had not conjured up images of other people and togetherness. Rather, it was just the opposite. John's meaningful experience of family had been one of absence, invisibility, and isolation. In addition, over time this family experience had had a profoundly detrimental effect on his health. He described how his experience of being invisible had provoked a deep sense of isolation and had heightened the gulf between himself and the rest of the world. As he concluded the conversation, John told the children how very important it was to acknowledge people and to include them. 'Even if it seems like they are different or don't care, the most important and caring thing you can do for a person you see sitting on the street is to look them in the eye and say hello just like you would if they were your family.'

What Habits of Knowing Do You Have About Family?

The experience recounted in the earlier story was another reminder of how my own habits of knowing have the potential to profoundly constrain my understanding of another's experience of family. My initial

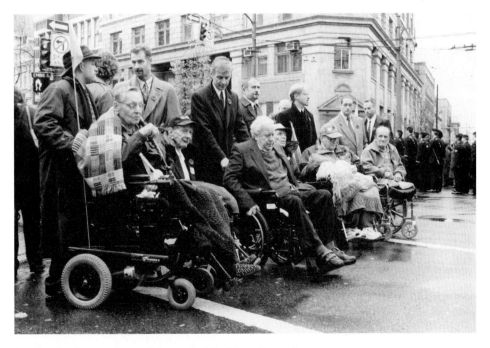

Another family experience. (Photograph by Fiona Raven.)

TRY IT OUT 1.1. **The Meaning of Family**

Take a few minutes and write a response to the following:

1. List four words that come to your mind when you think of the word 'family' and three defining features of your family.
2. Based on this reflection, what are two things you learned in your own family of origin that shape how you think of families? Can you think of other things that have influenced how you think of family (images depicted in advertisements, the geographic areas in which you have lived, experiences with friends, and so forth)?
3. Look at what you have written and ask yourself, What movie would I make about family? Who would be the central characters? Who would be the 'star'? What would the storyline be? Would there be heroes and heroines? Compare your 'movie' with the movie you think someone else in your family would make.
4. As you look over your responses to the earlier questions, consider how your personal view of family might be shaping your nursing practice.

---

thought that John wasn't addressing the children's questions was really a result of my own limited idea of family. Because *I* knew family to be a configuration of people, as he talked about *his* knowing of family I initially had difficulty making sense of what he was saying and more importantly did not immediately understand the significance of his family experience to his overall health and well-being.

It is probably fair to say that there is a dominant habit of considering family as a configuration of people. As discussed earlier, the particular images of family that are promoted in the Western world most often include a configuration of people in a typical Eurocentric form (for example, mom, dad, and the kids). However, given the multicultural, global community of the contemporary world, the differing values and customs, and the variety of life experiences people have, what constitutes family and how family is experienced is very diverse. Yet when we use the word family with each other there is often a built-in assumption that we are all talking about and meaning the same thing. Examine what family means to you using Try It Out 1.1.

What Habits of Knowing Do You Have About Health?

Another significant area of knowing that shapes our family nursing practice is our beliefs and habitual ways of thinking about health. Just as assumptions about what constitutes family have been shaped by dominant norms in Western society, your knowing of health likely has been influenced by dominant sociocultural norms. For example, as a result of the Cartesian view that has dominated Western biomedicine in North America, many people associate health with the absence of disease or limitation. Given the diversity of people, cultures, and experiences, however, health may mean very different things to different people. Yet as nurses set out to promote health, they often do so based on their own understandings and meanings of health. Stopping to examine one's beliefs and assumptions about health and to question how those beliefs and assumptions are shaping one's nursing practice

TRY IT OUT 1.2.   **The Meaning of Health**

Write

Take three pages of paper and describe an experience you have had living with some kind of health challenge of your own. It may be something acute like a flu, tonsillitis, or a sprained ankle; some chronic health challenge like depression or diabetes; or perhaps even something that has been seriously life threatening. As you describe your experience, include not only the details of what happened physically but also your feelings, thoughts, and actions at the time as well as the social forces or spiritual aspects that were relevant to your overall health experience (for example, family concerns, economic concerns, work demands, health care resource limitations, etc.).

Reflect

When you have finished writing, consider the following questions:

1. How was your life temporarily or permanently changed as a result of your health challenge?
2. What was of particular concern to you during that time?
3. What other factors in your life gave rise to particular concerns? For example, when I (Gweneth) had a back injury years ago, although I was concerned about my back and my physical healing, as a young mother with a new baby my most significant concern was my mobility—I needed to be able to move around enough to care for my son.
4. How did your particular concerns influence how you went about promoting your health and healing?

is vital if a nurse is to be responsive to families' particular experiences (see Try It Out 1.2).

Often we don't even notice our health until it is somehow impinged on. However, when we actually stop to think about health and what it means in our everyday lives, we begin to realize just what a multifaceted phenomenon it is. It becomes clear that health involves far more than the absence of disease. Health extends beyond the physical realm and involves a meaningful experience that is unique and particular to different people. For example, in my experience with my back injury that I (Gweneth) described in Try It Out 1.2, the physical limitations imposed by my injured back led me to see just how important choice and independence were to me as a person and to my everyday living. I became aware that health to me actually meant being able to exercise choice and to be independent. As a result, although I engaged in physiotherapy and other forms of treatment for my back, the reason I did so (my incentive, if you like) was not so much to have a strong back but to enable me to reclaim my independence and choice. A strong back was only significant within the more important *meaning* of health—which for me was choice and independence. This desire for choice and independence also led me to look for ways that would allow me (even with my back injury) to be independent and to exercise my choice to care for my son as I healed. That is, even when I was living with the health challenge of my back injury and limited independence, the way I 'lived and promoted my health' was to look for ways to express my independence.

What is Your Working Definition of Health?

As a unique individual you have your own definition of health. This definition 'operates' in your daily life and work regardless of the extent to which you are aware of it. However, if you are like most people, you may not have spent much time really thinking about what health means to you—how you meaningfully experience health. Without that conscious consideration and exploration, we tend to be influenced by the views that dominate our society. As a nurse working to promote health in families, it is vital that you are aware not only of your working definitions of family and health but also of how those definitions are shaping and perhaps constraining your practice. For example, when I (Colleen) was working in open-heart surgery, I employed very narrow definitions of health and family. In the recovery area, family was the immediate next of kin (usually, in my view, 'blood relatives' only), and as few people as possible, because I viewed family as extraneous to health in the immediate postoperative period. My view of health was pretty much limited to the physiological stability of the person who had the surgery. As long as heart rate and rhythm, blood pressure, hemodynamic pressures, and urine output remained within 'normal' limits, my ideas about health goals were met for any given patient. The 'busy-ness' of the unit, the speed with which I needed to discharge patients so that I could take new admissions, and my overall workload led me to give priority to these short-term, immediate goals. My goals for 'family members' were limited to them being co-operative with me and disrupting my work with the patient as little as possible. To accomplish this, I needed to help the family members deal with their worries and anxieties.

Over time, however, I began to see that even patients' physiological well-being was affected by the support of people whom they knew and trusted (the erstwhile bothersome family members). After some negative experiences with family members who were deemed 'legitimate' (a wife from whom a man was estranged) and positive experiences with ones who were not (a girlfriend with whom the patient in question had a deep and loving relationship), I began to pay more attention to what family meant to the people involved. I had to reset my priorities, reexamine my assumptions and stereotypes of family, and ultimately question exactly what I was doing as a nurse. This meant expanding my definition of health beyond the physiological to what I now would call 'relational', an understanding that encompasses family and the well-being of people in context. Box 1.1 offers some questions that can help lead you to expand your working definition of health.

BOX 1.1. **Questions Leading to Intentional Practice**

How is your working definition of health shaping how you engage with people, what you look for, what you find, and how you intervene?

What happens when your working definition differs from how family and/or health is meaningfully experienced and defined by the people for whom you are caring?

Do you ever stop to inquire into what health means to the people for whom you are caring?

How do you know you are in fact promoting their health?

● The Context of Knowledge That Shapes Our Habits

The reason we have begun the exploration of family nursing with this discussion about habits is because many of the ways we think and practice as nurses—our habits of conduct—are developed and shaped by the world in which we live. Many of the habits you have and will develop as a nurse are a result of living in the world of nursing. Similarly, the nursing profession exists within a larger sociopolitical world that shapes the norms and habits of the profession. So, for example, my (Colleen's) habitual way of seeing family in the open-heart intensive-care setting was shaped and supported by economic and political concerns about surgical waiting lists, operating room schedules, staffing levels, and nurse-patient ratios. I did not question how those economic and political concerns were limiting patient care and/or shaping my response as a nurse. Or to offer another example, in the Western world the health care emphasis on disease processes, pharmacology, and so forth makes sense when one considers how the Cartesian view (that separates mind and body) dominates Western society. From this view individual physical health is assumed to be distinct from other aspects of health.

Just as systemic forces shape practice they also shape the knowledge you have developed in nursing school. Yet the forces are often so hidden and taken for granted that we may not even be aware they are shaping us. For example, nursing knowledge development has been located in the dominant political ideology of liberalism (Browne, 2001). Individualism is the defining feature of liberalism, and advances the idea that people are rational, self-interested, autonomous actors who can be understood separately from their economic, political or historical context (Browne, 2001; Burt, 1995). Liberalism and individualism rest on ideas of individual freedom, egalitarianism (or the assumption that all people are socially equal), and neutrality (being unbiased and objective). Liberalism is linked to free-market economy in which each individual (regardless of their sociocultural position) is believed to have the same freedom to exchange goods and access resources. This location of nursing knowledge within the political ideology of liberalism has had a profound impact on how we think and practice as nurses. Browne (2001) contends that as a result of liberal individualist ideology as nurses:

- We focus on individuals in isolation from their family and/or their sociocultural world (our nursing knowledge and practice have been individualist in focus).
- We assume that society is essentially fair and equitable (that all people can access the resources they need).
- We prefer politically neutral knowledge (we don't actually scrutinize larger sociopolitical values that are constraining health care resources).
- We tend to support rather than challenge the status quo.

Overall liberal individualism has led nurses to assume that people are autonomous and that their behaviour and choices are independent of their relational, economic, historical, and political worlds. In assuming this liberal individualist perspective, nurses' abilities to know and respond to families in ways that are relational and health promoting has been severely hindered. For example, liberal individualism often leads nurses to put the responsibility for health on the individual without really considering how the person's context may be constraining his or her choice as an individual. For example, John's time of living on the street might be seen as a personal 'choice', rather than being seen as a result of complex relational, historical, economic, and political circumstances. This liberal individualist perspective has led to the development of habits of thought and action in nursing that are highly problematic. Therefore, throughout the book we create opportunities for you to examine how you might have taken up and/or might be taking up habits of practice that are grounded in liberal individualism. The family nursing approach we are advocating in this book challenges liberal individualism. The relational approach we propose seeks to understand, honor, and attend to people/families in context and views choice as a relational act that is profoundly shaped by contextual resources and constraints.

An Example: A Frustrating Man

Rosa, a friend of mine who started working at a diabetic clinic recently, told me (Colleen) about a young man, Artur, who attended the clinic on an irregular basis. The staff at the clinic told Rosa that Artur was 'difficult', 'frustrating', and 'noncompliant'. He only occasionally attended clinic, and his blood sugars were often high when he did, despite the staff giving him regular warnings and repeatedly explaining his prescribed regimen. Policies require that people who are insulin dependent must obtain a medical certificate in order to purchase needles from the pharmacy, but Artur had not attended the required education session so that staff could issue his certificate. The staff had a team meeting and decided someone should follow up with Artur regarding the choices he was making. Rosa volunteered.

Rosa reviewed Artur's chart and found that he had had diabetes since he was 11 years old. In addition to dealing with diabetes, Artur had a learning disability and dropped out of school 4 years earlier, at age 15. There was little other information on his chart except lab work, insulin orders, and his dietary 'prescription'. Rosa had difficulty in contacting Artur, as the phone number on his chart turned out to be a youth drop-in center. A week later, Artur called Rosa from the drop-in center where he had received the message.

Rosa asked how Artur was doing and told him that the staff were concerned that he had not turned up to get his certificate. Artur explained to Rosa that there was no point in him coming in because he had been cut off social assistance and could not afford new needles anyway. He told her that he currently worked at a McDonald's part time, and so he was 'eating better', but his scheduled work hours were the same times the clinic was open. Rosa asked Artur about his phone number and whether he had somewhere to stay. He explained that he was living with an aunt, but that they couldn't afford a phone.

This story provides a simple illustration of the contrast between seeing individuals as 'autonomous' and understanding people/families in their context. The staff who saw Artur as noncompliant and as making bad choices were drawing on liberal individualist ideas of Artur as a rational, autonomous actor. Drawing on objective, scientific knowledge, the staff know that following a diabetic regimen is logical and rational, and therefore they expect Artur to comply. In concert with liberal ideas about choice and free will, the staff focus on Artur's responsibilities for his own health and health care. When the circumstances of Artur's life come into view, however, his 'bad choices' can be seen as being shaped by a network of influences beyond objective knowledge of diabetes and beyond his own decision making and choice. For example, it is possible to see how his choices are strongly shaped by economics that limit his access to a phone, to nutritional food, to needles, and so forth. It is possible to see that his failure to attend the diabetic outpatient program is connected to his work and life context.

Liberal individualism shapes more than just nursing knowledge and how nurses view people. It also shapes public policy and the methodological presumptions made in policy analysis (Burt, 1995) and much of economics (Wilber, 1998). Indeed the Western free-market economy and liberal individualism are mutually sustaining. Cutbacks in social programs and an increasing emphasis on individual responsibility and self-reliance go hand in hand in free-market economies such as those increasingly dominating Canada, the United States, and Britain (Browne, 2001). So, social welfare policies, health care policies, and nursing knowledge are compatible, as they stem from the same philosophical roots. The policies that cut off Artur from social assistance are based in the same ideas that inform the policy governing how needles can be purchased and paid for, and the ideas that the nurses draw on in judging Artur's choices. Thus a seemingly simple matter of purchasing needles for insulin administration is shaped by the complex ways that sociopolitical and economic policies play out in the lives of families (in this case, Artur and his aunt).

As nurses we believe strongly that practice cannot be health promoting unless the contexts of families' lives are taken into account. *Therefore, the theoretical lenses and practice processes we offer in this book continually challenge notions of individualism.* Specifically, this book and the processes described in it

- are relational in focus,
- draw attention to sociohistorical contextual factors and inequities,
- lead to the development of political knowledge,
- support critique and challenge of the status quo.

● Beyond the Liberal Individualist View of Health

Nurses who have tried to move beyond the habit of focusing on individuals and their health problems and begin attending to people in context have commonly turned to ecological and environmental theories. Using

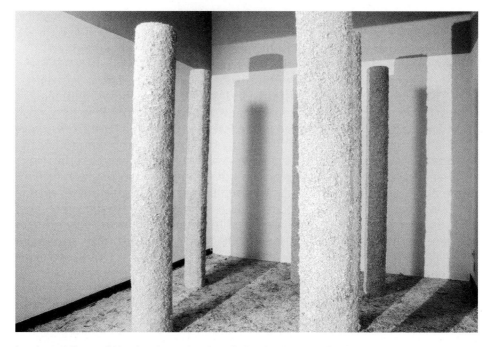

Lumbered Forest. (Wood and sawdust installation by Jocelyne Robinson.)

the idea that much of health care is like rescuing drowning victims without looking to see who is upstream pushing people in the water, Patricia Butterfield wrote an article in 1990 arguing that nursing had to 'think upstream'. She argued for using critical social theory to do so, but pointed to others, such as Chopoorian (1986), who has made similar arguments but proposes taking a broad environmental perspective in conceptualizing nursing as a way of 'thinking upstream'. More recently there have been further calls for nurses to take up environmental and ecological perspectives on health and health care (Hardin, 2001; Kneipp, 2000; Marck, 2000; Ribeiro & Bertolozzi, 1999). Integral to the relational approach to family nursing that guides this book is this socioenvironmental understanding of health and health promotion.

A Socioenvironmental Understanding of Health

If you read any nursing textbook you will come across the terms *health* and *health promotion*. If you pay close attention, however, you will notice that those terms are used in very different ways. As a result, in reading the nursing literature, the students we have taught have found themselves quite confused and uncertain about what health promotion is and what it actually looks like in practice. As we worked together to sort through the inconsistencies and clarify our understanding, we found a background paper by the Registered Nurses Association of British Columbia (RNABC, 1992) that addresses nursing practice in health promotion helpful. In this paper, three contrasting perspectives within health promotion are identified: the medical, the behavioral, and the socioenvironmental. Within each of these perspectives the definition of health varies, as does the focus of health promotion and nursing practice.

Distinguishing the three perspectives helps us understand how health promotion can refer to quite different forms of nursing practice. For example, if health is defined according to the medical perspective, nursing practice takes on a very different focus and purpose than if health is defined according to a socioenvironmental perspective. Unfortunately the perspective of health promotion that is governing the description of nursing practice in any given textbook or article is not always explicitly named. Similarly, many nurses who use the term health promotion to describe their practice have not clearly explicated the particular approach to health promotion that is guiding their practice. Yet if nursing practice is to be consistent and responsive to families, such explicit clarity is needed.

The first perspective, *the medical model*, defines health as the 'absence of disease or infirmity'. Based on this definition of health, nursing practice focuses on treating or preventing disease by correcting problems. The second perspective, *the behavioral model*, moves health beyond disease prevention and includes well-being. Subsequently, health-promoting nursing practice based on a behavioral perspective includes secondary and primary prevention and emphasis is given to changing behaviors and lifestyle (such as quiting smoking, increasing fitness) in order to decrease disease risks and maintain well-being. The third perspective, *the socioenvironmental model*, incorporates sociological and environmental aspects as well as the medical and behavioral ones. From this perspective, health is considered to be 'a resource for living . . . a positive concept . . . the extent to which an individual or group is able to realize aspirations, to satisfy needs, and to change or cope with the environment' (World Health Organization, 1984).

During the latter part of the 20th century, the dominance of medicine in health care was balanced by work conducted by The World Health Organization (WHO). The Ottawa Charter for Health Promotion (WHO, 1986) marked a shift from strictly medical and behavioral health determinants to health determinants defined in psychological, social, environmental, and political terms. This groundbreaking document that moved health promotion far beyond a disease and/or behavioral perspective to a socioenvironmental one emphasized that health was deeply rooted in human nature and societal structures (WHO, 1986). Subsequently, empowerment or the capacity to define, analyze, and act on concerns in one's life and living conditions joined treatment and prevention as an essential goal of health promotion (Labonte, 1993).

Living a Meaningful Life

Within the socioenvironmental perspective nursing practice is focused on enhancing the capacity and power of people to live a meaningful life. Although this capacity building may involve treating and preventing disease or lifestyle factors, the primary focus (for example, the reason disease is treated or certain lifestyles are promoted) is to enhance peoples' capacity and resources for meaningful life experiences. This socioenvironmental understanding of health is helpful in moving us beyond a liberal individualist view of health. That is, a socioenvironmental view of health moves us beyond thinking of health as an individual choice and responsibility and highlights how health is a sociorelational experience that is shaped by contextual factors.

Interestingly, the glue that binds the three perspectives of health together is the desire to help people live meaningful lives. For example, if one worked from a medical perspective of health promotion with a family who had a child living with juvenile diabetes, the focus would be on treating the diabetes and getting the blood sugars under control. The purpose in doing so, however, is so the child and family can live a *meaningful life*. Similarly, from a behavioral perspective one might teach the parents and child a diabetic regime and instruct them around certain lifestyle and behavioral changes. These behavioral changes, however, are intended to ensure the child does not end up with secondary complications that will put limitations on a meaningful life. What the socioenvironmental perspective does that is essentially different (and in our minds absolutely vital) is immediately shift the nurse's attention to the meaningful life and ensure it is always at the center of the nurse's focus and at the center of nursing practice. By shifting the attention to the meaningful life, the importance of context comes into focus. Whereas the medical perspective focuses the nurse's immediate attention on the disease and subsequent medical treatment, and the behavioral perspective focuses the nurse's immediate attention on lifestyle factors and disease prevention strategies, the socioenvironmental perspective immediately focuses attention on people's capacity to exercise their choice and their resources to construct and live a meaningful life. This includes an examination of the disease or limiting condition *and* the socioenvironmental capacities and limitations that are shaping people's choices. What is important about this distinction is that because the meaningful life is not the direct focus within medical and behavioral perspectives, quite often health care providers give precedence to disease treatment or prevention over what is significant to people in their everyday lives. Just as the physician at the breast cancer forum highlighted, disease and/or intervention to treat disease becomes the center of attention, rather than the people who are living with the disease. By focusing on the person's/family's life, the socioenvironmental perspective immediately draws attention to people/families, to what is particularly meaningful and significant to them, to how structural conditions shape capacity and resources, and to how all these need to be considered when determining how to intervene to promote health.

 To Illustrate

Diabetes care offers a good example of how the socioenvironmental approach directs our attention toward what is of meaning and significance to people and how such meaning must be understood in context. Based on a medical/behavioral approach to health promotion, the focus of diabetes care is typically on getting people to adhere to a diabetic regime. Most agencies have developed information handouts and standard protocols for nurses to follow when teaching 'a new diabetic'. Even an examination of the language that we use reveals what is given precedence. Diabetes is seen as an individual's disease and the individual is automatically labeled as a diabetic, thus putting the diabetes in the focus. It is the diabetes that monopolizes the conversation and becomes the focus of care and attention. Subsequently health is promoted by teaching individuals about the disease and instructing them on how to prevent complications by following a particular regime. This health promotion occurs without necessarily stopping to ask what is of particular significance to the people in their everyday lives, what living with diabetes will be like for them, what concerns they have, what capacities and resources they have to draw on as they live with this new health challenge, and so forth. Not only do nurses tend to overlook the importance of this vital context but many take for granted that what new diabetics need is instruction and information. It is standard practice for nurses to focus their attention on giving information they think the person needs, believing that if they offer this expert information the person will (or at least they should) follow it. When people don't follow their regimes, nurses become frustrated and wonder why.

A research project I (Gweneth) conducted a few years ago revealed that diabetic regimes are followed to the extent that they have meaning and significance for people (Hartrick, 1998). So, for example, an adolescent who is primarily concerned with 'fitting in' with a peer group and not being seen as 'different' will make decisions about diabetes care in accordance with that concern. If that means forgoing eating to not stand out as a 'freak' that may well be the choice that is made. Yet how often do we fail to stop and consider the context of peoples' lives? It is not uncommon for adolescents to be given the information about the regime and for parents to be given the responsibility to make sure their child follows the regime. Such an individualist, disease-care approach sets families up for struggle and frustration. If we are to promote health, we must first and foremost seek to know and understand what is significant and contextually meaningful to the people with whom we are working and ensure that any health promotion, including disease care and prevention, occurs in response to those concerns. For example, understanding and honoring the adolescent's concern to fit in informs us about what needs to be considered in helping him or her develop a relevant diabetes regime including contextually relevant strategies to both address the meaningful concern of fitting in while also attending to the diabetes and preventing future complications.

Implications of the Socioenvironmental Perspective for Nursing Practice

Perhaps beginning with the Ottawa Charter, the explicit articulation of the socioenvironmental perspective has had significant implications for how health professionals structure their practice. And these evolutionary changes in health promotion have substantial implications for the practice of family nursing. As we have just described, understanding health as a social and contextual phenomena means that health must be understood contextually, that is, understood to be shaped by social, physical, economic, and political environments.

Significance of Family

Understanding health as a social and contextual phenomena and knowing that family is the primary social structure in society highlights the significance of family to people's health. It reminds us that a person's health arises within and is shaped by the relational web in which they live (for example, family, community, society). It also underscores how important it is to consider this relational web in any health promoting activity. For example, health care today is most often structured according to the dominant norm of the dual-parent family that supposedly offers a loving, safe haven. One only has to look at the current move to deinstitutionalized care throughout the western world (for example, early post-op discharge, the decreased number of acute care beds, the rise in the number of surgical procedures being done as day surgeries, the move to community based mental health services) to see this norm in action. Underlying this whole trend is the generalized assumption that families are responsible, able and willing to look after their family members. This assumption has meant that people who do not live family according to this norm are disadvantaged. For example, some people who are discharged from hospital may be at home alone without care while still in a very acute state.

Structure of Family Nursing

Family nursing is typically structured as a service model type of practice. The nurse provides the services of assessing and intervening to treat illness and health problems. Yet the socioenvironmental perspective of health promotion informs us that the traditional service model of health care that focuses on the *servicing* of health problems lies in direct contradiction to the promotion of health and capacity (Bopp, 1989; Choi, 1985; Epp, 1986; Hartrick, Lindsey, & Hills, 1994; Labonte, 1993; Lindsey & Hartrick, 1996; Maglacas, 1988; McKnight, 1989; World Health Organization, 1984). According to the socioenvironmental perspective, if people are to develop and enhance their capacity to act on their living conditions, health promotion can no longer 'belong' to health professionals. If the health of people is to be improved, collaborative endeavors between people living health and those in the health care field are necessary. This means that the power and expertise for promoting health no longer belongs to professionals. Rather, people need to play a central role in their own health promotion and consequently power and expertise need to be shared and mutual.

The following are some of the central beliefs and assumptions underpinning a socioenvironmental perspective of health promotion. These principles, built on earlier work (Hartrick et al., 1994), can inform and direct family nursing practice.

1. All people have strengths and are capable of determining their own needs, finding their own answers, and developing their own solutions.
2. Every person and family lives within a social-historical context that helps shape their identity and social relationships. This sociohistorical context can lead to restriction of choices, limited resources, and a state of perceived powerlessness.
3. Diversity (race, gender, family form, age, sexual orientation, etc.) is positively valued.
4. People with fewer privileges (such as economic wealth, skill in the nation's official languages, education) have as much capacity as those with more privileges to assess their own needs (people are their own experts).

5. Relationships between people and groups need to be enacted with recognition of power dynamics and the intention to promote more equitable relationships. (This includes the 'professional' nurse-family relationship, about which we will say a lot more!).
6. The power of defining health problems and needs belongs to those experiencing the problems.
7. The people disadvantaged by the way society is currently structured must play a central role in developing the strategies by which to gain increased control over resources.
8. Empowerment is not something that occurs purely from within nor is it something that can be done for others. Rather power, and thus empowerment, is enacted in relationship.
9. Shared power relations do not deny health professionals their specialized expertise and skills. Rather, professional expertise and skills are used in new ways such that greater equity between families and nurses results.

These guiding principles not only require individual nurses to consciously and intentionally question the role they take with families and how they conceptualize family nursing practice, but also have implications for how health care is structured and perhaps needs to be restructured. Intentionally practicing from a socioenvironmental perspective of health promotion highlights the importance of never losing sight of what nursing assessment and intervention are fundamentally for and about—namely supporting people/families to exercise their power and choice to live meaningful lives.

As a result of taking a socioenvironmental approach to health promotion, family nursing moves beyond the treatment or prevention of disease and beyond working with people to address lifestyle factors. Family nursing becomes concerned with creating living conditions in which people's experience of health is increased. Although this may involve intervening to treat or prevent disease, the socioenvironmental perspective informs us that it is possible to promote health without necessarily reducing the prevalence of disease or specific risk factors. For example, health can be experienced and promoted in someone who is terminally ill or in someone who lives with chronic obstructive lung disease and continues to smoke. Viewing health as a resource for living and understanding choice and power as integral aspects of health moves us beyond the disease condition to promoting the meaningful experience of people in their everyday lives. Subsequently, central to any family nursing activity is the capacity of choice for people whose health is being promoted. Given the contextual nature of health (for example, health is determined through psychological, social, environmental, historical, and political factors), relational family nursing practice involves intentional efforts to create equitable relationships and to advocate for equity in resources, status, and authority for all people/families.

Moving Toward Health-Promoting Family Nursing Practice

During the past 2 decades this contextual understanding of health has led many nurses to take up a socioenvironmental perspective of health promotion. However, this change in practice has not been easy (MacDonald, 2002). Such a shift requires a major reconfiguration of the how, what, when, and who of practice.

An Example: Developing Health-Promoting Practices

A few years ago I (Gweneth) was asked to work with a multidisciplinary team of health practitioners who wanted to develop health-promoting practices with families. Administrators from a large acute-care hospital and a public health agency had collaborated on an initiative to address the needs of families and children living with asthma, allergies, and eczema. A principal goal of the project was to promote the health and well-being of children and families living with asthma, allergies, and eczema. The multidisciplinary team was formed to undertake this initiative. The nurse administrators at the two institutions asked me to conduct educational sessions with the team that focused on socioenvironmental health-promoting practice with families. As part of my involvement with the team, I conducted an educative-research project (Hartrick, 1998). My intent was to document how health promotion is experienced and enacted by practitioners in practice. In particular I wished to document the shifts in practice that occurred when the team members intentionally moved their practice from a medical- and behavioral-based approach to a socioenvironmental one.

The research project occurred over a 1-year period. During that time we held monthly education sessions to provide an opportunity for team members to share their everyday experiences of practice and critically think about the puzzling, paradoxical, and/or problematic features of health-promoting practice. Together we would sort through different practice possibilities that were consistent with a socioenvironmental perspective and that, more importantly, would promote the health and capacity of families.

The most predominant finding in the research was how, in very concrete and pragmatic ways, the team's focus of care moved from their overriding emphasis on reducing a child's asthma to focusing on enhancing the families' health experiences and capacity to live with asthma. Through their experiences the team developed an appreciation for the complexity of people's lives and how this influenced families' experiences of asthma. Overall they began working more collaboratively with families to address the broader determinants of health, and their practice changed in several ways. First, the participants' moved from thinking of themselves as experts in asthma care to seeing themselves as facilitators of health. This change is reflected in the following quotes. The first quote exemplifies the descriptions of the participants during the initial interview at the beginning of the project.

▶ *I'm the one that has the knowledge and I want to make sure that they can learn from that. Their role is first of all to learn something about their disease process and how to prevent it, or make it worse, or how to recognize signs when it is getting worse . . . just to recognize, not to be in so much denial about it.*

The next quotes are characteristic of the descriptions given during the final interviews and reveal the shift in their practice focus that took place.

▶ *Going to people and finding out what they need to know is the best way to go for it to succeed.*

> ▶ *Rather than having concrete goals the goals are more nebulous now, and the families are coming in when they want to, it's like a dance almost. You're trying to get them on this health promoting dance . . . they dance alone when they want to, or dance away. . . . I'm trying to make sure that the floor isn't slippery, they're not going to fall off the edge, that kind of stuff.*

A second change involved moving from focusing on asthma to focusing on children and families. For example, rather than focusing on giving asthma information and therefore giving the information that they thought families needed to know, the nurses began to inquire into the needs of particular families. As one nurse describes:

> ▶ *In the beginning I used to go with my big pile of papers and go in there and they'd barely say hello, and do you want a coffee, and I'd go into my thing about their asthma. And now I'm more relaxed about just letting them tell me what their needs are, and where I can help them and not just giving them information they need for the asthma part . . . listening to where they're coming from.*

Another fundamental shift was how the team members moved from an 'outsider' to an 'insider' perspective of illness. According to Conrad (1987) an outsider perspective of illness views illness from outside the experience. An insider perspective focuses directly on the subjective experience of living with and managing an illness. An insider perspective includes understanding the meaningful experience of the illness as well as knowledge of the disease process. As the team members strove to become more health promoting, they became aware of the significance of the personal meaning in peoples' health and illness experiences. Consequently, their care became focused on responding to the meaningful experiences of the families living with asthma.

This shift to an insider perspective meant that the team members moved from a stance of telling to one of asking. For example, rather than providing standard information to all families, the members began asking about the families' experiences and providing information and teaching within the context of those experiences. This is exemplified in the following quote:

> ▶ *My beliefs have come around a different way . . . and it wasn't until I realized that they weren't really listening to me . . . I could see where I wasn't looking at them as people, I was looking at them as a client and I had to give this asthma information and now I just feel totally different about it, I don't know how to explain it, I just feel totally different.*

One of most predominant themes within the final interviews was the profound shift that had occurred for the team members with regard to their views of health and health promotion. During the final interviews they all referred to social determinants of health and the importance of looking at 'the bigger picture'. They had moved from thinking of their work as individual focused to realizing the 'power of bringing people together'. They had come to see how a socioenvironmental perspective that focuses on enhancing peoples' sense of empowerment and choice was conducive to concrete outcomes such as decreasing the number of hospital admissions. This insight fostered their understanding of the relationship between the three models of health promotion (medical, behavioral, socioenvironmental) and enabled them to work more effectively with both families and their colleagues.

In relating their experiences of health promotion the team members' actions fell on a continuum ranging from individual family empowerment through to community organization and systemic change. The team members described realizing that they needed to move beyond individual families to system structures that got in the way of peoples' choice and the team's ability to effect change.

It is important to highlight the focus and effort it took on the part of the asthma team members to actually affect such shifts in their practice. For some of the members the move to a socioenvironmental perspective of health promotion required a complete reconfiguration of their practice. No longer the 'expert', they had to learn to look beyond their own preconceived ideas and knowledge to seek out the knowledge the family had to offer. They needed to learn how to follow the lead of the families rather than their own professional agenda. Their learning involved figuring out how to 'collaborate with' rather than 'do to' and 'do for' families.

Making the Shift in Practice

Purkis (1997) has demonstrated how even when nurses intend to practice in a socioenvironmental health-promoting way, their habit of practicing in a medically and treatment-oriented manner often dominates how they interact with people. For this reason, Purkis argues that to enact the values of health-promotion nurses must critically consider how they are living their expert knowledge in their everyday encounters with people. For example, Purkis' research showed that although public health nurses stated they were practicing according to a health-promotion model of practice they continued to practice in a very expert, power-over manner. During well baby visits, the nurses set the tone and focus of interactions by subtly cuing mothers about what was worthy of discussion. During the interactions the public health nurses continually prompted mothers on topics organized around 'childhood development'. The nurses deferred responses the mothers made that were outside the bounds of what they understood to be included in childhood development. Through this form of interaction the mothers received tacit yet clear instruction about what was normal, what was worthy of discussion, what they might need to learn more about, how they should proceed, and so forth. Purkis' research (which we discuss further in Chapter 2) demonstrated that even when nurses intend to move beyond an 'expert' approach to practice (as those public health nurses intended), their own concerns and habitual ways of practicing and existing institutional norms hindered their ability to do so.

To practice in ways that are consistent with a socioenvironmental perspective requires constant vigilance on the part of nurses. It requires that nurses

- continually examine their own habits of practice that might be constraining their ability to open up to families,
- consciously and intentionally focus their attention on what is of meaning and significance to families,
- incorporate an understanding of health as shaped by social conditions,

- critically consider the institutional working conditions and procedures that contravene such a focus (for example, certain policies, standard length-of-stay rules, standardized assessment tools).

In subsequent chapters we build on this socioenvironmental perspective of health, incorporating it within a relational approach to family nursing practice.

● Redescribing Family and Family Nursing

As you proceed through the chapters, you will have the opportunity to continue considering the ideas put forward in this chapter, and to critically look at how you are living your knowledge in practice. You will be invited to further examine how you are theorizing family and health and how your current theorizing is shaping your everyday practice. Because we believe family nursing knowledge is an active way of being in and approaching practice (not merely a set of abstract ideas or applicable techniques), it is our hope that through this book you will develop a greater ability to reexamine what you already 'know', step beyond your habitual ways of thinking and seeing, and use the perspectives presented here to begin to live and look at the world and at families in a new light.

In the following chapters you will be invited to question family nursing knowledge and practice and to refine your practice in order to become a *relational practitioner.* Whether you are an undergraduate student who has had little experience working with families or are a nurse with many years of practice experience, there are some fundamental questions regarding how one lives knowledge and relationally joins families that must never cease to be asked, questions that we hope to help you bring to the surface.

We are inviting you to join us on a journey of exploration and discovery into terrain that you may not have previously traveled. Similar to when one travels to a foreign country it is our hope that what you read and experience will not only expand your knowledge and understanding of family and family nursing but also perturb your thinking about new possibilities for your everyday practice.

THIS WEEK IN PRACTICE

Explicating Assumptions About Family Health

To determine the definition of family and health that is guiding your practice it is often helpful to actually look at your practice. For example, where you put your emphasis when caring for people, the role you play with families, and what you believe your responsibility to be offers insight into how you are implicitly defining both family and health and the relationship you see between them. To begin this process of explicating your definition of family and health and the values and beliefs that give rise to your nursing practice (in whatever that clinical area or setting might be) pay attention and ask yourself the following questions:

1. Where do I focus the majority of my time and energy in practice?
2. What concerns, goals, and/or purposes are directing me in practice?
3. What do I do to promote health in practice?
4. How am I (or am I not) attending to family in practice?

If you are not currently in a practice setting, think back to your most recent nursing experience to consider the questions.

CHAPTER HIGHLIGHTS

1. What habits were you able to identify in your own thinking as you read through this chapter?
2. What are two habits that you might want to intentionally alter in your practice?
3. What questions about family and health do you have after reading this chapter?

REFERENCES

Anderson, J., Perry, J., Blue, C., Browne, A. J., Henderson, A., Khan, K. B. et al. (2003). "Rewriting" cultural safety within the postcolonial and postnational feminist project: Toward new epistemologies of healing. *Advances in Nursing Science, 26*(3), 196–214.

Berman, M. (2000). *Wandering god. A study in nomadic spirituality.* Albany: State of New York Press.

Bopp, M. (1989, March). Spiritual barriers to health promotion. *Proceedings of the National Symposium on Health Promotion and Disease Prevention.* Victoria, British Columbia.

Browne, A. J. (2001). The influence of liberal political ideology on nursing practice. *Nursing Inquiry, 8*(2), 118–129.

Browne, A. J., & Fiske, J. (2001). First nations women's encounters with mainstream health care services. *Western Journal of Nursing Research, 23*(2), 126–147.

Burt, S. (1995). The several worlds of policy analysis: Traditional approaches and feminist critiques. In S. Burt & L. Code (Eds.), *Changing methods: Feminists transforming practice* (pp. 357–378). Peterborough: Broadview.

Butterfield, P. G. (1990). Thinking upstream: Nurturing a conceptual understanding of the societal context of health behavior. *Advances in Nursing Science, 12*(2), 1–8.

Choi, M. W. (1985). Preamble to a new paradigm for women's health care. *Image: The Journal of Nursing Scholarship, 17*, 14–16.

Chopoorian, T., L. (1986). Reconceptualizing the environment. In P. Moccia (Ed.), *New approaches to theory development* (pp. 39–54). New York: National League of Nursing.

Conrad, P. (1987). The experience of illness: Recent and new directions in the experience and management of chronic illness. *Research in Sociology and Health Care, 6*, 1–31.

Dewey, J. (1922). *Human nature and conduct.* New York: Henry Holt and Company.

Doane, G. (2003). Through pragmatic eyes: Philosophy and the re-sourcing of family nursing. *Nursing Philosophy, 4*(1), 25–32.

Elias, N. J. (1978). *The history of manners: The civilizing process* (Vol. 1). Oxford: Blackwell.

Elias, N. J. (1982). *State formation and civilization: The civilizing process* (Vol. 2). Oxford: Blackwell.

Epp, J. (1986). *Achieving health for all: A framework for health promotion.* Ottawa: Health and Welfare Canada.

Hardin, P. K. (2001). Theory and language: Locating agency between free will and discursive marionettes. *Nursing Inquiry, 8*(1), 11–18.

Hartrick, G. A. (1998). Developing health promoting practices: A transformative process. *Nursing Outlook, 46*(5), 219–225.

Hartrick, G. A. (2000). Developing health promoting nursing practice with families: One pedagogical experience. *Journal of Advanced Nursing, 31*(1), 27–34.

Hartrick, G. A. (2002). Transcending the limits of method: Cultivating creativity in nursing. *Research and Theory for Nursing Practice: An International Journal, 16*(1), 553–562.

Hartrick, G. A., Lindsey, E. A., & Hills, M. D. (1994). Family nursing assessment: Meeting the challenge of health promotion. *Journal of Advanced Nursing, 20*, 85–91.

James, S. M. (1907). *Pragmatism. A new name for some old ways of thinking.* New York: Longmans, Green & Company.

Kneipp, S. M. (2000). The consequences of welfare reform for women's health: Issues of concern for community health nursing. *Journal of Community Health Nursing, 17*(2), 65–73.

Labonte, R. (1993). *Health promotion and empowerment: Practice frameworks* (Issues in Health Promotion Series No. 3). Toronto: Center for Health Promotion.

Lindsey, E. A., & Hartrick, G. A. (1996). Health promoting nursing practice: The demise of the nursing process. *Journal of Advanced Nursing, 23*, 106–112.

MacDonald, M. (2002). Health promotion: Historical, philosophical and theoretical perspectives. In L. Young and V. Hayes (Eds.), *Transforming health promotion practice. Concepts, Issues and Applications* (pp. 22–28). Philadelphia: F.A. Davis.

Maglacas, A. M. (1988). Health for all: Nursing's role. *Nursing Outlook, 36*, 66–71.

Marck, P. (2000). Nursing in a technological world: Searching for healing communities. *Advances in Nursing Science, 23*(2), 62–81.

McKnight, J. (1989, Summer). Do no harm: Policy options that meet human needs. *Social Policy*, 5–15.

Papps, E., & Ramsden, I. (1996). Cultural safety in nursing: The New Zealand experience. *International Journal for Quality in Health Care, 8*(5), 491–497.

Paterson, J. G., & Zderad, L. T. (1988). Humanistic Nursing (NLN Publ. No. 41-2218, 2nd ed.). New York: National League for Nursing.

Polaschek, N. R. (1998). Cultural safety: A new concept in nursing people of different ethnicities. *Journal of Advanced Nursing, 27*, 452–457.

Purkis, M. E. (1997). The "social determinants" of practice? A critical analysis of the discourse of health promotion. *Canadian Journal of Nursing Research, 29*(1), 47–62.

Registered Nurses Association of British Columbia (RNABC). (1992). *Determinants of health: Empowering strategies for nursing practice. A background paper.* Vancouver, British Columbia.

Reimer Kirkham, S., Smye, V., Tang, S., Anderson, J., Blue, C., Browne, A. et al. (2002). Rethinking cultural safety while waiting to do fieldwork: Methodological implications for nursing research. *Research in Nursing and Health, 25*, 222–232.

Ribeiro, M. C. S., & Bertolozzi, M. R. (1999). Nursing and the environmental matter: A proposal for a theoretical model for the professional practice. *Revista Brasileira De Enfermagem, 52*(3), 365–374.

Rorty, R. (1999). *Philosopy and social hope.* London: Penguin.

Smye, V., & Browne, A. J. (2002). Cultural safety and the analysis of health policy affecting aboriginal people. *Nurse Researcher, 9*(3), 42–56.

Tanner, C. (1988). Curriculum revolution the practice mandate. In *Curriculum revolution: Mandate for change* (pp. 201–216). New York: National League for Nursing.

Thayer-Bacon, B. (2003). *Relational (e)pistemologies.* New York: Peter Lang.

Tomlinson, A. (1988). Communication skills. *Nursing, 3*(27), 1006–1009.

World Health Organization. (1984). *Health promotion: A discussion document on the concept and principles.* Geneva: World Health Organization.

World Health Organization (1986). *Ottawa charter for health promotion.* Ottawa: Health and Welfare Canada.

Wilber, C. K. (Ed.). (1998). *Economics, ethics and public policy.* Lanham, MD: Rowman & Littlefield.

2 Family Nursing Knowledge: A Living Process

OVERVIEW

In Chapter 2 we begin to consider what family is and what family nursing is. We offer a series of theoretical lenses and perspectives for your use in considering these questions.

A s we described in Chapter 1 our intent in this book is to provide an opportunity for you to enhance your conscious and intentional living of knowledge. We want to enable you to try out different ways of knowing 'family' and to develop wider possibilities for responding to families. To that end, in this chapter we briefly look at the ways of knowing that have traditionally dominated family nursing practice and introduce other possibilities that we believe have the potential to both expand the knowing of family and enhance the capacity for respectful and responsive family nursing practice. In a way we are attempting to act as travel guides. The journey into the terrain of family nursing is yours to take. As guides we draw your attention to different possibilities that you might try out while on the journey. This chapter can be thought of as the overview tour that provides a synopsis of theoretical perspectives to which we will continue to refer and draw on throughout the rest of the book.

● What Is Family?

Although there is a range of definitions of family offered in the nursing literature, most definitions tend to contain similar elements. The majority of definitions describe 'family' according to structure (who is in the family) and function (what the family provides or does). The definitions offer a conceptualization of family as a configuration of people who are connected in some way (for example, legally, socially, biologically) and who provide some kind of function for each other. Hanson (2001) has also offered the following distinctions between definitions of family: legal (relationships through blood ties, adoption, guardianship, or marriage), biological (genetic, biological networks among people), sociological (groups of people living together), and psychological (groups with strong emotional ties).

During the past decade, theorists from numerous academic disciplines such as sociology, women's studies, anthropology, and nursing have challenged the definitions that perpetuate the norm of the two-parent nuclear family and have called for new definitions of family that address the varied family forms that exist in the contemporary world. Two examples of definitions that have been created in nursing in response to that challenge include Wright and Leahey's (1994) definition 'the family is who they say they are' (p. 40) and Hanson's (2001) 'two or more individuals who depend on one another for emotional, physical and economic support. The members of the family are self-defined' (p. 6).

However, as new definitions arise and family is retheorized in an effort to attend to family diversity, the focus continues to be on family in its *literal* form. The definitions continue to conceptualize family as an *entity* that can be demarcated in some way (such as by form, 'who they say they are' or function, 'emotional, physical support'). As we have worked with families we have experienced 'family' in ways that are not revealed through literal conceptualizations. In particular we believe what is missing from many of the definitions is the understanding of family as a complex relational experience. That is, we have come to see family as a complex process where economics, emotion, context, and experience are interwoven and multilayered. And, we have come to believe that limiting our understanding of family to its literal, surface form (as an entity or a configuration of people) hides aspects of family that are integral to addressing the complexities within families' health and healing situations. Subsequently we want to offer the opportunity for you to consider other possibilities when constructing your working definition of family. We create this opportunity by briefly describing theories that are currently used as the conceptual foundation for understanding family in nursing and then exploring other perspectives that offer expanded views from which to consider the question: What is family?

● Family in Its Literal Form

The question What is family? has been largely addressed in family nursing by drawing on theories from other disciplines such as sociology, anthropology, and psychology. Three borrowed theories that have had a particularly strong influence on the conceptualization of family in nursing include:

- Structural-functional theory,
- Developmental theory,
- Systems theory.

Structural-Functional Theory

Structural-functional theory, as the name implies, conceptualizes family in structural and functional terms. This theory has been used in nursing to provide a framework for assessing how families are organized (structured) and what the family does (functions) to maintain and promote the health of its members.

Developmental Theory

Developmental theory also conceives of family in its literal form (for example, two heterosexual parents with children). This theory posits that families progress through a relatively predictable sequence of stages and at each developmental level there are particular tasks in which a family engages (for example, childbearing, childrearing) (Duvall, 1977; Duvall & Miller, 1985). This developmental perspective has been used in nursing to understand and assess the family's evolution through the lifecycle and the accomplishments in each of the stages.

Systems Theory

Perhaps the most influential of the three borrowed theories has been general systems theory, originally proposed by Karl von Bertalanffy, a biologist and philosopher. Systems theory focuses on the organization of the family and not surprisingly conceptualizes the family as a system of interacting parts. Similar to structural-functional theory, systems theory emphasizes interaction and integration among various parts of the system (rather than on the individual functions of the parts). The intent of family systems theory is to explain how parts of the family system (family members) affect the family as a whole and, simultaneously, how the whole affects each part (how the family affects individual members) and how the sum of the parts is greater than the whole (a family is more than a collection of individuals). General systems theory has been used to expand understanding of living systems in fields such as biology and subsequently has been used in numerous fields including business, engineering, cybernetics, education, communication, and family nursing.

Influence of Grand Theories

Structural-functional theory, developmental theory, and systems theory can be thought of as 'grand theories', that is to say, theories that are used to explain phenomena generally, in many, if not all contexts. These three grand theories have not only helped shape how families are understood in nursing but also have had a profound impact on family nursing practice. Even what is thought of as 'family nursing' (often associated narrowly with childbearing families) has been influenced by these theories. They have been used in various combinations to develop many of the assessment tools and approaches that currently dominate the family nursing field. Each has influenced and often been integrated into family nursing approaches. If you examine assessment tools and/or models of practice in other family nursing textbooks in some detail, you will probably be able to identify elements of one or more of the above grand theories. For example, you will find that most family nursing assessment models contain questions about the structure and function of the family, the developmental stage of the family and the way in which the whole and parts interact and influence the family overall.

Criticisms of Grand Theories in Family Nursing

Although these theories have been extremely helpful in ensuring that nurses (a) move beyond an individual focus and come to understand the important influence and role of family in health and healing, (b) understand the complexity within families, and (c) have a direction for practice, they have also been criticized during recent years. These criticisms are in concert with criticism of grand theories in general. Two interrelated areas of critique have arisen regarding the use of these theories in family nursing.

First the theories themselves, and the way they have been applied in nursing, have met with criticism. For example, although developmental theory has been helpful in highlighting the developmental transitions families experience, the stages and transitions that are identified within the theory (childbearing, childrearing, empty nest, and so on) reflect the idealized heterosexual, middle-class family that consists of a married couple and the requisite couple of children. As a result, developmental theory has been criticized for mirroring a certain social class and cultural perspective and not reflecting the reality of families today. Sociologists and feminist theorists have argued that the theory does not reflect the reality of many families in the world today (Cheal, 1993) and that families are far more complex and diverse than what is proposed in developmental theory (Collins, 2000). Clearly all families do not develop in the same way and, commonly, the developmental needs of individuals in the family may not always be 'in sync' with the developmental needs of the family unit. Similarly, although systems theory has served to highlight the relational and complex nature of families, the theory has been critiqued as having mechanistic roots (Parse, 1990). Parse maintains that the application of theories such as systems theory has often led nurses to practice in a fashion similar to fix-it mechanics (that is, there is the assumption that the 'machine' can be fixed by carrying out maintenance). Using preconceived assessment tools nurses set out to determine how the system is functioning and what they need to do to change and improve 'it'.

In addition to critiquing the theories themselves and identifying the limitations of the theories and how they have been applied, structural-functional, developmental, and systems theories have been criticized because they are 'borrowed theories' (Hayes, 1997). Nursing theorists in particular have leveled this critique, arguing that because these theories are borrowed from other disciplines they do not constitute nursing theory and/or reflect nursing knowledge. As Hayes (1997) highlights, 'consideration of theoretical patterns having to do with family nursing is rare' (p. 58). Along this vein, Cody (2000) emphasizes the importance of using 'nursing's own science to guide practice with families' (p. 284). Consequently such nurse theorists question the validity of structural-functional, developmental, and systems theory when it comes to nursing practice.

● Broadening Our Understanding of Family

Both of these areas of critique are important for you to consider when expanding your understanding of family and theoretically informed practice. However there is another crucial aspect to theory in family nursing that needs to be addressed—namely, *how* theory is used to inform practice. Specifically we are concerned with, and want to challenge, the authority that nurses may give to theory over families. For example, as the above grand theories have become solidified truths, they have dominated and profoundly shaped the art and science of family nursing practice. The theories and models of practice that have been developed from them have become what we described in Chapter 1 as habits of conduct. Nurses have developed the habit of looking at families as systems and assessing families in terms of their structure and function and their interactive processes. In this way the theories have gained authority over families. For example systems theory has become what White and Epston (1990) describe as a 'normalized truth' (Hartrick, 1995). The conceptualization of family as a system has come to dominate most, if not all, family nursing theory and practice. Most nursing students who have gone through educational programs during the past two decades would have learned the truth that family is a system of interacting parts. This truth has become so taken for granted that it goes unquestioned—and therein lies the problem (Hartrick, 1995). As White and Epston (1990) describe, normalized truths end up restricting and constraining our view. By 'normalizing' family as a system, we become blinded to other possible ways of thinking about family (Hartrick, 1995).

When theories are given such authority, it is the theories that to a large extent determine what questions nurses ask and what they focus on. That is, theories shape what we described in Chapter 1 as our selective interests. Nurses then interpret the answers to the questions through the theoretical constructs. The theories, in concert with wider social understandings of family, development, health, and so on, end up determining the truth of the family. Because nurses often lead their interactions with families and are the ones asking the questions, following the lead of the nurse, families often construct their answers according to these questions and underlying theories.

 To Illustrate

As discussed in Chapter 1, Purkis (1997) demonstrates how nurses working in a public health clinic constructed relationships with parents and children by providing parents with 'cues' regarding when to talk and what to talk about. Purkis offers the following example in which Fran, a nurse, having weighed and measured 4-month-old Lorraine, assesses the 'changes' that have occurred since the last visit by her and her mother, Erica. In looking at the example, one can hear growth and development theory dominating and shaping the entire interaction and assessment:

Fran: OK, and what sort of things do you notice her doing now, developmentally, that she wasn't . . . when you were in here at 2 months [looks briefly at the nursing record on the desk in front of her].

Erica: She's talking a lot . . . she's quite vocal sometimes . . . she's not too vocal today [laughs]. She seems to be grabbing at things a little bit. She learned how to pinch real good! She pinched me . . . and . . . I've given her some toys to play with, and she's really fascinated by those.

Fran: Is she pick . . . is it the toys that she's picking up, or more that she's watching?

Erica: She's got a thingamajiggy [points at the ceiling] . . . a mobile. And she really likes that, and I've given her a mirror to look in, so the Playskool thing has a mobile on it, she loves that. She rolls it and she looks at herself and talks and [laughs].

Fran: OK. Is she rolling yet?

Erica: She's trying to. She's really trying to turn her back and her hips but she can't quite get the leverage to push herself over.

Fran: Well, she'll probably surprise you.

Erica: She rolled over, actually.

Fran: Oh, really!

Erica: A month ago, like from a . . . front to back, but she doesn't know how to do it back to front.

Fran: OK.

Erica: But she only did it once for me. She hasn't done it since, so I think she maybe had a little spurt of energy that day of something [laughs].

From Purkis, M. E. (1997). The "social determinants" of practice?
A critical analysis of the discourse of health promotion. Canadian Journal of Nursing
Research, 29(1), 47–62. Used with permission of the Canadian Journal of Nursing Research.

Looking at this example one can see how authority has been given to growth and development theory (over the family) and how that theory determines the questions that are asked and the information the mother provides. Basically the nurse's understanding of the family is limited by a growth and development lens. In addition the way the nurse uses this theoretical lens puts her in charge of the entire interaction. It is the nurse who is positioned as the 'legitimate' questioner, and the mother is allotted the role of the responder who is meant to follow the lead of the nurse. The mother, following the cues of the nurse, quickly cues into, and in some ways already knows, how the conversation is to be organized (that is, according to the indicators of verbal, fine motor, and gross motor development) and with minimal prompting she joins in accordingly, thus demonstrating her 'good parenting' (Purkis, 1997).

This example shows how as nurses take up habitual ways of practicing and viewing families, their views become constrained by the limitations of the theory they take up. Although growth and development theory may well inform the understanding of this child/family's health experience, by giving authority to that theoretical lens, other aspects of the child/family did not have a chance to been seen. For example, had Fran been able to see through or around her taken-for-granted emphasis on child growth and development, the interaction might have gone quite differently. Fran might have been able to move beyond the topics that she deemed important, open up to other ways of engaging with this family and might have come to know other aspects of the family's life situation that were particularly significant to them. We explore this 'opening-up process' in much more detail in subsequent chapters.

● Theories as Instruments at Our Disposal

As we discussed in Chapter 1, theories are merely instruments at our disposal to help us understand family and to enable us to practice in knowledgeable ways. Theories help us challenge and expand our selective interests. Yet theories can also serve to constrain our view. For example, by only drawing on developmental theory, Fran's view of Erica and Lorraine was severely limited. If Fran had drawn on bonding and attachment theory, the interaction between her, Erica, and Lorraine would have looked different. However, we are not suggesting simply exchanging one theory for another—in either case the theory might or might not have coincided with what was of significance to the particular family. Rather, we are suggesting that as nurses we need to scrutinize theory in light of the families we meet to ensure they are actually helping us to *attend to what is of concern and significance to family,* and ultimately be more responsive and health promoting. For example, families are not really 'systems'; rather theorizing family as a 'system' is just a way of trying to help nurses see and attend to the complex and mulitfacted nature of families.

Overall the value of a family theory lies not in its 'truth value' but in how it enhances our ability to know and understand actual family experiences—how it informs our knowing of family in ways that are meaningful and relevant to the people with whom we are working. Therefore, rather than determining which is a more valid or true theory for guiding family nursing practice by comparing different theories (such as by comparing family theory from other disciplines to theory that has been developed within the science of nursing), theory needs to be interrogated in light of family and nursing experiences. Because all theories and truths have limitations, we believe that in order to heighten awareness of how theories are governing nursing practice and to be able to make more conscious choices about which theories will enhance practice, nurses must continually ask how adequate any theory is for guiding practice. As suggested in Chapter 1, the important question is: *How do these theories sensitize me to particular families and how will they enhance and/or constrain my ability to responsively attend to particular families at particular times?* In order to be more responsive and health promoting, we need to move beyond taken for granted views of family. We require perspectives that help us challenge taken for granteds and offer alternative views.

This understanding of theory as 'just a tool' can be both exciting and disconcerting. For those of you who have felt constrained by particular theories or have wondered how theory might be more relevant to everyday practice it may be quite liberating to approach your practice in this pragmatic way. For others who have assumed that a theory presents a 'truth' that can serve as the foundation for practice it might be unsettling to say the least. We want to be very clear that we are not diminishing the importance of theory. In fact it is just the opposite. Rather we are advocating for more critical consideration of how theory informs practice. As you contemplate this pragmatic perspective within the context of your own particular theoretical practice, you can rest assured that throughout the book it is our intent to provide lots of opportunity for you to consider and reconsider theory as you evolve your own family nursing practice.

● Beyond the Cartesian 'Literal' View of Family

The Cartesian worldview (described in Chapter 1) has dominated science in the Western world and has resulted in a reductionist approach to human beings and human *being*. Cartesian science functions at the level of what can be measured, observed, and quantified. Phenomena are reduced to the status of objects resulting in other modes of existence being reduced or lost altogether because they are not observable or quantifiable. For example, people are viewed in terms of their objective exteriors, and other aspects of existence such as their introspective and spiritual lives are either not seen or are ignored.

Impact of a Decontextualized View of Family

Perhaps one of the most problematic effects of Cartesian science has been the way that human life and people have been decontextualized. Seeing people as distinct entities separate from one another and their world does not allow us to see how people as relational beings are integrally connected and shaped by everyone and everything else in their world. As Kreiger (1999) describes, such a view fails to recognize how social experiences are literally incorporated biologically and are reflected in population patterns of health and disease. Social experiences intricately shape how people biologically 'develop, grow, age, ail and die' (Kreiger, 1999, p. 296). Failing to see the relationality of human life results in people being treated and approached as separate, self-sustaining, and self-creating entities. A good example of the impact of this decontextualized view was recently offered by an anthropology colleague of ours who remarked on how health care practitioners went about measuring the efficacy of Viagra. Looking at Viagra and Viagra users in a decontextualized way, the questions of efficacy centered around men's physical response to the drug (the men are objects whose response can be seen and quantified). Our colleague commented on the multitude of unexplored aspects that were crucial to know about if we were to actually understand the drug's efficacy. These other aspects included the experiential, historical, and sociocultural aspects (for example, what had taking the drug meant for the man? How had the man's *life* been affected by the Viagra? If the man had a partner, how had this person's life been affected? What had it meant for their relationship? Had there been an impact on how he related in his larger community? Were there sociocultural aspects that were significant to how the drug had affected him and his life?). This example highlights the limitations of the Cartesian view and the reasons we felt compelled to develop a relational view of family and family nursing.

Developing a Relational View of Family Health

As Kleffel (1996) argues, in order to account for the conditions that compromise health and to identify the interrelationships between social, political, and economic structures and the origins of health and illnesses, nurses need an "ecocentric" view. Rather than seeing humans as central and the environment as either irrelevant or something to be controlled, we need a view in which 'everything is (understood to be) connected to everything else' (Kleffel, 1996, p. 4). Kleffel points out that nursing theorists such as Parse, Rogers, Newman, and Watson have based their work on such a paradigm. Using such a perspective, nurses attend not just to individuals and families-in-context, but to individuals and families as situated in, shaped by, and continuous with their social, economic, historical, political, and physical contexts. That is, the relational nature of human beings and health is recognized and attended to. It is understood that people live within a relational web and consequently any health care intervention must not only be understood relationally but also must be evaluated from a relational vantage point.

The theories and processes that we draw on in this book are consistent with such an understanding. We are calling the approach we are taking 'relational' because the theories or lenses we offer later in this chapter emphasize the interconnectedness of people and their world and offer insight into the importance of sociocontextual structures in

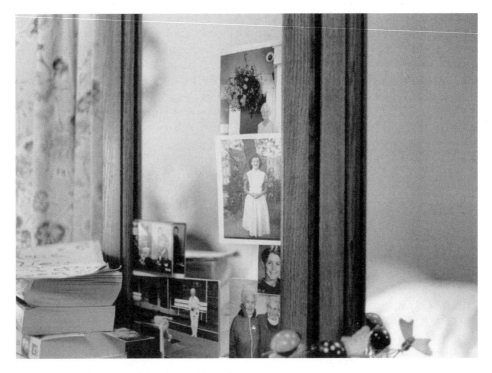

Mirror image. (Photograph by Gayle Allison.)

understanding family. In addition, although the theoretical lenses we present are in many ways distinct from each other, they each view the knower as central to knowledge and truth. That is, from the relational view, objective and subjective knowledge are inseparable. As described in Chapter 1, the relational view assumes that even objective 'facts' are interpreted by subjective people.

● A Relational Approach to Family Nursing Practice

One of our biggest challenges in writing this book has been putting what we want to say into language that will communicate what we are intending. Although the term relational seems to us to point to what we want to highlight, we have found that when we speak of 'relational practice' people do not hear the contextual aspects that we want to highlight. Many people think we are merely talking about and emphasizing nurse-family relationships. Similarly, when we use the term 'contextual' people think we are focusing on sociocontextual structures and somehow do not hear the interconnected relationality we are intending to emphasize. For that reason we want to explicitly clarify that in this book we use the term relational to describe the complex, relational nature of human life, the world, and nursing practice. Although relationships between people are certainly part of this relational understanding, relational nursing practice refers to far more than nurse-family relationships. In describing our approach as *relational nursing practice* we are saying that *we view and approach the world through a relational lens, always assuming and looking for how people, situations, contexts, environments, and processes are integrally connecting and shaping each other.*

Quantum Physics, the 'New Science', and Complexity Theory

The move beyond Cartesian science that has occurred throughout the past few decades has enhanced our understanding of the relational nature of human existence. One body of knowledge that has contributed to this relational understanding is quantum physics (Capra, 1976; Gleick, 1987) and in particular complexity theory (Prigogine & Stenger, 1984). Quantum physics has shown how all things in nature are interrelated. This new science provides an understanding of the universe as interdependent and relational, where the observer cannot be separated from the observed. 'In the quantum world, relationships are not just interesting; to many physicists, they are *all* there is to reality' (Wheatley, 1994, p. 32). Ray (1994) contends that reexamination of nursing practice within the new science theory has the potential to revolutionize nursing science. We have found complexity theory to be particularly helpful in broadening our view beyond the Cartesian—to see and understand people/families relationally (Hartrick, 2002; Miller, McDaniel, Crabtree, & Stange, 2001).

We have drawn on the principles and ideas within complexity theory that have particular relevance to family nursing and reconstituted them to enhance the view of relational practice. Subsequently, we do not provide an understanding of complexity theory but rather draw on complexity theory to articulate what we believe to be integral to relational family nursing practice.

People Are Relational Beings

Pause for a moment and try to think of a time when you are not in-relation. Although you might start to think of solitary activities that you engage in, probably if you think carefully about those activities you will see that in each of the activities you are still in-relation with something or someone. During a walk in the forest you are in-relation with nature, while reading a book you are in-relation with the text. Even during meditation people are in-relation with larger forces of energy. This relational nature of life is one of the foundational principles of complexity theory. According to complexity theory nothing exists independent of its relationship to something or someone else. The result of this relational connection may be subtle or profound.

To Illustrate

A good example offered in discussions of complexity theory is the 'butterfly effect'. Complexity theory demonstrates that the beat of a butterfly's wing could trigger a breath of breeze that eventually, through a series of initially minute and unforeseeable changes, could become a tornado (Vicenzi, White, & Begun, 1997). The path and force of this 'breath-tornado' is determined by a complex number of variables. Minute changes to any of the conditions or to one or more of the variables could drastically change the path and force of the breeze. The actual outcome of the beat of the butterfly's wing is ultimately determined by an infinite number of variables and their relational interactions.

This example depicts the sensitivity of living beings to other living beings and the world and the unpredictability and nonlinearity of cause and effect. One small variation can dramatically change the outcome yet the variables are so many and the complexity of interactions so great that the actual outcome can never be fully known or predicted. When we think about this butterfly effect within the context of family nursing practice several things are highlighted. First, it highlights how people's experiences of health are interrelated and affected by everything else in their world (Hartrick, 2002). So for example, the impact of Viagra is not a linear cause-effect process. The impact of Viagra is mediated by all of the other aspects of a man's relational existence including his particular inner physiological relationships, his familial and community relationships, environmental aspects, and so forth. This is why even with measurable interventions such as a medication dose one cannot assure a cause-effect response. The impact of even a medication is determined by a multitude of variables and relationships.

This butterfly effect has great significance for family nursing practice. In particular it highlights the nonlinear nature of change and the impossibility of nurses 'producing specific outcomes'. Although the Cartesian, reductionist view of science guides us to believe in a cause-effect model of practice, complexity theory informs us that outcomes are determined by people and their relational webs. If you stop and think about your nursing experiences, this butterfly effect is probably evident. For example, as nurses we have found there have been times when our deeply concerted efforts have had little impact on the people with whom we are working. No matter what we have done we have not been able to produce the outcomes for which we are striving. At the same time we have had experiences where a seemingly brief connection or minor effort on our part has had a profound effect on a family. Realizing the nonlinear, relational nature of human life and change helps us understand this variation in outcomes and highlights how the outcomes of our actions are always relationally determined. That is, as nurses we do not have the power or potential to make actual changes in families. Rather, any change that occurs will be the result of a multitude of relational factors. However, because our actions impact the relational outcome, complexity theory underscores the importance of being thoughtful about how we relationally engage with families. Because even a breath of a butterfly wing can spark a tornado, we must tread lightly as we enter in-relation with people/families and be deeply mindful of how we may be impacting the relational flow we are entering (Hartrick, 2002).

People and Human Experiences Are Dynamically Connected

A second principle of complexity theory is that people and human experiences are dynamically connected (Jantsch, 1980). As the Viagra example above depicts, every aspect of one's life is dynamically connected with the other aspects. This is why family is so important in nursing. As we discussed in Chapter 1 all people live family because they live in a society where family is a central social organizer. Even if they do not have a literal family, they experience family just by living in the everyday relational world—when they turn on their television, when they read a newspaper or walk in a park. Explicitly recognizing this dynamic connectedness underscores the importance of looking at the whole of people's lives. As nurses we have found this principle directs us to listen beyond the 'separateness' (or solitary nature) of the individual who may be sitting before us describing a health concern (Hartrick, 2002). As we listen with our 'relational ears' we begin to hear the larger life experience, how his or her health concern is related to his or her personal aspirations, life patterns, and life challenges. For example, listening to a family living with asthma, we listen for how the changes necessary to create an allergen-free environment will impact their overall life. What will the extra housework that is required to maintain a dust-free environment mean to a busy family or a single mother who is working full time? What of the family for whom an allergen-free environment is beyond possibility, such as the millions of underhoused families in our world today? For example, in Canada, many Aboriginal people are required to live on reserves in homes (the size, shape and materials firmly dictated by law) that are infiltrated with mould.

People Always Act in Relation to Something Else

A third principle of complexity theory is that people always act in relation to something—or someone—else (Zohar, 1990). This means that each person/family will present different aspects of themselves in different situations and in different relationships. Wheatley (1994) emphasizes that this does not mean people are inauthentic, rather they are merely 'quantum'. For example, take a minute and think about this idea in relation to your own life. Do you find that you are different in different situations and with different people? Have you ever had the experience of getting a report about a patient or reading his or her medical chart and then finding when you meet that person she or he is quite different from what you had heard or read about? Complexity theory contends this is because of the relational nature of matter. That is, quantum matter develops a relationship to that with which it comes in-relation and is changed in the process of that relational connection. So when we join in-relation with a family, what we observe is the family presenting *in response to us.* This means that we influence and in some way determine who we meet and what we observe in people just as they somewhat determine who and what they meet in us. For example, can you think of people or environments who 'bring out the best' in you? This relational nature of being and observing underscores the influence that you have as a nurse on the health-promoting process, what you experience and what you draw forth in others. As we have come to understand this relational nature of human existence, we have found ourselves much more mindful and intentional in our work. In particular, we seek to join in-relation and look at families in ways that will draw forth their health and capacity. For example, when we meet families we purposefully look for the capacities that are living within them rather than the problems that need to be serviced. This does not mean that we ignore the problems. Rather, it means that relationally we attempt to focus on, draw forth, and connect with capacities and potential in people rather than with their deficits. And, it means we focus on understanding and enhancing the relational capacity between us.

To Illustrate

    I (Colleen) have found this understanding of complexity and connection most helpful in my approach to smoking and mothers. In my work in the area of violence against women, I noted that many women smoked. As a reformed ex-smoker, I had a very judgmental attitude toward smokers, particularly mothers. I would look askance at women smoking wherever I went: playgrounds, grocery stores, and so on. Fortunately, I chanced to read some of Hilary Graham's research in which she described the meaning of smoking to women who had been battered (for her more recent work see Graham & Der, 1999a, 1999b, 1999c). She explained that although the women had little control in their lives, smoking was one area in which they did. In the context of coercive control by their partners, they were 'allowed' to smoke without question. Having a smoke also meant 'time out'—from their work and childcare, and sometimes from battering. Very poor women who had absolutely no other 'luxuries' could have this small source of relief, pleasure, and control for a very small price. Although I had previously understood the physiological relief afforded by smoking, I had not considered how smoking might be connected to other aspects of a woman's life within a family context. This knowledge helped me to shift my stance toward the women with whom I came in contact and to more intentionally seek to understand what smoking meant in the context of what was of significance to *them* and their families. In doing so, I found that I was able to open up conversations that my previous narrow understanding had prevented.

Relational Lenses

As we have developed a relational approach to knowing and worked with people/families, we have found three particular perspectives helpful. Thinking of these perspectives as similar to lenses on a camera we find that by intentionally viewing families from these different vantage points (through these lenses), our overall knowing and understanding of family health is enhanced. The lenses we have found particularly helpful in approaching family and family nursing relationally include a hermeneutic phenomenological lens, a critical lens, and a spirituality lens. Within what we are calling a critical lens, we discuss three overlapping perspectives—the feminist, the postcolonial, and the poststructural—that are concerned with power and the social context. In concert with a pragmatic approach, in which theories are seen as tools that can enhance our knowing and response to family, we take up the hermeneutic phenomenological lens contextually, use a critical lens to deepen our understanding of the context, and employ a spiritual lens to deepen our understanding of both context and meaningful living experience. Some of the key ideas within each of the perspectives are summarized in Figure 2.1 and Boxes 2.1 and 2.4.

Seeing Family Through a Hermeneutic Phenomenological Lens

Hermeneutic phenomenology focuses on how phenomena present themselves in lived experience (Heidegger, 1962; Merleau-Ponty, 1962). We do not intend to describe hermeneutic phenomenology in any full way (to really know and understand phenomenology as a philosophical perspective requires advanced and in-depth study) so keep in mind that hermeneutics and phenomenology as philosophical perspectives and as methods of inquiry have far more to them than what we describe here (for a more thorough overview of hermeneutic phenomenology, see Moules, 2002).

A phenomenological approach has been used by some nursing theorists in ways that focus on the individual, abstracted from context. For example, Browne (2001) points out that phenomenology has been used in concert with the ideas of individual free will and choice in the theories of some nursing authors such as Newman, Parse, Mitchell, and Cody. However, we are using a hermeneutic phenomenological lens in ways that take the context of experience explicitly into account. Thus, for example, choice and free will are understood to be constrained by life circumstances and possibilities, by culture, and by relationships with others and communities. What we offer below is a brief description of how *we* have found some of the central concepts within this perspective to be relevant in enhancing our understanding and view of family. A summary of the key concepts, assumptions, and ideas within 'our' hermeneutic phenomenological lens are included in Box 2.1.

BOX 2.1. **Hermeneutic/Phenomenological Lens**

Key Ideas

Living Experience
Meaning
Concern
Significance
Situated
Constituted

Assumptions and Ideas

- Our views of other people, situations, and the world can never be deemed objective or 'truth or fact'.
- People are not separate from their world but are *situated* in and *constituted* by it.
- People are influenced and shaped by the world because we are an integral part of it and it is an integral part of us.
- People have life experiences that are unique and at the same time have shared meanings with others.
- People can only be understood in relationship to their world, for it is only within their context that what people value and find significant is visible.

 An Example: A Disobedient Boy

A neighbour once told me (Gweneth) about an experience her son had had at school. The school had decided to put on a live theatre production of one of Charles Dickens' stories. All children in her son's class were expected to participate. My neighbour described how distressed her 10-year-old son was at what he saw as violent parts in the story. He had grown up in a family where strong concerns about how violence is condoned in our society were regularly expressed. To him, participating in this play was comparable to participating in a violent act. As a result he had refused to be involved in the play. His teacher viewed his refusal as uncooperative behavior, which she interpreted as disobedience. The school principal viewed the problem as an educational concern, in that by not participating in the play the boy would miss an essential learning experience. In relating this story to me, the boy's mother was expressing her pride in her son's obvious ability to make his own decisions and assert himself with authority figures.

From this description it is easy to see that the 'truth' of this situation and the knowledge that each person took away from the situation was different. Each person's understanding arose from his or her own personal expectations and beliefs and contextual location. For the teacher the truth was a disobedient boy; however, for the mother the truth was an assertive boy who acted from his convictions. For the principal the truth was a missed educational experience. As individuals they each made meaning of this same situation (interpreted and experienced the situation) in very different ways.

This story exemplifies many of the central concepts within hermeneutic phenomenology. First, hermeneutic phenomenology assumes that our views of other people, situations, and the world can never be deemed objective or truth or fact. As what we know and experience arises from who we are, our knowledge reflects our own interpretation of a particular person, family, or situation. What I take notice of in a family and the meaning I make of a family (my interpretations) are always funnelled through my person—through what I believe and value, what I am expecting or anticipating, what I have experienced, what theoretical knowledge I have learned, and so forth. This is because, according to phenomenology people are not separate from their world, but are *situated* in and *constituted* by it.

Situated in the World

Situated means that people do not just live in an environment but they inhabit their world (Benner & Wrubel, 1989). Being situated means that we live in a meaningful world that is informed by our experiences with family, culture, school, work, friendships, and a myriad of other influences. Our everyday smooth functioning in the world is facilitated by sharing a common language and understanding customs and practices. Phenomenology focuses on the relationship of the person 'in' the world, not separate from it. 'World' in this sense goes beyond the physical environment to include the meaningful sets of relationships, practices, and language that we have by virtue of being born into cultures (Leonard, 1989). From this perspective it is impossible not to be influenced and shaped by the world because we are an integral part of it and it is an integral part of us. People and their world are one.

Constituted by the World in Us

Phenomenology also views people as *constituted*. People become who they are as a result of their evolutionary history, their experiences, as well as the teachings/learnings handed down by previous generations (including cultural dos and don'ts and family norms and standards). Just as we embody the genetic biology of our parents, as we live in the world we begin to embody the evolving sociocultural norms of our society. We take up experiences, knowledge, and teachings bodily and they become part of us. Overall the notion of 'constituted' refers to the world that is in us—the world that we have taken up and that has become an integral part of us.

The young boy in the earlier story had grown up *situated* in a family that abhorred violence. Being situated in his particular family, he had become *constituted* as a person who was deeply *concerned* about violence. How he was situated in the world (for example, in his particular family who abhorred violence and in a society that condoned violence in the media) and how he was constituted by the world that was in him (for example, the family values and attitudes that had become a part of him) directly shaped the *meaning* he made of Dickens' play, how he *experienced* the school project, and how he was compelled to act. Similarly, how his teacher and the school principal were each situated and constituted gave rise to different meanings and truths about the same situation.

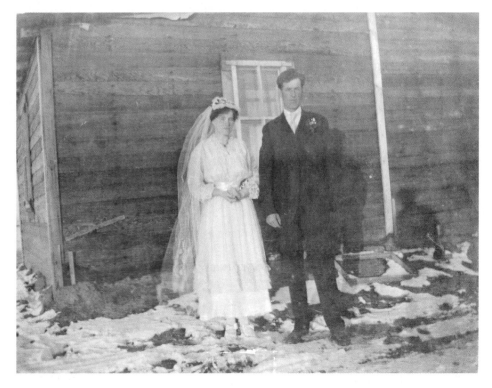

A homesteading family experience. (Photograph courtesy of Gweneth Doane.)

An Example: Work Before Play

    In the early 1900s my (Gweneth) grandparents immigrated to Canada with a few dollars in their pockets and homesteaded on the Saskatchewan prairies. The rugged life of homesteading required constant hard work. To survive one had to be reliable and accountable to those close by, be honest and forthcoming, and had to know how to get by with very little. Although when I was a child my grandparents were retired and living in a comfortable home on a city street, they were still constituted by their homesteading values and way of being. Growing up *situated* in that homesteading milieu, that way of being became a living process through which I was shaped. Living amid my grandparents who were *constituted* by their homesteading experience and my mother who had been their young child during the 1930s Depression, I was constituted by those values and attitudes. Just as I inherited their genetic structure, I inherited their homesteading culture and way of being. Even though I am now an adult and have lived away from my extended family and from Saskatchewan culture for many years, the values, way of being, and work attitudes of the homesteading culture are clearly living in and through me. Phenomenologists would say that I am *constituted* by them. For example, if I don't pay close attention I find that at times my sense of responsibility about my work can override my leisure time. The homesteading work ethic is 'in my bones'. That homesteading constitution shapes how I experience situations and other people with whom I work including my interpretations, my expectations, and so forth. Currently living in (*situated in*) the 'West Coast' culture of British Columbia, which is far more 'play' focused, I find I continually bump up against myself and my constituted way of being that says work before play. Although I can make conscious choices and live a more play-full life, that Saskatchewan history is part of my constitution and will forever be in me.

Because people are situated and constituted they will have life experiences that are unique. At the same time there may be *shared meanings.* For example, I (Gweneth) grew up with three siblings. As adults we have discussed experiences we had as a family during our childhood. Through these conversations it is evident that at times we made meaning in similar ways (for example, we share a knowing and understanding of our mother) and at other times we made quite unique interpretations (we each experience and relate to our mother in somewhat different ways).

Shared and Unique Meanings

This idea of *shared and unique meanings* applies to health and illness. A simple example is the experience of having a cold. The actual course of the illness for each of us is unique (for example, what exact symptoms we get and how they affect us) and what the cold means for us varies (it might give us a valid reason to get some much-needed rest or it might mean missing out on something we really wanted to do). As well as unique meanings, each of us shares an understanding of what it is like to have a cold. Because we have had the experience we are sensitized to *what it is like* to have a headache, runny nose, cough, and fatigue. However, a vital distinction is that we can't really know what it is like for another person in a particular moment of time unless that person tells us of their experience.

Different Values and Concerns

Because people are situated and constituted, in the phenomenological view, people are beings for whom things (events, actions, objects, experiences, people, and so on) have particular significance and value. Because people have qualitatively different concerns and priorities based on their situatedness and constitutedness, what is valuable and significant varies for each person, and for each person over time. For example, as a nurse interested in children, public policy that has an impact on young families may be of more interest and concern to me than would public policy about gerontology. This is not to say that such concerns or interests are mutually exclusive but only that one stands out as being more or less important, more or less significant depending on my consitutedness and my situatedness. Similarly in the example of the cold, within the same experience different things will be of concern and significance to different people. For a mother with a new baby, giving the cold to her baby might be of particular concern. For a mother *situated* in a low-paying job without paid sick leave, being unable to work might be of greatest concern; if she visits a physician for treatment, the physician's particular concern might be preventing the cold from turning into a pneumonia. For the woman in prison, a cold might be of little significance in contrast to her other concerns. For this reason, phenomenologists contend that to gain an understanding of people they must be considered in relationship to their world, for it is only within their context that what people value and find significant is visible. This is an important concept that we will be revisiting throughout the book.

Family As a Meaningful Experience

Overall when we look at family through hermeneutic phenomenology lens we are reminded that there is no one truth of family but many possible interpretations. Whether we are working with a literal family or an individual person who has no current ties to a literal family, *all people meaningfully experience family* (remember John in Chapter 1). The aim is to gain a greater understanding of the meaning of family in the everyday lives of people. From a phenomenological perspective to know family is to know how family is meaningfully experienced in the everyday lives of particular people in particular situations. Rather than focusing on determining the structure or function of a family or the truth or facts of a family situation, a hermeneutic phenomenological lens focuses our attention on illuminating the *meaning* those facts and the situation have for the people experiencing them. As nurses guided by a hermeneutic phenomenological lens, we want to know what meaning family has in the lives of the people with whom we are working.

Through a phenomenological lens, we understand family as *situated* and *constituted*. Subsequently, we view each family as unique. This means that, for example, although five families may have a child with juvenile diabetes, we recognize that the diabetes will likely have different meanings for the different families and consequently be experienced differently. Depending on how the family is constituted and situated, what diabetes means in their everyday lives and what is *significant* and/or of *concern* will vary. Although nursing research into families' experiences can inform us about what might be part of a family's experience and biomedical research can offer knowledge of the treatment and prevention of the disease, such knowledge only becomes relevant *within the context of family knowledge and experience.* For this reason we intentionally try to ensure that our 'expert' nursing knowledge does not overshadow or obscure the meaning and experience of diabetes for each family with whom we work. We explore this 'use of knowledge' in more detail later.

Seeing Family Through A Critical Lens

Although a hermeneutic phenomenological lens points to the social context as important to understanding meaning, a critical lens focuses on the social context itself. Using a critical lens draws explicit attention to power, social inequities, and structural determinants of health. 'Structural' refers to basic structures in society such as the state, local, and global political economies; globalization; racialization; and dominant institutions such as health, legal, educational, and government systems (Browne, 2001). A critical lens helps us to focus on how structural conditions shape social inequities, health, and health care and how they provide the basis for political knowledge and change beyond the level of particular families. Some of the major concepts from the critical perspectives are summarized in Figure 2.1 and Box 2.2.

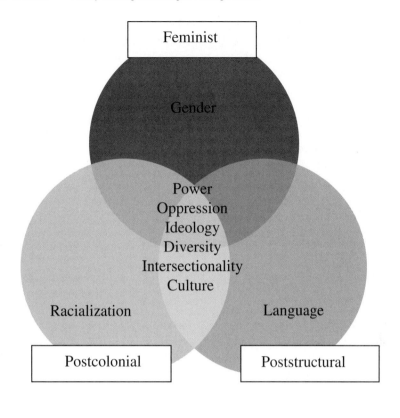

Three Perspectives in the Critical Lens: Key Ideas

F I G U R E 2.1. Three Perspectives in the Critical Lens: Key Ideas.

A critical lens is concerned with power, oppression, culture, the economic conditions of life, social change, and emancipation. This lens encompasses many perspectives and sociological theories that aim to challenge and disrupt what is taken for granted ('the status quo') by digging beneath the surface of society and examining the assumptions and masks that shape our understanding of how the world works. From early roots in Marxist analyses, critical theories have developed in many ways and are now understood to be concerned 'with issues of power, and justice and the ways that the economy, matters of race, class and gender, ideologies, discourses, education, religion and other social institutions, and cultural dynamics interact to construct a social system' (Kincheloe & McLaren, 2000, p. 281). As with hermeneutic phenomenology, we do not intend to describe critical theories in any complete way. We offer a brief description of some of the central concepts and perspectives within a critical lens that *we* have found relevant to understanding family health, concepts and perspectives that offer us an expanded view and a broader base for increasing our responsiveness to family.

> ### BOX 2.2. Critical Lens: Assumptions and Ideas
>
> - All knowledge is shaped by socially and historically shaped power relations.
> - Facts (or 'truth claims') can never be separated from values or ideology; there is no foundational knowledge that can be known outside of human consciousness, values, and history.
> - Every form of social order involves some form of domination and power.
> - Belief systems presented and treated as 'facts' by those in power act as barriers to conscious action and freedom.
> - Mainstream research and practice generally maintains and reproduces (perhaps unwittingly) systems of race, class, and gender oppression.
> - Certain groups in any society are privileged over others; oppression is most forcefully reproduced when people who are subordinated accept their social status as natural, necessary, or inevitable.
> - Language is central to developing knowledge and creating meaning.
> - A critical lens can help see through objective appearances and expose underlying social relationships.
> - By explaining and critiquing the social order, critical social theory serves as a catalyst for enlightenment, empowerment, emancipation, and social transformation.
> - Critically oriented knowledge ought to offer cultural or social critiques with a view to transforming the status quo.
>
> *(Browne, 2000; Kincheloe & McLaren, 2000)*

An Example: An Irresponsible Daughter

Yesterday, Bulbir, a nurse on a medical-surgical unit of a small urban hospital, told me (Colleen) about a kafuffle on her unit. The staff were furious with the daughter of a woman who had been recently discharged following a hip replacement. The 82-year-old woman was readmitted with bedsores, dehydration, and severe pain. Bulbir had been working on the day the woman had been discharged, and Bulbir recalled that at the time her daughter had said very clearly that she could not look after her mother. However, the staff had insisted that her mother 'had to go' as there were other patients awaiting admission, and thus there was no bed for her. Both at discharge and on readmission of the woman various staff members expressed considerable anger, wondering 'what kind of daughter' would refuse to care for her mother. Bulbir said that the daughter (Lena) was very upset at the staff and their treatment of her. Lena felt extremely guilty about her mother's condition, and even more guilty in the face of the staff's anger (apparently expressed both indirectly with accusatory glares and head shaking, as well as directly, when one staff member asked 'How could you let this happen?'). Bulbir asked Lena what was going on for her. She explained that they live in a very small mobile home, but that the rent is quite high. They need to live in the area because Lena's son (age 43) has schizophrenia but has been doing very well at a day program nearby. Lena has a weekend housekeeping, care-taker job in a wealthy community two bus rides from her home. The job requires Lena to stay overnight, and during the weekend, her mother's condition deteriorated.

In this story, Bulbir helps us 'dig beneath the surface' using a critical lens. Bulbir inquired about the context of this family's life, and thus surfaced how economic conditions (among other things) were shaping the family's experience of health and health care. One of the central values of a critical lens is the way it helps us penetrate the world of objective appearances in order to expose the underlying social relationships that are often concealed. Critical theorists 'try to demonstrate that what appears to be common sense, to be natural and necessary, really rests on conditions that are *socially produced*' (Osmond, 1987, p. 110, emphasis added). Thus, a major goal of critical theory is to reveal how surface reality often contradicts the underlying reality. Donning a critical lens we begin by questioning and uncovering how family nursing is being constructed out of dominant, stereotypical notions. On the surface, to some of the staff this family's 'reality' was an uncaring, neglectful daughter refusing to take on her social and family responsibilities. What is not so readily evident (until you use a critical lens) is that the staff's assumptions (about what a family and a good daughter are) work with health care system policies (such as length of stay for a hip replacement) to create this detrimental situation.

Belief Systems as Barriers

The staff's assertion that Lena's mother 'had to go' is an example of a central notion in critical theory—that belief systems presented and treated as 'facts' by those in power act as barriers to conscious action and freedom. The staff apparently did not question whether Lena could afford (in financial terms) to take care of her mother. In addition to being in a position of power (relative to their patients) because of their professional status, in Western countries health care providers often have a greater income and more education than their patients. Thus, health care providers are often operating on assumptions that do not match the reality of families' lives. Definitions of and assumptions about family that merely reflect mainstream, middle-class, White, Eurocentric, heterosexual family structure treat that structure as 'normal' and serve as barriers to families who do not fit that structure. In the face of the staff's directive that her mother must go home, and despite her misgivings, Lena took her mother home and then felt guilty at being unable to care for her properly. This points to another idea within critical perspectives—that oppression is most forcefully reproduced when people who are subordinated accept their social status as natural, necessary, or inevitable.

By examining how our nursing practice is socially produced through taken-for-granted norms and stereotypes, a critical lens helps us identify and then reject all forms of truth that may be subordinating human consciousness and action (Giroux, 1983). Critical theorists remind us that human consciousness, particularly self-consciousness, is vital to human liberation. A critical lens fosters more self-consciousness in us as we go about our nursing work and thereby the opportunity and freedom to more consciously choose the truth that we will follow. For example, a critical lens draws our attention to the authority that we are giving to any theory and/or to predetermined family assessment tools and leads us to question how those theories and tools may be subordinating a family's own perspectives and constraining our ability to be responsive to what is meaningful and significant to families. For example, if Fran, the public health nurse in Purkis' (1997) study described earlier, had brought a critical lens to her interaction with the family, she would have been compelled to look beyond the dictates of growth and development theory and listen for the sociopolitical aspects of the family's situation. If it transpired that the mother (Erica) was struggling to find childcare and work to support her daughter Lorraine, that struggle, and the social conditions that produced that struggle, would be a nursing concern for Fran.

Knowledge Creates Change

This points to another central premise of critical theory—that knowledge should be used toward social change and for emancipatory political aims. Critical theorists argue that critical thought must be combined with critical action (praxis) to bring about change in what we criticize. Osmond (1987) explains that whereas interpretive, hermeneutic sciences aim at understanding meaning without necessarily influencing it, 'critical sciences aim to both understand the world and to change it' (p. 107). The goals of a critical perspective are to provide a critique of the societal status quo and to effect social change. Critical theorists argue that knowledge should be used toward the alleviation of social problems and draw attention to families as social, political, and economic units. This is not to say that Fran would 'fix' Erica's childcare and employment problems, but that Fran would understand what was of significance and concern to Erica and act toward the alleviation of such problems. In this example, actions might take the shape of referrals for childcare or supporting a community initiative for improved childcare.

From Bulbir's story it is clear that simply discharging Lena's mother back home into the same set of circumstances will not be health promoting. A critical lens and its emphasis on emancipatory political aims works at both the level of the individual and at a social level. For example, at the individual level, Bulbir might share her understanding of Lena's family with the rest of the staff to help broaden their understanding of this particular family. The staff might then see if some home support or alternative care was possible for Lena's mother. At the social level, they might challenge the discharge 'rules' that dictate a proscribed length of stay regardless of the patient's condition or the availability of suitable care after discharge.

Knowledge and Values Are Interrelated

A critical lens is based on an assumption that knowledge can never be separated from values or ideology; scientific research and theories (and the practices to which those give rise) are embedded in societal norms, values, and expectations. Knowledge is value-laden because those who have developed the theories have lived and participated in society and thus have been influenced and shaped by taken-for-granted societal truths and expectations. For example, family development theory mirrors dominant dual-parent, White, middle-class societal values. Therefore, critical theorists contend that theories and models need to be scrutinized and questioned so that we do not (in the name of scientific practice) inadvertently lay oppressive societal values and expectations on people/families who may not fit those norms.

Within the family literature Duffy and Leeds (2001) offer examples of two societal narratives that dominate our assumptions about family and oppressively shape social expectations of family. The first narrative depicts family as the mainstream societal 'cop' having the responsibility to mould and shape its members into normative behavior that conforms to the larger societal script. This dominant narrative leads to the expectation that a central family function is to socialize children to become functional adults who fit the mainstream mould. Certainly as mothers we have both routinely felt pressure from others (for example, in stores, at school) to make our children conform to society's image of the nonquestioning, quiet, obedient well-behaved child.

The second dominant narrative Duffy and Leeds (2001) identify is that of the family as a 'safe haven'. In this narrative the family is expected to function as a source and center of interpersonal life and fulfillment. For example, Stajduhar (2001, 2003) studied palliative caregiving by family members and found that health care providers and families uncritically took up the narrative of family as a safe haven in the shared ideology that home is the best place to be and die. Health care providers assumed that families wanted to and were obligated to provide this safe haven. This assumption worked in concert with pressures arising from the health care system such as health care reform and rationing of resources. Ultimately it meant that families felt pressured to provide home care to their dying relatives and that family caregivers felt that health care providers exploited their sense of family obligation.

As the examples cited earlier begin to illustrate, all theories are embedded with certain social values and those social values may or may or may not be conducive to a particular family's well-being. This means that (a) any theory and knowledge must be scrutinized for its limitations and blind spots and (b) no single theory can offer a sufficient and comprehensive view of family. A critical lens helps us to consciously consider the view of family any theory is providing, to scrutinize the societal values and assumptions we may be perpetuating in our practice if we live that knowledge, and to more intentionally choose how we will live knowledge-in-practice.

Family as a Sociopolitical Experience

When we look at family through a critical lens we are compelled to question the everyday *taken for granteds* (ideologies) that shape our understanding of family and that shape people's experiences of family. Donning a critical lens positions us to expose the underlying *sociopolitical structures* that are advantaging some people/families and disadvantaging others. It reminds us that *social conditions* are not natural or constant and that existing structures (for example, health care structures) may need revising in order to be *equitable* and responsive to families, particularly to those families who do not (or cannot) conform to dominant values. Although the hermeneutic phenomenological lens draws our attention to how families are situated and constituted, the critical lens draws our attention to the sociopolitical, economic, and language contexts within which families are situated and constituted. Within the critical lens, particular perspectives draw attention to different aspects of the contexts within which families are situated and constituted. Next we turn your attention to three different perspectives within a critical lens: the feminist, postcolonial and poststructural.

A Critical Feminist Perspective

A feminist perspective brings to the critical lens a concern for how power is gendered, and conversely, a critical lens brings to a feminist perspective a concern with how gender relations are socially produced. A critical feminist perspective is concerned with gender equity and focuses on the necessity of restructuring societal roles and relationships to create equal rights and power for both women and men. Such a perspective also draws attention to how gender roles are deeply imbedded within Western capitalist society. For example, in her study of men in nursing, Evans (Evans, 2002; Evans & Frank, 2003) illustrates how men are trapped into certain forms of masculinity. She shows how as a result of these socially sanctioned masculine roles, men in nursing are at greater risk than their woman counterparts for being ridiculed, devalued, and unsupported for their choice of career and of engaging in gender-inappropriate behaviour. According to Evan's research, male nurses are routinely assumed to be gay and, paradoxically, often feared to be sexual predators in relation to women and children. Evans found that men in nursing were continuously defending their career choices, behaviours, and sexuality. Not surprisingly, sexual stereotypes are the greatest deterrent to men from entering nursing (Hanvey, 2003).

Viewing families through a critical feminist lens draws explicit attention to the gendered context of families and provides an avenue for discovering the subtle ways that dominant societal values prescribe gender roles and responsibilities and for exploring the power these gender roles have in families. Feminists argue that male-female relations are socially constructed and that the family is the prime site for the reproduction of relations of domination and subordination between the sexes. Mandell and Duffy (1995) tell us that 'Feminist analyses have clarified the contradictions contained within family life. They have exposed women's ambivalent relationship to the family as chief family labourer, as principal victim of family violence, as embodiment of family sentimentality and romance' (p. 2). Thus, a critical feminist lens highlights how the experience of family is gendered, how roles within the family are gendered, and how such gender roles are shaped by larger social forces.

 ## To Illustrate

In her study of palliative caregiving, Stajduhar (2001, 2003) used a critical perspective that she saw as encompassing a feminist perspective to analyze family caregiver experiences within a larger sociopolitical and economic context. She showed how caregivers did not necessarily choose to engage in home-based palliative care but that their engagement often stemmed from an obligation to care, especially if they were women. She also showed how health care providers reinforced the taken-for-granted assumptions that women would make this choice freely and that they were available and able to take up the caregiving role. Stajduhar illustrated how the health care system, driven by cost containment and efficiency models, reinforced the idealization of dying at home, leaving the caregivers feeling pressured to conform, disadvantaging many, particularly women and other marginalized groups.

Think back for a moment to the example of Lena in the story provided by Bulbir earlier. To what in that story does a critical feminist perspective draw attention? What similarities do you note between the example provided by Bulbir and the dynamics identified in Stajduhar's research?

Family as a Gendered Experience

Looking at family from a critical feminist perspective draws attention to the way in which being in a *family is a gendered experience* and the way *power* within the family is gendered. Looking through a critical feminist lens it is possible to see that the way *gender roles* and inequalities are played out in family are continuous with the wider fabric of society. So, gendered family roles and experiences are not merely 'choices' made by individuals, but rather are enactments of wider social values, expectations, and ideologies.

When we look at family from a critical feminist perspective we are compelled to question how gender shapes our understanding of family and shapes people's experiences of family. Further, we are compelled to question how our practices are being shaped by gendered assumptions and how those practices might reinforce gendered inequities. For example, research has consistently shown that the most caregiving is done by women, and that caregiving has a tremendous impact on women's health. Rather than either a burden or fulfillment, caregiving can be both destructive and renewing (Wuest, 2001). However, researchers such as Stajduhar (2003) and Wuest (1997, 2001) have shown that health care providers reinforce expectations that women are caregivers, often overlooking the burden of that care, and can create and intensify problems for caregivers. A simple example is a sign with visiting instructions on a wall in a unit for children with eating disorders. The top two lines of the sign read 'Moms! No food from home'. In subtle and not-so-subtle ways gendered expectations are conveyed. These expectations advantage and disadvantage both women and men. Often women are handed responsibility while fathers are left out or overlooked. For example, as nurses do we assume a single mother would have more knowledge and better nutritional practices than a single father and shape our practice accordingly? Similarly, are we more likely to assume that an elderly patient will be discharged from hospital into the care of her daughter or daughter-in-law rather than her son or son-in-law?

It is important to note that Western feminism (or certain forms of feminism—often labelled 'liberal White feminism') is often critiqued as focusing on gender as though gender is experienced in the same manner by all women. Other feminists, notably those who sometimes call themselves 'Black feminists' such as hooks (for example, 1984, 1990), Collins (1990, 1993), and Brewer (1993) have offered analyses of power and oppression that distinguish feminist perspectives that foreground gender from those that emphasize the 'intersectionality of oppressions'. 'Intersectionality' refers to the interaction between forms of oppression (for example, racism, classism, sexism) in ways that magnify one another (Brewer, 1993; Collins, 1993). That is, for example, the experience of being poor (or subjected to racism, or disabled, or aged) is not simply an 'added' form of oppression for a woman, rather, being poor magnifies the oppression inherent in being a woman. Similarly, being subjected to racism amplifies poverty, as does disability, and so on. Intersectionality addresses the ways in which various forms of oppression reinforce each other and interact. Thus, for example, an Aboriginal family whose members cannot find employment because of racism is forced to remain poor, and so on. This form of feminism overlaps with a postcolonial perspective, which draws particular attention to the continuing legacy of colonialism and to the impact of ongoing neocolonialism.

A Postcolonial Perspective

Although some strains of feminism draw attention to forms of inequality beyond gender, postcolonial theory helps us bring our attention to the social conditions occasioned by colonialism and its constant companion, *racism*. Colonialism encompasses the processes by which a foreign power dominates and exploits indigenous groups and more specifically refers to these processes enacted by European powers between the 16th and 20th centuries (Henry, Tator, Mattis, & Rees, 2000). Neocolonialism refers to similar domination and exploitation, but rather than being accomplished through physical settlement and military domination, as was the case in the earlier European colonialist expansion, neocolonialism is accomplished through trade agreements and diplomacy backed up with military threat. For example, although the country of Ghana has a wealth of resources and a progressive government and achieved independence from Britain in 1956, hunger and deprivation are widespread as the county continues to struggle under the debt load of international loans initially made from the International Monetary Fund and more recently from the World Bank.

Racism is a constant companion to colonialism because assumptions of racial superiority justify and facilitate domination of indigenous peoples. Throughout the history of colonialism, colonizers have seen indigenous peoples as 'backward', 'savage', less civilized than the colonizers, and in need of taming, education, or civilizing. The values and practices of the colonizers were (and continue to be) imposed as superior, and cultural hegemony, as well as political, economic, and military dominance by Europeans, was achieved throughout much of Africa, Asia, and the Americas (Henry et al., 2000). One of the most notorious examples in Canada is that of the residential schools imposed on Aboriginal people. Over many decades, Christian churches in concert with the state forced Aboriginal families to send their children to residential schools. In addition to separation from community and family and loss of language and culture, these children were often subjected to emotional, physical, and sexual abuse. Today, lawsuits related to such abuse are widespread throughout Canada and ongoing.

Such domination by Western powers continues today through neocolonialist practices, facilitated again by racism. A current example is the trafficking in women from countries such as the Philippines, another country labouring under enormous foreign debt. The economy of the Philippines is such that many citizens immigrate around the world in search of income with which to support their families. Some women (often educated as nurses) emigrate to Western countries (including Canada, the United States, Britain) to work as nannies and caregivers, whereas many others are marketed as 'brides' or as sex trade workers in these same countries.

Postcolonial theory draws attention to the historicity (or historical development) of social conditions and draws attention to people who have been, and continue to be, marginalized by colonialism and racism. Smye & Brown (2002) explain that the 'post' in postcolonial does not mean the notion of 'after' colonialism but rather refers to the importance of engaging in a purposeful examination of colonialism as it existed and continues to exist both locally and globally. Drawing on the work of Bhabha (1994) and Quayson (2000), Smye & Brown explain that postcolonialism takes us back and forth between ideas of the past to solutions in the present and the structures that create them.

An Example: Pap Smears in Reserve

A group of nurses in a remote community recognized that Aboriginal women had very high rates of cervical cancer. They discovered that the women typically did not have Pap smears done routinely or sometimes ever. Rather than adopting a finger-wagging, blaming sort of approach (you must have a Pap smear every year, my dear), the nurses realized that, given the history of the church school in the area, many of the women may have been sexually abused. They also considered that the history of race relations in the community had not created an atmosphere of trust between the Aboriginal women and the predominantly White nurses. Accordingly, they sought the input of female elders and offered a 'women's clinic' where Pap smears were only suggested as a possibility after dealing with a range of other issues that the women raised. The elders were enlisted as healers/supporters during the exams, and although some women continued to decline to have Pap smears, the number of women doing so tripled within a year.

A postcolonial lens reminds us that we are situated and constituted, not only within an immediate local culture, but also within a global culture and within a historically determined context. As illustrated in this example, a postcolonial lens draws our attention to the ways in which power and privilege associated with nation and 'race' have shaped families and individuals and continue to shape them. By donning a postcolonial lens, our attention is drawn to historical locatedness and a consideration of how existing practices and policies may be colonizing rather than decolonizing in their consequences. And as evidenced in this example, a

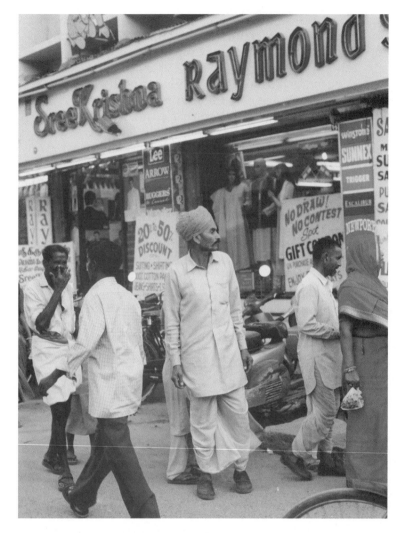

The Postcolonial. (Photograph by Len Budiwski.)

postcolonial lens encourages an analysis of, and thus more possibility of redressing, specific instances of local oppression.

 An Example: No Fighting

A while ago I (Colleen) was in an emergency unit doing research on how nurses deal with violence against women (Varcoe, 2001). As I arrived one day, a number of the staff greeted me excitedly. 'We've got one for you', said one of the physicians. The staff pointed out a young woman who was in with paralysis and aphasia. The staff said that she had been admitted before and that both organic and psychiatric explanations for her paralysis and aphasia had been ruled out. The staff said they suspected her husband was violent toward her, because during the woman's previous admission, the husband had been very angry, shouting and abusive toward the psychiatric nurse who was doing an assessment, and because on this admission, he seemed angry and hostile toward the staff. Relevant to this situation was the fact that the family was from a particular group whom many of the staff identified by race and previously told me that they saw as more violent than the majority (White) population. The woman (I will call her Fatima) was accompanied by two men: her husband and brother-in-law.

Partly because the staff indicated the woman to me, the brother-in-law approached me. He was very frustrated with the staff for not having any explanations for his sister's condition and for assuming violence was an issue. I asked him what he thought was the problem. I had a little difficulty following his English. He told me that Fatima had paralysis and quit talking before and explained that she was afraid of ghosts. The nurse with whom I was working joined us and asked him if anything happens at home prior to her becoming paralyzed. A wary light shone in his eyes, and he said defiantly, 'It has never happened. No fighting'. I asked what he meant, and he said, pointing to the nurse 'that's what she means, fighting at home'. He went on to explain that the last time they were here, his brother (the woman's husband) became very angry, and now everyone thinks that it is 'fighting' that causes her behavior.

Stop for a minute and think about this situation. As a nurse what stands out for *you*? Certainly if we don a phenomenological lens we can see how different people are making meaning of the situation in very different ways. From a phenomenological view it is obvious that what is of meaning and concern to the nurses is different from what is of meaning and concern to the family. Yet they both have the welfare of Fatima at the forefront of their experience. Again, a critical lens can help us understand what is giving rise to such strong differences, and a postcolonial lens illuminates certain features.

One of the first things that becomes apparent is how the staff are seeing the family in terms of their racial and ethnic background and applying stereotypical beliefs (for example, how violence is a norm in a particular group of people). Based on these stereotypical beliefs they reach the conclusion (or should we say jump to the conclusion) that the husband is abusive toward his wife. In dealing with Fatima, the staff drew on the idea of race to identify Fatima and her family, thus engaging in the process of racialization (see Box 2.3).

The story of Fatima's experience illustrates how a postcolonial perspective draws attention to certain features of the social context as nursing concerns. For example, nurses operating from a critical postcolonial perspective would be concerned with the social problem of racialization (that is, making judgments based on stereotypical notions of race) that is constraining Fatima and her family's experience in the emergency department. Similarly, operating from a postcolonial perspective, a nurse would also be concerned about how stereotypical thinking might shape understanding of family. For example, drawing on their own Eurocentric understanding of 'family', the nursing staff said that they thought it was 'weird' that Fatima's brother-in-law accompanied her to the hospital and this seemed to give further evidence that something wasn't right here— that something sinister was being covered up.

Fatima's situation also points to the importance of emancipatory political aims at the social level. In this case, actions might include

BOX 2.3.	**Race, Racialization, Racism, and Postcolonial Theory**

Racialization refers to the social process by which people are labelled according to particular physical characteristics or arbitrary ethnic or racial categories, and then dealt with in accordance with beliefs related to those labels (Agnew, 1998). People are racialized according to physical characteristics (labelled Chinese, African Americans, East Indian, and so on) and stereotyped according to this racialization 'Chinese are good at mathematics', 'Blacks are athletic'. Racializing, or treating race as a biological or genetic 'truth' or reality, is a precursor to racism. Racism is the use of genetic or biological background as a basis for assumptions about individuals or groups. In racism, racialized groups are seen as different from other individuals or groups and are treated differently through daily practices (Shaha, 1998). In the case of Fatima's family the staff drew on assumptions about certain (racialized) groups being more violent than others.

This is where postcolonial theory can be helpful. Postcolonial theory emphasizes that the concept of race has no basis in biological reality. Race is a "socially constructed phenomenon based on the erroneous assumption that physical differences such as skin color, hair color, and texture, and facial features are related to intellectual, moral or cultural superiority" (Henry et al., 2000, p. 4). Race is not a biological trait but a socially constructed phenomenon. As such, race has no relevance independent of its social definitions. Confusion often arises between the idea of race and the fact that people are genetically linked. Although UNESCO released its first statement on race in 1951 dispelling its validity as a biological category and has continued to do so as recently as 1997, there is still the tendency for nurses and other health professionals to confuse race with genetic characteristics. For example, the incidence of sickle cell anemia among African Americans is often offered by health care providers as evidence of race even though it is a genetically linked health problem like any other such as cystic fibrosis or Hodgkin's disease. And, unfortunately, the distinguishing of people according to race continues to be practiced widely in the contemporary social world.

Although race is a social construction and has no basis in biological reality, 'as a social construction, race significantly affects the lives of people/families of color' (Henry et al., 2000, p. 5). In Canada, the United States, and indeed most Western countries, despite policies to the contrary, race affects such important and diverse aspects of life as educational opportunities, employment opportunities, health, and health care. For example, if you consider the assumptions the emergency staff made regarding Fatima and her family, you can see how race influenced how they were seen and in turn affected their caregiving experience.

In Western countries, racism continues to function in the subjugation of both indigenous peoples and people of colour. And racism is a daily practice in the world of health care. Although Fatima may or may not have been being abused by her husband, the staff, already in a powerful position relative to the family, drew their conclusions based on both privileging the truths of medicine and psychiatry and stereotypical, racist thinking. It is possible that the family members were angry and hostile because of the assumptions being made about them and because they did not think they were getting the help that they needed.

strategies to counter stereotypical assumptions based on race and the dominant power dynamics in operation. For example, as a nurse observing this situation I (Colleen) felt compelled to question the basis of the staff's assumptions and address the way that the family members were at a particular disadvantage in relation to the health care providers because they were brown-skinned people who spoke little English in a community dominated by white-skinned people with medical knowledge.

Family As A Cultural Experience

When we use a postcolonial perspective to consider families we are required to attend to the ways in which *colonization* has shaped and continues to influence families around the globe. Through colonial rule, many cultures have had to cope with the imposition of Christian-European family norms and with the values of their colonizers. Although forms of family practiced by people in Asia, Africa, and the Americas often were not compatible with the imposed ideals of the heterosexual, male-dominated family, colonized peoples responded to such imposition by using a wide variety of family forms (Potthast-Jutkeit, 1997). Today, for example, many new immigrants to Western countries continue to live in extended groups with several generations and families of adult siblings living together in the same home. Former colonial powers in turn have been exposed to this greater variety of family forms, particularly through immigration from their former colonies. Thus diverse forms of family have persisted despite colonial and neocolonial dominance. A postcolonial perspective further directs us to challenge the ways in which colonialism is enacted through theory and question the use of theories based on Eurocentric norms as a basis for practice with families in multicultural societies. For example, we pointed out earlier in this chapter that developmental theories have been criticized for such biases. To take another example, the idea of 'self-esteem', a common construct in Western countries, has been based on Eurocentric norms and may have limited relevance to many people. What about the idea of 'sibling rivalry'? What meaning might this have for a family whose culture is deeply rooted in ideas of filial piety, such as, for example, traditional Chinese cultures influenced by Confucian thought?

Postcolonial theory compels us to pay particular attention to the ways in which race and racism function in our understanding of family and in shaping people's experiences of family. For example, the term 'extended family' is sometimes used only in relation to people who are racialized—that is, rather than see habitation as an extended family arising from particular economic, social, and historical conditions the family form signalled by extended family is seen as related to race or ethnicity. Postcolonial theory extends the idea that families are constituted and situated by drawing attention to particular social, historical, political, and economic conditions. Postcolonial theory also focuses attention on the ways in which our own experiences of power and privilege based on nation and 'race' shape our understanding and practice.

A Poststructural Perspective

The term poststructuralism is generally applied to the work of a variety of scholars including Derrida (1973), Foucault (1979a, 1979b, 1981), Kristeva (1986), and Lacan (1977). Although the ideas of these different writers are distinct and varied, they share certain fundamental assumptions about language, meaning, and subjectivity (Weedon, 1987). Many critical theorists, most notably Habermas (for example, 1984), share a concern with language and some of the poststructuralist assumptions. An essential assumption underlying poststructural thought is that language creates social reality as opposed to reflecting or describing it.

Poststructuralist theory contends that language is not a neutral tool we use to describe something, rather there are inherent meanings and rules embedded within language that limit the meaning a person can make and subsequently communicate (Cheek, 2000).

LANGUAGE SHAPES EXPERIENCE

The power of language lies in how it is used. By using and joining in with the discursive practices of society (ways of using language and the meanings embedded within that use), each person experiences what it *means* to be a person and how to *be* as a person. For example, phrases such as 'Don't cry like a girl' or 'She's a real tomboy' give clear messages to children about what boys and/or girls are. A rugby coach criticizing boys by yelling 'You're playing like a bunch of *girls*' reinforces these ideas. It is in this way that people are literally spoken into existence as they participate in the everyday language and discourse of their culture (Davies, 1990a; Weedon, 1987)

As people acquire language they learn to give meaning to their experience and to understand it according to particular ways of thinking and believing that are embedded within existing discourses. In Western culture, for example, by participating in, and integrating the discourses that outline mothering, women are provided with specific and select options for how they become a mother and live out the life of mother. The specific ways of talking of and about mothers (social discourses) such as 'You must be so thrilled to be a new mother'; 'There is no more important work than raising children'; 'A woman's true fulfillment is through motherhood'; 'When are you planning to start a family?'; and 'How could a mother let her children run around so unsupervised?' provide women with specific information about what it means to be a mother, what being a mother should look and feel like, and how to enact the role of mother (Hartrick, 1998).

Bakhtin (1981) contends that discourses are so powerful because as people participate in the discursive practices of their culture, they forget that the discourses are separate from who they are. Weedon (1987) provides the example of how existing discourses of motherhood can spark feelings of inadequacy for a new mother. The embedded messages that a new mother receives from existing discourses of motherhood tell her 'she is supposed to meet all the child's needs single-handed, to care for and stimulate the child's physical, emotional and mental development and to feel fulfilled in doing so' (Weedon, 1987, p. 34). The language and discourse surrounding the institution of motherhood shape, constrain, coerce, and potentiate a new mother's experience, the meanings she assigns to the experience, to her new child's behavior and to herself, and the action she engages in as a mother (Davies, 1990b). It is little wonder that feelings of inadequacy often accompany new motherhood!

LANGUAGE SHAPES GENDER ROLES

Gender roles offer an example of how paying attention to language can alert us to societal norms that may be subtly constraining families. The tradition of women's responsibility for domestic labour and childcare and men's responsibility in the world of work are views that are embedded within discursive practices. For example, we often speak of men 'helping out' with household chores or 'babysitting' their children when their

---

TRY IT OUT 2.1.   **Media Messages About Family**

Look at a 'parenting' magazine.

If you live in Canada or the United States, *Parenting*, and *Parenting Magazine* are available at supermarkets and newsstands. *Little Treasures Magazine* or *Kiwi Parent* are available at the same places in New Zealand, or if you are in Australia you could pick up *Practical Parenting—Australia's favourite parenting magazine* or *Junior*. Other publications such as *Redbook* target women more generally, but have a subemphasis on parenting. Some publications target certain groups. For example, *Christian Parenting* is billed as a 'magazine that targets real needs of the contemporary family with authoritative articles based on fresh research & the timeless truths of the bible'. *Essence* is described as the 'magazine for today's black woman. Edited for career-minded, sophisticated and independent achievers. Highlights career/education opportunities, fashion, beauty, money management, fitness, parenting, and home décor'.

Pick any one of these magazines and examine the cover, the table of contents, or an article that relates to family. What does the magazine convey as the answer to the question What is family?

Now, don the lenses that we have just described and the ideas they draw to your attention. What taken for granteds can you see? What truths do the images and text convey? What stereotypes are reinforced? What is conveyed as meaningful and significant? What is conveyed about gender, race, culture, and so on? What families would fall outside of the images, stereotypes, ideas, and truths?

---

wives are out somewhere, while women dominate the covers of magazines such as *Good Housekeeping*. Or, to take another example, the language of 'parenting' can be seen as gender-neutralizing language that obscures the gendered work of 'mothering'.

Family As a Discursive Experience

Looking at family from a poststructural perspective offers a view of how family is spoken into existence by the everyday discourse in which each of us participates. This perspective highlights the power of language in shaping families and their experiences. As we look from this vantage point we can see the potential in moving beyond the general discourse of family to listen to how a particular family is 'languaging' their experience. At the same time we can create opportunities for families to disrupt dominant discourses that are constraining them. The poststructural perspective also reminds us as nurses to pay attention to how we are speaking families into existence—how what we say to families is enhancing their capacity of choice or perpetuating stereotypical norms and expectations. At this point, consider the activities in Try It Out 2.1

Seeing Family Through a Spiritual Lens

The significance of spirituality to people's health and healing has been recognized since the days of Florence Nightingale. Barnhum (1996) describes how Nightingale emphasized the spiritual as well as the biological aspects of nursing care. But what are the spiritual aspects of nursing care? In reviewing the conceptualization of spirituality within the nursing literature, McSherry and Draper (1998) contend that there are as many definitions of spirituality as there are thinking, reflecting theorists. Although spirituality commonly tends to be perceived as an offshoot of religion, writers such O'Murchu (1998) emphasize the importance of distinguishing between religion and spirituality. According to O'Murchu, spirituality has always been more central to human experience than religion. Whereas religions are constituted by formally institutionalized structures, rituals, and beliefs, spirituality concerns the primal search for meaning. Simmington (2004) describes that the word 'spiritual' is derived from the Latin word *spriritualis*, meaning to breathe, wind, air, or spirit. Citing Burkhardt and Nagai-Jacobson (1994) and Keegan (1994), Simmington reports that within the health care literature spiritual has been defined by such phrases as 'the current of life' and 'that part which gives meaning and purpose' (2004, p. 474). Because spirituality is concerned with the primal search for meaning, a spiritual lens complements a hermeneutic-phenomenological lens, to which meaning is central, and a critical lens as people/families search for meaning within the social, political, economic, and historical contexts of their lives.

In delineating a spiritual lens that is consistent with a relational approach to family nursing, the following descriptors best capture what we refer to when we speak of spirituality:

1. A quality that goes beyond the religious affiliation, that strives for inspirations, reverence, awe, meaning and purpose, even in those who do not believe in any god (Murray & Zentner, 1989).
2. Spirit is a vital force: When spirit-power flows into the practical activity a person is inspired, filled with spirit (Kovel, 1991).
3. Inspiration is a state where people become capable of acting beyond their normal range. Spirit connotes hidden power. When speaking of "the spirit of the agreement" one speaks of the hidden and real force of the agreement, beyond what is apparent (Kovel, 1991).
4. Spirituality cannot be distinguished from other aspects of human existence. Spirituality has to do with fundamental matters, with our lives at their deepest (Wagner, 1988).
5. Spirit enlivens, empowers and motivates, and spirituality has to do with what takes place within, between and beyond people (Wagner, 1988).

A summary of the key concepts, assumptions and ideas we are using as part of a spirituality lens is included in Box 2.4.

Reconciling the Spiritual and the Scientific

According to Simmington (2004), a literature review reveals that nurses are the most prolific writers on the concept of spirituality when compared with any other professionals. 'Nursing authors adamantly remind their colleagues of their roots and of their commitment to healing and wholeness and beseech their readership to recognize that people's spirituality has a significant influence on their health and well-being' (p. 471). However, in spite of this large body of literature on spirituality, when examining how spirituality is integrated into nursing work Nolan and Crawford (1997) maintain that spirituality is rarely addressed in academic and clinical education or in the daily practice of nursing. Moreover, according to these authors, nurses who do contemplate spirituality in nursing work often experience cognitive dissonance in attempting to

---

BOX 2.4. **Spiritual Lens**

Key Ideas

Spirit
Life Force
Ultimate Concern
Power
Vision
Hope

Assumptions and Ideas

- Spirituality is not synonomous with religion.
- Spirituality is about 'the current of life' and 'that part which gives meaning and purpose' (Simmington, 2004, p. 474).
- Spirituality cannot be distinguished from other aspects of human existence.
- Faith is central to spirituality and is what orientates people's lives.
- Faith is the state of ultimate concern.
- Faith as ultimate concern shapes people's goals, hopes, and strivings.

---

integrate spiritual care into science-based nursing practice. It seems nurses have difficulty reconciling the spiritual with the scientific.

This difficulty in reconciling the spiritual and the scientific is also evidenced in the larger world. Wilbur (1998) describes that although science and spirituality are inextricably linked in their search for answers about the nature and mystery of life, they have come to be viewed as somewhat dichotomous domains (Clark, Cross, Deane, & Lowry, 1991)— as a polarity of opposites (Wilbur, 1998). In his book *The Marriage of Sense and Soul*, Wilbur (1998) discusses how this polarity arose and provides a vision of how spirituality and science might become an integrated whole. The following is a brief and very simplified interpretation and reconstruction of some of Wilbur's ideas. The discussion is intended as a foundation for considering how spirituality and science may be brought together in family nursing. For a full view of Wilbur's ideas, readers will need to visit his original work.

Wilbur (1998) describes that in the premodern world there was no differentiation between religion and science. For example, a scientist could be prevented from pursuing scientific investigations because they clashed with the prevailing spheres of religious morals. The "battle cry of the Enlightenment" was a call to end the oppression effected by premodern religion (Berman, 1981, 2000). Where religion and science had been previously fused, modernity differentiated the spheres, letting each proceed in its own way, unencumbered by intrusions from the other (Wilbur, 1998). As a result of this differentiation, the connection between the spiritual and the scientific was severed and over time a dissociation and alienation occurred. According to Wilbur (1998), this dissociation of the spheres set the stage for 'a dramatic, triumphant, and altogether frightening invasion' by an explosive science. (p.11).

'Within a mere century, objective, empirical *science* completely dominated serious thought in the Western World. Science became scientisim, and the belief that there was no reality except that revealed by objective science became the prevailing view. The result was a flatland view of people and human life' (Wilbur, 1998, p. 11). That is, as we have discussed earlier we were left with a view or lens that only allowed us to access exteriors and that blinded us to the interiors of self expression, subjectivity, lived awareness, first-person accounts, and the integral connection of people to each other and to their world, including their experience of the transcendent. Basically Wilbur contends that objective scientism advocates for only one field of vision—that of the physical flesh and human senses. Although this empirical lens of science can offer a view into physical structures and processes like atoms, brain synapses, DNA structures, or body pathology, other lenses are necessary to access domains of existence that are not seen through the empirical lens— through 'the eye of flesh'. Just as the hermeneutic and critical lenses address and expand this flatland view of people/family and move beyond the eye of flesh, a spiritual lens provides yet another expanded view. The spiritual lens provides what Wilbur terms the eye of contemplation. A spiritual lens transcends the logical and the rational, seeing beyond the objective (empirical lens), beyond the interpretive (hermeneutic lens), and beyond the contextual (critical lens) to illuminate the soulful 'spirit' or life force of people/families. As we look through a spiritual lens we see beyond the physical, psychological, and social health of families to see the strength and life force that constitutes, inspires, and shapes them. And, looking through all three lenses (a hermeneutic phenomenological, a critical, and a spirituality lens) it is possible to glimpse the interplay among families' interpretations, the contexts of their lives, and their life force.

An Example: Losing 'Spirit'

A few years ago, a friend of mine (Gweneth) was admitted to the hospital with flulike symptoms that had progressively worsened and were perplexing his physicians. Initially his admission was for investigation purposes and he anticipated his stay in the hospital would be brief. I saw Don the day he was admitted to the hospital just prior to my leaving for a holiday. When I returned from my trip, I was surprised to hear that he had been in the hospital for the entire 3 weeks I had been away and there was still no conclusive diagnosis. When I went to see Don, the first thing I became aware of as I entered his hospital room was the silence. Although there were announcements being made over the hospital intercom and I could hear the background noise of the nursing station, the room was completely soundless. Poking my head around the corner, I saw Don lying in his bed and his wife Lynn sitting in a chair beside him. I was immediately struck by their 'flatness'. Don had obviously lost weight since I had last seen him and his physical appearance had changed dramatically; however, there was an even greater change in his demeanour. The man I knew who exuded life and whose 'spirit filled a room' was nowhere to be seen.

As I greeted Don and Lynn I found myself in a state of disbelief—could these be the same people I had seen only 3 weeks earlier? As I looked around the room I realized that the room seemed to mirror their lifelessness. There was nothing in the room to reveal that this couple had lived there for even a minute, let alone an entire 3 weeks. There were no personal effects, no flowers, no radio, no family pictures— there was no sense of life or presence.

Commenting that they 'had had a long haul of it', I asked Don and Lynn how they were, given the 3 long weeks they had spent living in the hospital. In a resigned voice, Don responded that the time in the hospital hadn't really involved living, rather it had been a period of waiting—'waiting to start living again'. That statement was an apt descriptor of what I saw—as they waited for a diagnosis and Don's physical symptoms worsened, they had become 'patients' stripped of the activities, experiences, and backdrop that symbolized who they were in the world. In their waiting they had gone 'on hold', entering a space void of life and spirit. In so doing the connection to their life force—to their spirit—was obviously waning. The image that came to mind as I stood in the room with them was that of a candle whose flame was slowly flickering out. As Don's friend I worried about the flame getting smaller and smaller and ultimately extinguishing all together.

As a nurse I had witnessed many people's life force and spirit wane in the face of illness and adversity. But knowing Don so well 'in life' and seeing the profound impact the situation had had on him in such a short time highlighted, yet again, the importance of the spiritual aspect of health and healing and of nursing practice. As I stood in-relation with Don's spirit and experienced the heaviness within him, I wondered about the nurses who cared for Don. Had they noticed his waning spirit? Did they see care of 'Don's spirit' as integral to any and all of the nursing care they were providing? How had they attempted to intervene, or had they? Perhaps not knowing him they did not realize the significance of the flat energy and his 'low' spirit? As his friend I could see how Don's waning spirit was as important a symptom of his illness as his nausea. Yet I wondered, would I have recognized this in others who I did not know 'in life'? Might I have ignored or overlooked it or viewed it as someone else's domain of responsibility? Perhaps the nurses had noticed but were unsure how to attend to his spiritual distress—how to care for his life force as he lived in this illness situation.

Attending to Spirit: A Question of Faith

> We are endowed at birth with nascent capacities for faith. How these capacities are activated and grow depend to a large extent on how we are welcomed into the world and what kinds of environments we grow in.
>
> Faith is interactive and social; it requires community, language, ritual and nurture. Faith is also shaped by initiatives from beyond us and other people, initiatives of spirit or grace. How these latter initiatives are recognized and imaged, or unperceived and ignored, powerfully affects the shape of faith in our lives.
>
> —Fowler (1981, p. xiii)

So how might we as nurses 'attend to and care for spirit'? How might we recognize, honor, and care for the life force of people/families? As I (Gweneth) have contemplated these questions, read within the spirituality literature, and worked with people/families, I have found that inquiring into people's faith is a beginning step (Hartrick, 2002). Faith is the most primary force in human nature, human politics, relationship, and thought (Lynch 1973). Although faith is most often thought of within the context of religion, faith is not always religious in its content or context (Fowler, 1981). Fowler describes faith as a generic, universal feature of human living. Similarly, Lynch (1973) contends that faith provides a structure for composing or recomposing our thinking and our experiences. It 'is a form of imagining and imaging the world' (Lynch, 1973, p. 5). Faith exerts an ordering force and is the way of discerning and committing to values and power (Fowler, 1981). It is for this reason that attending and inquiring into people/families' faith can support the care of spirit.

Although faith varies between people/families, the content of faith does not matter for the formal definition of faith (Fowler, 1981). For example, regardless of whether faith is tied to a religion, and one is Protestant, Muslim, Catholic, Buddhist, or adheres to some other form of religious doctrine, regardless of whether one is agnostic, or atheist, all people are concerned with how to put their lives together and with what will make life worth living (Fowler, 1981). As such, Tillich (1958) offers the definition of faith as a state of being ultimately concerned. According to Tillilch, faith is the most centered act of the human mind providing an orientation of the total person, giving purpose and goal to one's hopes and strivings, thoughts, and actions (Fowler, 1981). Faith shapes how people invest their deepest loves and their most costly loyalties (Fowler, 1981). The Hindu term for faith, 'sraddha', means *to set one's heart on*. Faith involves an alignment of the will, a resting of the heart in accordance with one's ultimate concern. Fowler describes faith as involving a commitment of loyalty and trust. It illuminates what one is loyal to and in what one puts one's trust. Faith also involves vision and is a mode of knowing. What we envision for ourselves and how we 'know' and make meaning of our experiences is shaped by our faith—by that which ultimately concerns us.

An important distinction theologians make is the difference between belief and faith. Faith is not a matter of holding a certain belief system (Tillich, 1958) nor does it act on pure evidence (Lynch, 1973). Rather, faith 'is the evidence of things not seen, the substance of things hoped for' (Lynch, 1973, p. 51). Fowler (1981) contends that when faith is reduced to belief (as in credal statements), the essence of faith is lost. Fowler distinguishes belief and faith by characterizing the different questions that emerge from each. For example, if one constitutes faith as belief, the central question becomes: What do you believe? In contrast, faith as ultimate concern sparks questions such as: What do you set your heart on? To what vision of right-relatedness between humans, nature and the transcendent are you loyal? What hope and what ground of hope animates you and give shape to your life and to how you move into life?

Overall faith is a way of finding coherence and giving meaning to the experiences and relations in our lives. Niebuhr (1972) contends that faith is present in the shared visions and values that hold groups (and we would add families) together. According to Fowler (1981) 'faith is a person's or group's way of moving into the force field of life' (p. 4). For some people, faith takes the form of religion. At the center of their lives are particular religious beliefs and practices that shape the basic structure of their lives and the choices they make in terms of food, clothing, living arrangements, health care practices, and so forth. Other people live their faith in a nonsectarian manner and are not affiliated with any religious belief system or practice. Thus attending to spirit involves inquiring into what it is that is of 'ultimate concern' to particular people/families and attending to the particular faith that is central in their lives.

Family As a Spiritual Experience

Viewing family as a spiritual experience leads us to inquire into the ultimate concerns that are shaping people's lives. It guides us to pay attention to how people/families are moving into and through life, at how they are 'presencing' themselves within their world, and what commitments are guiding their life choices and decisions. Looking through a spiritual lens, we are compelled to ask what it is that this person/family has 'set their heart upon'. A spiritual lens makes us curious about the loyalties that are at the center of their lives and in what they are putting their trust—their faith. It raises the question: What leaps of faith are being taken? And what is hoped for in taking those leaps of faith? At the same time it sparks questions about how as nurses we might attend to spirit—how we might nurture the spirit-power. Given Kovel's (1991) claim that spirit connotes hidden power and people become capable of acting beyond their normal range when in-spirit (inspired), we are reminded of the significance of spirit during illness and adversity. A spiritual lens directs us to ask how we might help people/families tap their hidden spirit power. Overall, understanding family as a spiritual experience highlights that spirituality cannot be distinguished from other aspects of human existence. We are reminded to seek to know what fundamentally matters to families at the deepest levels of their lives. And finally, looking through a spiritual lens motivates us to 'care-fully' pay attention and attend to what is taking place within, between, and beyond people.

Bringing the Lenses to Our Work With Families

We believe that the hermeneutic phenomenological, critical, and spiritual lenses outlined earlier offer vitally important windows into 'family health' and that these lenses complement empirical knowledge. The flatland views that have dominated our 'knowing' of people/families health and healing can be transformed into multidimensional ones. To illustrate both the use of these lenses and the relationship of their use to family nursing practice, we offer the following example.

An Example: Shopping for Junk Food

During a nursing practice seminar a student described a dilemma she was facing with a family with whom she was working in practicum (Hartrick, 1997). The practicum focused on family health promotion and involved working with a 'healthy' family in the community. The family with whom this particular student was working consisted of a mother and three school-aged children. During one of the student's visits, she accompanied the mother to the grocery store. While there, the student watched as the mother (who was on social assistance and therefore had a very limited budget) filled her grocery cart with what the student described as 'expensive junk food'. In seminar, the student expressed her feelings of both dismay and uncertainty about what she 'should have done' and what she 'needed to do now' to be a health-promoting nurse with this 'single mother' and her family. The student stated that her knowledge of nutrition and children's nutritional needs made her cringe at the thought of the family eating the prepackaged processed food the mother had purchased.

Let's take a few minutes to consider this situation and think about what would be the most responsive way to proceed in 'family nursing practice'. First, it is important to begin by recognizing that we only have one person's experience and interpretation of the situation—the student nurse's. This distinction is important because (according to phenomenology's notions of situated and constituted) how the student interpreted the experience (for example, even what she deemed to be nutritional food) may be quite different from how the mother and/or children might interpret the experience. At the same time because we cannot inquire into the family's experience we are missing vital knowledge. What is of significance and concern for the student may not be the same as what is of significance and concern for the mother and her children. For example, because the student nurse is situated in a health-promotion practicum and constituted by her nursing knowledge and nursing identity, she has particular concerns about the nutritional needs of the family as well as concerns about her own professional responsibility and action with regard to how to be a health-promoting nurse. Because we cannot speak with the mother, we do not know what was of significance to her in her shopping experience, how those concerns were similar or different from the student's, how those concerns shaped the items she chose, and how this particular shopping venture is relevant within the larger context of her life.

Using a Hermeneutic Phenomenological Lens

Looking through a phenomenological lens we are compelled to *know* more about the experience of the mother and the rest of the family members. Although we too share concern for health promotion, the phenomenological lens reminds us that we need to understand what is meaningful to the mother and her children in order to understand and respond to what is significant to them. One of the first questions that comes to mind is whether nutrition is even something that is meaningful to them and if so, how is it meaningful? Is it even something they think about? We are also curious about the *meaning* the groceries have—whether they are everyday staples, special treats, and so forth? Remembering that the family is on a limited income we wonder *what it is like* for this mother to try to feed a family on such a small budget? What *concerns* guide her as she goes about buying food for her family? For example, as a mother also working outside the home one of my (Gweneth's) overriding concerns is getting something that is both nutritional and easy to prepare because I am often rushed for time and tired at the end of the day. Sometimes if I am having a particularly busy week I am most concerned with making sure that what I buy will be fast to prepare. At other times I might decide to let my desire to buy treats for my children override my concern for nutrition. As I understand that meaning and concern are contextual and therefore dynamic and changeable, I would be curious not only about what guided the mother's shopping that day, but also about her overall experience of nutrition and feeding her children.

Using a Critical Lens

When we consider this situation through a critical theory lens we are immediately struck by the *sociocontextual factors* that shape the situation. For example, we are reminded (and disturbed) by the societal values that led to this family having to be on a limited income. In Canada, social assistance is routinely inadequate to meet the necessities of living, and this situation is getting worse (e.g., Klein & Long, 2003). We are curious about whether there are contextual factors that are supporting and/or constraining the family from accessing adequate resources to meet their nutritional needs. For example, is there an accessible and reasonably priced grocery store close by that has good quality produce? We are also curious about what informs the student's and the family's understanding of nutrition. For example, how has their understanding been shaped by marketing of products (for example, by the beef and dairy industries)? How has the mother's shopping choices been influenced by media (for example, by aiming television ads at children so they will pressure their parents to buy certain cereal and so forth)? The critical lens also leads us to question what the student's role is in this situation—including what her rights and responsibilities are and how she might best support the rights and concerns of the mother.

A critical feminist lens leads us to think about how the majority of economically disadvantaged single parents are women. We are curious how *gender* influenced the student's interpretation of the situation, her interpretation of the mother, and the expectations she holds of both herself and the mother. For example, would she have the same expectations of a father with regard to what he should know about nutrition and how he should be feeding his children? Would we assume that 'a good mother' should be buying proper food yet give more latitude to a father because that is not typically men's work? How does the student's gender shape the way she interacts with the mother and the different gendered children? Similarly, a feminist lens highlights the importance of ensuring that there is a power-with relationship between the mother and the student.

Bringing a poststructural lens to this situation, we are curious about the way in which the idea of 'single mother' is speaking this family's experience into existence even in advance of any contact with the family. We wonder how our perspective and that of the student is shaped by societal images of single mothers as 'failed women' or as 'social liabilities', or even as contemporary heroines.

Finally, using the concept of 'intersectionality' from postcolonial and feminist perspectives, we are curious about what 'intersecting forms of oppression' this woman might be facing. Has her family endured poverty over many generations? Did she have access to education? Has she experienced racism? Heterosexism? Is she able-bodied and able-minded?

Using a Spiritual Lens

Bringing a spiritual lens to this situation we are curious about the larger life situation of this family and of the family members. What ultimate concerns shape their lives? What is the life force that guides them? How does this larger life force shape what they set their hearts on and what they hope for (e.g., during a particular day or this particular shopping expedition)? Do they adhere to particular religious beliefs or practices that shape their choice of food? How do they presence themselves and relate to others, to the world around them, and perhaps to some form of the transcendant? What in-spirits (inspires) them and what depletes their spirit energy? Although these may or may not be questions that you directly ask a family, using a spiritual lens helps us 'listen for' cues and aspects related to spirit. And, using a spiritual lens reminds us to ask ourselves how we might best inspire and recognize the hidden power of spirit in this particular family.

As we use the different lenses to expand our understanding and knowledge it very quickly becomes evident that before we can answer the question of how the student could possibly proceed in nursing practice we need a lot more knowledge and information from the family. This points to one of the most important guiding principles of family nursing. For nurses to practice in a knowledgeable, competent, and ethically responsive manner they must work in-relation with families because it is families who are most knowledgeable about themselves. Nursing knowledge becomes relevant and useable in the context of family knowledge. Therefore, families are always at the center of any clinical decision making in nursing practice.

The understanding that families bring one form of 'expert' knowledge and nurses bring another form has major implications for the how, what, when, why, where of family nursing. In later chapters, we offer a more in-depth discussion of how this 'collaborative sharing of knowledge' guides and directs nursing practice.

An Invitation

As previously discussed the different lenses and perspectives we use to understand family have the potential to help us expand our understanding and also to constrain it. No one lens is sufficient to reveal the depth and richness of family. For that reason, we have described a number of lenses and perspectives that offer somewhat different views of family. As you continue on in the book, we invite you to engage in an inquiry process of your own. It is our hope that you will try on some of the lenses we have offered and see what new and perhaps different things you begin to notice, what new questions you begin to ask, what new observations you make. To support you in that process we have created some activities you might undertake to foster your inquiry process. To begin, try the activities we have suggested for This Week in Practice.

THIS WEEK IN PRACTICE

Exploring Difference

This week we invite you to seek out someone whose experience of family is different from your own and someone whose experience is similar to your own. In preparation, spend a few minutes thinking about how you might go about this. What comes to mind with regard to how you might choose someone? For example, how would you identify someone who would potentially have had a different family experience than your own? What criteria of difference would you use? It may occur to you to choose someone from a different ethnic or racial background. However, are you sure that those characteristics would mean they had a different family experience? Is it possible that someone who looks different from you physically may have experienced family in ways closer to your own than someone who 'looks' the same as you?

After you have decided how you will choose the two people, consider how you might approach them. How would you talk to them to come to know their experience? For example, how would you engage in order to move the conversation beyond the factual description of their literal family to the experience of family? What questions might you ask?

After your conversation with the chosen people, have a discussion with your classmates or colleagues. For example, it might be interesting to discuss how many people you each had to go through to find someone 'similar' or 'different'. What were the differences? The similarities? How did the experience of talking with the person inform your understanding of family? What questions were raised for you? What were the 'surprises'?

CHAPTER HIGHLIGHTS

1. How might your nursing assessment and/or intervention practice change if you were to intentionally bring a hermeneutic phenomenology lens to your practice?
2. What is one 'ah ha' that you had as you read and critically thought about your own current taken-for-granted assumptions about family, nursing, or health care?
3. How do you currently attend to 'spirit' in your nursing practice, and how might a spiritual lens enhance that?

REFERENCES

Agnew, V. (1998). *In search of a safe place: Abused women and culturally sensitive services.* Toronto: University of Toronto Press.

Bakhtin, M. (1981). *The dialogical imagination: Four essays* (M. Holquist, Ed., and Trans.). Austin: University of Texas Press.

Barnhum, B. S. (1996). *Spirituality in nursing: From tradition to new age.* New York: Springer.

Berman, M. (1981). *The reinchantment of the world.* London: Cornell University Press.

Berman, M. (2000). *The wandering god.* Albany, NY: State University of New York Press.

Bhabha, H. (1994). *The location of culture.* London: Routledge.

Benner, P. & Wrubel, J. (1989). *The primacy of caring: Stress and coping in health and illness.* Menlo Park, CA: Addison Wesley.

Brewer, R. M. (1993). Theorizing race, class and gender: The new scholarship of Black feminist intellectuals and Black women's labour. In S. M. James & A. P. A. Busia (Eds.), *Theorizing Black feminisms: The visionary pragmatism for Black women* (pp. 13–30). London: Routledge.

Browne, A. J. (2001). The influence of liberal political ideology on nursing practice. *Nursing Inquiry, 8*(2), 118–129.

Browne, A. J. (2000). The potential contributions of critical social theory to nursing science. *Canadian Journal of Nursing Research, 32*(2), 35–55.

Burkhardt, M. A., & Nagai-Jacobson, M. G. (1994). Reawakening the spirit in clinical practice. *Journal of Holistic Nursing, 12*(1), 9–12.

Campbell, J., & Bunting, S. (1991). Voices and paradigms: Perspectives on critical and feminist theory in nursing. *Advances in Nursing Science, 13*(3), 1–15.

Capra, F. (1976). *The tao of physics.* New York: Bantam Books.

Cheal, D. (1993). Theoretical perspectives. In G.N. Ramu (Ed.), *Marriage and the family in Canada today* (2nd ed., pp. 18–34). Scarborough, ON: Prentice-Hall Canada.

Cheek, J. (2000). *Postmodern and poststructural approaches to nursing practice.* London: Sage.

Clark, C., Cross, J. Deane, D., & Lowry, L. (1991). *Spirituality: Integral to quality care. Holistic Nursing Practice, 5*(3), 67–76.

Cody, W. (2000). Nursing frameworks to guide practice and research with families: Introductory remarks. *Nursing Science Quarterly, 13*(4), 277.

Collins, P. H. (1990). *Black feminist thought: Knowledge, consciousness, and the politics of empowerment.* New York: Routledge.

Collins, P. H. (1993). Toward a new vision: Race, class and gender as categories of analysis and connection. *Race, sex & class, 1*(1), 23–45.

Collins, P. H. (2000). It's all in the family: Intersections of gender, race and nation. In U. Narayan & S. Harding (Eds.), *Decentering the center: Philosophy for a multicultural, postcolonial and feminist world* (pp. 156–176). Bloomington: Indiana University Press.

Davies, B. (1990a). The problem of desire. *Social Problems, 37*(4), 501–516.

Davies, B. (1990b). Positioning: The discursive production of selves. *Journal for the Theory of Social Behavior, 20*(1), 43–63.

Derrida, J. (1973). *Speech and phenomenon.* Evanston, IL: Northwestern University Press.

Doane, G. (2003). Through pragmatic eyes: Philosophy and the re-sourcing of family nursing. *Nursing Philosophy, 4*(1), 25–32.

Duffy, M., & Leeds, M. (2001). Which story shall we tell? In P. Munhall & V. Fitzsimmons (Eds.), *The emergence of family into the 21st century* (pp. 27–37). Sudbury, MA: Jones & Bartlett.

Duvall, E. M. (1977). *Marriage and family development* (5th ed.). Philadelphia: Lippincott.

Duvall, E. M., & Miller, B. (1985). *Marriage and family development.* New York: Harper & Row.

Evans, J. (2002). Cautious caregivers: Gender stereotypes and the sexualization of men nurse's touch. *Journal of Advanced Nursing, 40*(4), 441–448.

Evans, J., & Frank, B. (2003). Contradictions and tensions: Exploring relations of masculinities in the numerically female dominated nursing profession. *The Journal of Men's Studies, 11*(3), 277–293.

Foucault, M. (1979a). *Discipline and punish.* Harmondsworth: Penguin.

Foucault, M. (1979b). What is an author? *Screen, 20*(1),13–33.

Foucault, M. (1981). *The history of sexuality. Volume I, An introduction.* New York: Vintage Books.

Fowler, J. (1981). *Stages of faith.* New York: Harper & Row.

Giroux, H. A. (1983). *Theory and resistance in education: A pedagogy for the opposition.* S. Hadley, MA: Bergin & Garrey.

Gleick, J. (1987). *Chaos: Making a new science.* New York: Viking.

Graham, H., & Der, G. (1999a). Influences on women's smoking status: The contribution of socioeconomic status in adolescence and adulthood. *European Journal of Public Health, 9*(2), 137–141.

Graham, H., & Der, G. (1999b). Patterns and predictors of smoking cessation among British women. *Health Promotion International, 14*(3), 231–239.

Graham, H., & Der, G. (1999c). Patterns and predictors of tobacco consumption among women. *Health Education Research, 14*(5), 611–618.

Habermas, J. (1984). *The theory of communicative action.* Boston: Beacon.

Hanson, S. (2001). *Family health care nursing: Theory, practice and research* (2nd ed.). Philadelphia: F.A. Davis.

Hanvey, L. (2003). *Men in nursing.* Ottawa: Canadian Nurses Association.

Hartrick, G. A. (1995). Part 1: Transforming family nursing theory: From mechanism to contextualism. *Journal of Family Nursing, 1*(2), 134–147.

Hartrick, G. A. (2002). Beyond interpersonal communication: The significance of relationship in health promoting practice. In L. Young & V. Hayes (Eds.), *Transforming health promotion practice. Concepts, issues and applications* (pp. 49–58). Philadelphia: F.A. Davis.

Hayes, V. E. (1997). Searching for family nursing practice knowledge. In S. E. Thorne & V. E. Hayes, (Eds.), *Nursing praxis knowledge and action* (pp. 54–68). Thousand Oaks, CA: Sage.

Heidegger, M. (1962). *Being and time* (J. MacQuarrie & E. Robinson, Trans.). New York: Harper & Row.

Henry, F., Tator, C., Mattis, W., & Rees, T. (2000). *The colour of democracy: Racism in Canadian society.* Toronto, ON: Hartcourt Brace.

hooks, b. (1984). Feminist theory: From margin to center. Boston: South End Press.

hooks, b. (1990). Yearning: Race, gender and cultural politics. Boston: South End Press.

Jantsch, E. (1980). *The self-organizing universe.* Oxford: Pergamon.

Keegan, L. (1994). The nurse as healer. Albany, NY: Delmar.

Kincheloe, J. L., & McLaren, P. (2000). Rethinking critical theory and qualitative research. In N. K. Denzin & Y. S. Lincoln (Eds.), *Handbook of qualitative research* (pp. 279–313). Thousand Oaks, CA: Sage.

Kleffel, D. (1996). Environmental paradigms: Moving toward an eccentric perspective. *Advances in Nursing Science, 18*(4), 1–10.

Klein, S., & Long, A. (2003). A bad time to be poor: An analysis of British Columbia's new welfare policies. Vancouver: Canadian Centre for Policy Alternatives and Social Planning and Research Council of BC.

Kovel, J. (1991). *History and spirit. An inquiry into the philosophy of liberation.* Boston: Beacon Press.

Krieger, M. (1999). Embodying inequality: A review of concepts, measures, and cmethods for studying health consequences of discrimination. *International Journal of Health Services, 29*(2), 295–352.

Kristeva, J. (1986). The Kristeva Reader (Toril Moi, Ed.) Oxford: Blackwell.

Lacan, J. (1977). *Ecrits.* London: Tavistock.

Leonard, V. W. (1989). A Heideggerian phenomenological perspective on the concept of person. *Advances in Nursing Science, 11*(4), 40–55.

Lynch, W. (1973*). Images of faith.* Notre Dame, Indiana: University of Notre Dame Press.

Lyotard, J. (1984). *The postmodern condition.* Minneapolis: University of Minnesota Press.

Mandell, N., & Duffy, A. (1995). *Canadian families: Diversity, conflict and change.* Toronto: Harcourt Brace.

McSherry, W., & Draper, P. (1998). The debates emerging from the literature surrounding the concept of spirituality as applied to nursing. *Journal of Advanced Nursing, 27,* 683–691.

Merleau-Ponty, M. (1962). *Phenomenology of perception* (C. Smith, Trans.). New York: Humanities Press.

Miller, W., McDaniel, R., Crabtree, B., & Stange, K. (2001). Practice jazz: Understanding variation in family practices using complexity science. *The Journal of Family Practice, 50*(10), 872–878.

Moore, T. (1994). *Soulmates: Honoring the mysteries of love and relationship.* New York: Harper Collins.

Moules, N. (2002). Hermeneutic inquiry: Paying heed to history and Hermes. An ancestral, substantive and methodological tale. *International Journal of Qualitative Methods, 1*(3), article 1. Retrieved Oct. 15, 2003 from http://www.ualberta.ca/~ijqm/.

Mumford, L. (1957). *The transformations of man.* London: Allen & Unwin.

Murray, R., & Zentner, J. (1989). *Nursing concepts for health promotion.* London: Prentice-Hall.

Niebuhr, R. (1972). *Experiential religion.* New York: Harper & Row.

Nolan, P., & Crawford, P. (1997). Towards a rhetoric of spirituality in mental health care. *Journal of Advanced Nursing, 26,* 289–294.

O'Murchu, D. (1998). *Reclaiming spirituality.* New York: Crossroad.

Osmond, M. W. (1987). Radical-critical theories. In M. B. Sussman & S. K. Steinmetz (Eds.), *Handbook of marriage and the family* (pp. 103–124). New York: Plenum.

Parse, R. (1990). Health: A personal commitment. *Nursing Science Quarterly, 38*(3), 136–140.

Potthast-Jutkeit, B. (1997). The history of the family and colonialism. *History of the Family, 2*(2), 115–121.

Prigogine I., & Stenger, I. (1984). *Order out of chaos*. Toronto: Bantam Books.

Purkis, M. E. (1997). The "social determinants" of practice? A critical analysis of the discourse of health promotion. *Canadian Journal of Nursing Research, 29*(1), 47–62.

Quayson, A. (2000). *Postcolonialism: Theory, practice or process?* Cornwall: Polity Press.

Ray, M. (1994). Complex caring dynamics: A unifying model of nursing inquiry. *Theoretic & Applied Chaos in Nursing, 1*(1), 7–14.

Shaha, M. (1998). Racism and its implications in ethical-moral reasoning in nursing practice: A tentative approach to a largely unexplored topic. *Nursing Ethics, 5*(2), 139–146.

Simmington, J. (2004). Ethics for an evolving spirituality. In J. Storch, P. Rodney, & R. Starzomski (Eds.), *Toward a moral horizon. Nursing ethics for leadership and practice* (pp. 465–484). Toronto: Pearson Prentice Hall.

Smye, V., & Brown, A. (2002). "Cultural safety" and the analysis of health policy affecting aborijinal people. *Nurse Researcher, 9*(3), 42–56.

Stajduhar, K. (2001). *The idealization of dying at home: The social context of home-based palliative caregiving*. Unpublished doctoral dissertation, University of British Columbia, Vancouver, BC.

Stajduhar, K. (2003). Examining the perspectives of family members involved in the delivery of palliative care at home. *Journal of Palliative Care, 19*(1), 27–35.

Tillich, P. (1958). *Dynamics of faith*. New York: Harper & Brothers.

Varcoe, C. (2001). Abuse obscured: An ethnographic account of emergency nursing in relation to violence against women. *Canadian Journal of Nursing Research, 32*(4), 95–115.

Vicenzi, A., White, K., & Begun, J. (1997). Chaos in nursing: Make it work for you. *American Journal of Nursing, 97*(10), 26–32.

Wagner, J. (1988). Spirituality and administration. *Weavings, 3*(4), 15.

Weedon, C. (1987). *Feminist practice and poststructuralist theory*. New York: Basil Blackwell.

Wheatley, M. J. (1994). *Leadership and the new science*. San Francisco: Berrett-Koehler Publishers, Inc.

White, M., & Epston, D. (1990). *Narrative means to therapeutic ends*. New York: Norton.

Wilbur, K. (1998). *The marriage of sense and soul. Integrating science and religion*. New York: Random House.

Wright, L. M., & Leahey, M. (1994). *Nurses and families: A guide to assessment and intervention* (2nd ed.). Philadelphia: F.A. Davis.

Wuest, J. (1997). Illuminating environmental influences on women's caring. *Journal of Advanced Nursing, 26*, 49–58.

Wuest, J. (2001). Precarious ordering: Toward a formal theory of women's caring. *Health Care for Women International, 22*(1/2), 167–194.

Zohar, D. (1990). *The quantum self: Human nature and consciousness defined by the new physics*. New York: William Morrow.

3 All Practice is Theoretical

OVERVIEW

In Chapter 3 we make the case that
rather than theory being something that
one 'applies' at particular times, theory
is inherent in all practice. Therefore the
question is not whether to use theory in
family nursing practice, but how better
to theorize practice. As a contribution
toward this process, in this chapter we
explore how the work of nurse theorists
from the human science paradigm can
enhance the 'knowing' of family health
and the enactment of relational nursing
practice.

● Forms of Knowledge and Ways of Knowing That Shape Nursing Practice

Throughout the past two decades there has been an intense interest in the question of 'knowing' in nursing (how we know and what we know). This interest in many ways was initiated by Carper in 1978 who proposed that there are at least four 'ways of knowing' in nursing: empirical, aesthetic, ethical, and personal knowing. She described the *empirical* pattern of knowing as the dominant form and as involving factual and descriptive knowing aimed at the development of abstract and theoretical explanations. Carper saw the *aesthetic* pattern of knowing as related to understanding what is *of significance to particular* patients (and we would say, particular families) and identified empathy—'the capacity for participating in or vicariously experiencing another's feelings' (p. 15)—as a central mode of aesthetic knowing. She described the *ethical* pattern of knowing as requiring knowledge of different philosophical positions regarding what is good and right and as involving the making of moral choices and actions. Finally, Carper drew on Buber to describe *personal* knowing as encompassing knowledge of the self *in-relation* to others and in-relation to one's own self.

Carper's typology challenged empirical knowledge as the knowledge base for nursing and widened understanding of knowledge and knowing in nursing. Carper's work stimulated lively investigation and debate about knowing in nursing (for example, see Benner, Tanner, & Chesla 1996; Chinn & Jacobs-Kramer, 1988; Wainwright, 2000; White, 1995) and inspired nurses to consider ideas about knowing that authors in other disciplines had generated. Chinn and Jacobs-Kramer offered a detailed critical analysis of Carper's work to facilitate integration of these patterns of knowing into clinical nursing practice (White, 1995).

Another Typology of Ways of Knowing

Simultaneous with Carper's work, other disciplines were considering the idea of knowing. In 1986, a group of psychologists (Belenky, Clinchy, Goldberger, & Tarule, 1986) published a book entitled *Women's Ways of Knowing*. Based on their research regarding intellectual development of women in the United States, they described how women's self-concepts and ways of knowing are intertwined and illustrated how women's intellectual development is both hindered and developed within two most influential institutions: the family and schools. They posited that women variously employed a range of ways of knowing that varied from silence to constructed knowledge. Some women were locked into a world of *silence* that was the extreme absence of voice and independent thought. Others operated primarily from *received knowing*, that is, they were dependent on the voice and views of others for their own 'knowing', whereas others also listened to their own inner voices, with some intentionally seeking their own knowledge. Some women took up *reasoned reflection* as their mode of knowing, with some questing for knowledge and understanding, which Belenky and colleagues defined as two different types of *procedural knowledge* (purposefully developed knowledge). Finally, these authors described how some women moved toward what they called '*constructed knowledge*'. In this way of knowing, the women integrated what they thought was personally important with what they learned from others, 'weaving together the strands of rational and emotive thought and . . . integrating subjective and objective knowing' (Belenky et al., p. 134).

Schultz and Meleis (1988) saw the work of Belenky and colleagues as particularly salient to nursing. They said that 'many nurses have contented themselves with using the words of others to express and guide their knowing' (p. 219) and called on nurses to use more than empirical research as a path to developing knowledge. They suggested that in addition to empirical knowledge, clinical and conceptual knowledge are also foundational to nursing.

Subsequently, nurses continued to modify and develop understandings of 'knowing' in nursing through both theoretical- and research-based investigations (see for example Banks-Wallace, 2000; Grant, 2001; Liaschenko, 1997; Liaschenko & Fisher, 1999; Schaefer, 2002). Fully discussing this rich literature is beyond the scope of this book, but there are two developments that are of key importance to relational nursing practice:

1. the position of personal knowledge
2. the importance of sociopolitical knowing

Notice as you read further how these developments complement the lenses that we introduced in Chapter 2.

The Position of Personal Knowledge

Personal knowledge has only recently come to be valued in nursing. Since Carper's (1978) description of patterns of knowing in nursing, increased attention has been focused on personal knowing. Nursing scholars have divided into at least two camps regarding what they think about personal knowledge in nursing. In one camp are the followers of Carper, who have accepted her notion that personal knowing is a separate category and one of at least four fundamental patterns of knowing in nursing.

In another camp are those such as Benner (1984), Smith (1992), and Sweeney (1994) who build from Polanyi's (1962) work on personal knowledge and argue that personal knowing is not a separate category but penetrates all forms of knowing. For example, Smith asserts that knowing is the weaving of threads that may originate from sources such as science, the arts, life experiences and encounters. She says that although the sources of knowledge may be similar or different, the threads we select from those sources are personal choices. Consequently, all knowing is personally shaped. We agree with Smith that 'in this way *all knowing is fundamentally and primarily personal knowing*' (p. 2, emphasis ours). As we described in Chapter 2, as a person you bring different 'knowledges' together in your own unique way—filtering them through your own personal framework of understanding, your past

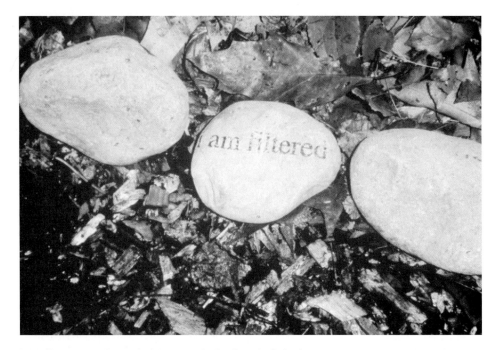

I am. (Leaves, rocks and photo transfer by Connie Sabo.)

experiences, your values, your beliefs, and so forth. Subsequently, all knowing is personal because it arises from your own particular perspective.

In concluding that all knowing is personal knowing Smith (1992) and Sweeney (1994) both argued that the category of knowledge that Carper called personal knowledge is actually *self-knowledge*. Self-knowledge involves knowledge of oneself including awareness of one's values, beliefs, socioenvironmental location, and so forth. Self-knowledge allows us a clearer view into how we are making our personal choices of knowing. Cultivating self-knowledge is part of the process of 'reflexivity', which is active, purposeful reflection on one's beliefs, values, thoughts, and actions, and thoughtful action as a consequence of that reflection. (We explore the skills of self-knowing and reflexivity more fully in Chapters 5 and 7.) As we develop and pay attention to self-knowledge, we have the opportunity to see how we personally shape all our knowledge and to question reflexively, and perhaps move beyond, the habits of mind (habits of knowing) that constrain our understandings. That is, by developing and paying attention to self-knowledge we can begin to see and more purposefully decide how we are personally shaping knowledge. At the same time, as we open to knowing ourselves more fully, we simultaneously expand our knowing of others. We are able to expand and move beyond our own selective interests and to better see the taken-for-granted assumptions and contextual elements that may limit our view of families and of the world.

Understanding that all knowledge is personal suggests that 'lived experience' cannot be seen as incontestable knowledge or 'truth'. For example, just because we experience a family as 'challenging' does not mean they *are* challenging. As hermeneutic phenomenology informs us our lived experience is interpreted within and through our own ideology, our values, our taken-for-granted rights and wrongs, our personal interests, and so forth. For this reason, it is important to critically examine our experiences as well as the ideology and contextual forces that are shaping our experiences. This inquiry process of reflexively scrutinizing our experiences and how we are knowing those experiences promotes our ability to expand our interpretations and know in new ways.

The Importance of Sociopolitical Knowing

Whereas this reflexive consideration of personal knowing is vital to nursing practice, reframing one's own knowing may be insufficient for transforming larger practice patterns that are shaped by the dominant societal interests and ideologies. For example, one nurse alone cannot change a policy that dictates the service model of health care that we discussed in Chapter 1. Personal interests can lead to individual resistance to practices and policies that constrain socioenvironmental health promotion, but collective changes are required to transform the structures that are dominating practice. It was this understanding that led White (1995) to argue for adding sociopolitical knowing to Carper's original typology.

Adding Sociopolitical Knowing to Carper's Typology

White (1995) noted that the context appeared to be missing from both Carper's (1978) analysis and Chinn and Jacob-Kramer's (1988) analysis and extension of Carper's work. White remarked that Chinn and Jacob-Krammer's reconceptualization was an adequate description of the nurse-patient relationship and the persons of nurse and patient, but that the sociopolitical context of people and their interactions was missing. Thus, White advocated adding 'sociopolitical knowing' to the typology of ways of knowing in nursing. She argued that the other patterns address the 'who', 'how', and 'what' of nursing practice, but sociopolitical knowing addresses the 'wherein', drawing attention to the broader context of practice and causing 'the nurse to question the taken-for-granted assumptions about practice, the profession, and health policies' (pp. 83–84).

Importantly, White pointed out that the sociopolitical context of relations fundamentally concerns cultural identity. She noted that one's cultural location influences one's 'understanding of health, disease, language, identity and connection to the land' and that such knowing 'is related to deeply embedded historical connections to and dislocation from land and heritage' (p. 84). Similarly, Banks-Wallace (2000) argues that racial/ethnic identity and class are significantly influential on women's ways of knowing. For example, she points out that although the women Belenky and colleagues interviewed were diverse, they potentially overrepresented both women of color who were socially or economically disadvantaged and Euro-American women who were advantaged. Thus she concludes that Belenky and colleagues' description of 'women's ways of knowing' is not adequate, for example, to diverse African American women. Banks-Wallace draws on a 'womanist' understanding of ways of knowing to suggest how health interventions can be made far more effective in assisting African American women to incorporate health promoting behaviours. By womanist she means understanding based on women's experiences of the combined effects of being both an African American and a woman. This is a specific example illustrating the importance of understanding the intersectionality of oppressions as discussed in Chapter 2. Banks-Wallace points out that most "cultural-based" interventions in health care focus attention on appropriate language, rather than considering whether the knowledge being offered is relevant and valid for the group being targeted. She uses the example of health-promotion interventions to address issues such as cardiovascular disease, obesity, and hypertension (e.g., weight loss, diet, blood pressure monitoring) for African American women that do not take into account the experience of living under the chronic stress of 'feeling like they are nothing' in American society. To us this highlights the importance of informing our practice through sociopolitical knowing—of intentionally inquiring into and taking the context of families, nurses and health care into account.

Bringing Knowledges Together

Throughout this book, we continually draw your attention to the context and to the importance of personal and social location to both families' and your own understanding of health and health care. We agree with White (1995) that a sociopolitical understanding can be a frame within which to understand other patterns of knowing and that this frame is essential to the future of nursing in the increasingly economically driven world. At the same time we agree with writers such as Benner (1984), Smith (1992), and Sweeney (1994) that all knowledge is personally shaped. Overall this means that we approach practice with the understanding that all knowledge is dynamic and contestable and that to practice in an informed and knowledgeable manner requires paying attention and inquiring into self/other/context 'all at once'. From a relational perspective it is not simply a matter of being intentional toward families. You are not just trying to understand families—you are trying to know families in context, yourself in context, and yourself and families in context relationally. Said another way, in a relational approach, intentional practice means intentionally inquiring into self/other/context all at once and bringing multiple ways of knowing and forms of knowledge together simultaneously. One useful tool to aid you in this process is nursing theory.

Becoming Intentional Theoretical Practitioners in Nursing

Although it seems logical to expect nursing theory to be evident in nursing practice, in observing clinical nursing practice Liaschenko and Fisher (1999) noted that one rarely hears practicing nurses use language of nursing theory unless they have been mandated to do so by accrediting bodies or institutional practices. Similarly, we have found that not only do many nurses tend to be unaware of the theoretical nature of their actions, they often do not understand or recognize the significance of nursing theory to their everyday practice (Hartrick, 2002). This failure to see the relevance of theory to everyday nursing practice is a consequence of how nursing has tended to think about or not think about theory (Hartrick, 2002). For example, nursing theory has often been taught in isolation from practice. Theory tends to be viewed as an abstract body of knowledge that is learned outside of the practice arena. Subsequently, it is not uncommon to hear nurses declare that theory has no relevance in the 'real world' of nursing work. Thinking of theory as something separate from practice has led many nurses to overlook the practice-theory connection in their everyday actions. And, as a result they are not aware of how their existing theories may be constraining their actions.

Yet if you stop for a moment and try to think of a time when you are not practicing theoretically you will find it difficult to do so. For example, when you set off down the corridor to respond to patient call bells, making a decision about which of two patients to respond to first involves 'theorizing' which one requires the most urgent attention; when you make a bed with clean linen your action is informed theoretically; similarly, doing a dressing change using sterile technique is theoretical action. Although the act of theorizing your everyday work may not be conscious, each of you brings beliefs, assumptions, and hypotheses to each moment of your practice and those ingredients constitute a theoretical base for action. Although this theory may not be a formal nursing theory, it *is* theory.

Even though all practice is theoretical, often nurses are not aware of the theories that are shaping their actions and do not consciously or intentionally choose the theories that will guide their practice. Thus nurses can unintentionally allow theory to have authority over their practice and over families. For example, as we discussed in Chapter 1 as a person/nurse each of you has a definition of health and a particular view of family guiding your practice. Those definitions and views strongly shape how you go about your work—how you promote health, engage with families, and so forth. Yet many nurses are not consciously aware of the theories of health and family they bring to their practice.

Overall we have found that this lack of conscious and critically reflexive theorizing profoundly limits nurses' choices and decision making and their capacity for ethically responsive practice. Practicing without a conscious theoretical intent is comparable to setting off on a trip into unknown terrain without a roadmap or compass. Although you might eventually get somewhere and you might see interesting things along the way, it is far more difficult to make one's way randomly and/or to know if you are heading in a direction that is worthwhile. Also, without theoretical tools, your knowledge of the terrain may be lessened, the choices of routes you see will likely be fewer, and you might not realize when you have stepped off the road you wish to take.

As the discussions in Chapter 2 highlighted, by purposefully bringing different theoretical lenses to your practice you can greatly expand your knowledge of and responsiveness to families. And, conscious awareness of the theories that are guiding you allows you to be more intentional in how you are guided by those theories as you work with families. For example, each time you listen to a report about a family or patient you are 'listening for' certain things—and it is the theories guiding your practice that determines what you listen for. If you are consciously aware of the theories guiding you and choose theories that will expand your knowing of families' experiences, your listening can be simultaneously focused yet expansive. Intentional theorizing expands the number of ways of viewing any family and offers more choices for how you might engage, what you might look for, and how you might respond. This conscious awareness of your theoretical intent also creates the opportunity for you to learn from your experiences with families and continually be retheorizing your practice (Hartrick, 2002). That is, rather than unconsciously giving theory authority over families or over your own practice, theorizing in a conscious and intentional manner makes it possible for you to 'follow the lead of families' and respond to what is meaningful and significant in their particular health and healing experience. At the same time, what you learn from families can inform your own family nursing theory.

● Theorizing Your Practice

From a pragmatic perspective relational practice requires continual and explicit theorizing. It requires that nurses continually ask themselves: *What theories are informing and shaping my practice, how aware am I of the theories that are guiding me, and how might I intentionally retheorize my practice to enhance my responsiveness to families?* As discussed in Chapter 1 relational practice from a pragmatic perspective involves a continuous scrutiny, questioning the adequacy of all theory, knowledge, and practice. For example, as we turn to theory to inform our practice we need to ask:

- How does this theory define the focus of family nursing?
- What does the theory, idea, or concept draw my attention to?
- What does it take for granted or assume about family, health, and/or nursing?
- How does it expand my view and help me move beyond my own selective interests?

Similarly, to consider a theory's adequacy in terms of its usefulness with a particular family it is important to ask:

- How does this theory inform and/or constrain my knowing?
- What does it overlook?
- What does it lead me to question?
- What does it lead me to doubt?
- What does it lead me to take for granted?

And, because knowing is a form of active practice, we need to consider the adequacy of any theory in terms of the direction it provides for practice. Useful questions related to adequacy that we might ask are:

- What does this theoretical understanding lead me to do?
- What actions am I compelled to take?
- Are those actions 'adequate', 'responsive', and the 'best' in this particular moment with this particular family?

To support the development of critically reflexive theorizing, in this chapter we invite you to further your own theoretical practice and to inquire into the theories that are currently governing your nursing actions. As students you have probably been exposed to a number of existing nursing theories that may be shaping your understanding of nursing practice. At the same time you will have personal experiences and/or nursing experiences that have shaped how you view people, health, healing, and so forth. Throughout this book our intent is to create opportunities for you to examine the integral relationship between theory and practice and to more explicitly theorize your practice. To aid you in this process, we now present some existing nursing theories that we see as falling within nursing's human science paradigm. These theories offer a view of nursing as a human-centered process. As with all of the ideas we present in this book, it is not our intent that you take these theories up and apply them, but rather we offer them to you as food for thought to be drawn on as you more explicitly articulate your own theory of nursing practice. As Watson (1988) describes, theory is 'an imaginative grouping of knowledge, ideas and experience that are represented symbolically and seek to illuminate a given phenomena' (p. 1). This definition highlights how theorizing is a living process that involves imagination, creativity, curiosity, a stance of unknowing and personal exploration, and meaning making. It is this imaginative process we would like to invite you into. As you read the discussion of the theories following, read with a *reflexive curiosity* about yourself. That is, continually ask yourself:

- What do *I* think about this?
- How do *I* see this?
- How are *my* beliefs similar and/or different from this?
- What have *I* experienced, read, or learned about that is in keeping with this theory and/or contradicts it?

Keep a pad of paper next to you and write down any thoughts that arise, any ideas, concepts, assumptions, and/or beliefs from the theories that particularly resonate with you and any 'ahas' you have. And remember, this is just the beginning of an ongoing process of explication, so don't worry about how much you are able to identify. What is most important is that you begin to ask yourself the questions!

● Nursing Theories in the Human Science Paradigm

As discussed in Chapter 2, nurse theorists have expressed concern that many of the theories that dominate the family nursing world are borrowed from other disciplines. In addition to this borrowing of theory, Newman (1994) describes how in attempting to establish itself in the scientific arena, the discipline of nursing initially focused on meeting the criteria established and expected by 'hard' scientists. As a result many nursing theories were firmly grounded in a Cartesian worldview. However, during the past 3 decades a new paradigm of nursing science has developed. Beginning with Martha Roger's (1970) theory of unitary human beings, nurses turned their attention to articulating the 'human science' of nursing. Theories within the human science paradigm move beyond Cartesian science to consider the meaning and experience of people, health, and nursing.

Watson (1988) summarizes the human science paradigm in nursing as being based on:

- A philosophy of human freedom, choice and responsibility
- A biology and psychology of holism (nonreducible persons interconnected with their world)
- A knowledge development process that includes not only empirical science but also esthetics, ethics, values, intuition, and process discovery.
- A way of being that is relational and process oriented
- A scientific worldview that is open and ever changing

The nursing theories we include here arise from this human science paradigm. We have chosen particular ones that we believe offer relational views of family and family nursing practice. As we have previously mentioned in Chapter 2, the theories within the human science paradigm have been identified as congruent with an ecological approach to nursing practice (Kleffel, 1996). Yet Browne (2001) has argued that the assumption of individual free will and choice that underpins these theories is problematic in that it does not attend to the way in which choice is contextually shaped. From the points that these two authors raise, it becomes evident that they have each critically considered the theories in light of their own experience and practice. And the two differing perspectives highlights that there is no 'truth'. After thoughtfully and reflexively considering the theories in light of her own location and practice, each author came to a somewhat different conclusion about the theories. As you read, we invite you to engage in your own reflexive consideration of these theories. Read the theories with a reflexive eye. That is, consider the theories in terms of the questions of adequacy we identified earlier. Try to think of people/families with whom you have worked as a nurse or with whom you might currently be working and think about how these theories might have informed and reshaped your nursing practice with those people/families. Just as Kleffel and Brown have done, consider what *you* see of value in the theories and what you see as limitations.

Paterson and Zderad's Humanistic Nursing Theory

In 1976 Josephine Paterson and Loretta Zderad published their classic book *Humanistic Nursing*. Describing nursing as 'an experience lived between human beings' (Paterson & Zderad, 1988, p. 3), these nurse theorists inspired us to move beyond the technical 'doing' of nursing and open ourselves up to the feeling and 'being' of nursing. Believing that nursing theory should be rooted in practice, Paterson and Zderad turned to a phenomenological method of inquiry to support their theory development process. Their theorizing began with the knowledge that as nurses they themselves were 'knowing places' and as such were integral to the knowledge development process. They contended that knowing was cultivated from within an experience and consequently it was the responsibility of each nurse to contribute to the evolution of nursing theory by paying close attention to their everyday practice experience and inquiring into that experience. Borrowing from R. D. Laing, they defined theory as 'the articulated vision of experience' (Zderad, 1978, p. 45). To develop and evolve their theoretical practice, therefore, these theorists believed that as nurses engaged in everyday work, they needed to ask questions of their practice such as—what, why, how, how better, ought, and ought not. Theoretically sound practice required that nurses tune into themselves as knowing places and reflect on new possibilities within their everyday work.

Nursing As a Happening Between People

O'Connor (1993) suggests that perhaps the major contribution Paterson and Zderad's humanistic nursing theory offers is the view of nursing as a particular kind of human relating. At the center of their theory is an understanding of nursing as a 'happening between people'. The theory emphasizes a particular way of being that involves presence and awareness to support a 'withness' between nurse and patient. They emphasize the importance of this way of being within the doing of nursing. Said another way, their theory gives direction to the 'how' of nursing as well as the 'what'. By articulating the being of nursing, their theory takes nursing practice beyond the subjective/objective dualism to a way of being and approach that is objective, subjective, and intersubjective all at once. They distinguish objective reality (what occurs 'out there' and can be observed, pointed at, and examined), subjective reality (what is known from the inside out, reality that is the awareness of one's own experience), and intersubjective reality (what is experienced in the between space when two or more people come together). These theorists emphasize that humanistic nursing dwells primarily in the intersubjective realm while simultaneously recognizing the trifold (objective, subjective, intersubjective) reality of the nursing world (O'Connor, 1993).

Although these theorists do not directly address family in their theoretical descriptions, because of the strong phenomenological roots of this theory and the focus on human experience and being, from the description of the central concepts following we believe that the theory has the potential to inform family nursing. O'Connor (1993) describes the following central concepts:

- *Freedom*: people have an inherent capacity to choose to respond and to choose how to respond to situations in life.
- *Uniqueness*: every person (and we would add, family) is unique and holds his or her own "angular view" (Paterson & Zderad, 1988, p. 37) through which he or she sees the world.

- *Adequacy*: people have the capacity of hope and the capacity to envision possibilities.
- *Relatedness*: people have the capacity for relationship including a capacity for being with another human being. As people relate to each other they 'become more' and learn more about their uniqueness.
- *Historicity*: people are their history and this history affects their inner responses. Awareness of the meaning of personal history enables people to be 'in charge of it' (Paterson, 1978, p. 63).

Promoting the More-Being of People

A central premise of humanistic nursing theory is that the nursing concern goes beyond the well-being of patients to the 'more-being' of both patients and nurses. From the simplest greeting of a person to the most advanced resuscitation, nurses act to call forth the potential in people (Paterson & Zderad, 1976). This calling forth involves both the assessment and intervention processes. This calling forth is accomplished by presencing (being attentively present) with people—by joining people in their situations, sharing knowledge and experience, and nurturing 'responsible choosing'. Throughout this process the patient and nurse work together to search for the meaning of the health and illness situation. One particular process these theorists suggest is listening to people and living past events through with them (O'Connor, 1993). An example might be when a child is admitted to hospital with an acute asthmatic attack. Instead of 'telling' the parents what they need to do to prevent another attack, the nurse would begin by asking about their experience, including how it seemed to transpire and their own experiences during the situation, and then using that knowledge and understanding to collaboratively consider options for future management of the child's asthma.

In articulating how nurses proceed in practice these theorists offer the following descriptors of nursing:

- Nursing as doing and being
- Nursing as dialogue
- Nursing as here and now
- Nursing in situations
- Nursing all at once
- Nursing as complementary synthesis

Nursing As Doing and Being

Paterson and Zderad (1976) highlight the inextricable link between nursing doing and being. Moving beyond the level of nurses 'doing to' and/or 'doing for' people, these theorists call for nurses to focus on 'being with and doing with' (Paterson & Zderad, 1976, p. 13). Being with involves 'turning one's attention toward the patient, being aware of and open to the here and now shared situation and communicating one's availability' (Paterson & Zderad, 1988, p. 14).

Nursing As Dialogue

Paterson and Zderad (1988) contend that nursing is a mutual, two-way process that happens in the 'between' space. Nursing practice must therefore occur in response to particular people and particular situations or needs. In this way nursing involves 'a purposeful call and response' (p. 24). The central goal of this responsive, human-centered nursing is to nurture the well-being and more-being of people. Nursing as dialogue is not merely communication through words but involves meeting, relating, presence, and call and response, or mutual back and forth between people. For dialogue to occur there must be an openness that is revealed directly and indirectly 'in a glance, a touch, a tone of voice' (p. 28).

Nursing As Here and Now

Paterson and Zderad (1976) highlight the connectedness between one's past, present, and future. Subsequently they contend that humanistic nursing is always inclusive of both the nurses' and the patients' history, meanings, hopes, fears, and possibilities (O'Connor, 1993). From a here-and-now perspective, each moment is significant, irreplaceable, and imbued with potential.

Nursing in Situations

Humanistic nursing theory highlights how all nursing occurs against the backdrop of a situation and the intersubjective 'dialogue' of patient and nurse is subjected to 'all the chaotic forces of life' (p. 29) and the complex and conflicted realms of the health care world (O'Connor, 1993). The situational nature of nursing practice means that both patients and nurses are affected by other people and the network of relationships and social structures within which they exist.

Nursing All at Once

All at once is the way that Paterson and Zderad (1976) convey the paradoxical, complex, and multifaceted nature of nursing practice. It speaks to how people are simultaneously strong and vulnerable, how nurses are simultaneously being with and doing with, how when patient and nurse meet they are simultaneously alone and in the world, and so forth. Within their discussion of nursing all at once, these theorists purport that a central skill of nurses is the ability to balance the myriad of forces and situational elements to be present in the nursing act.

Nursing As Complementary Synthesis

Closely related to the concept of all at once, nursing as complementary synthesis highlights how nurses traverse both the objective world of biomedicine and the subjective and intersubjective realms of people and situations (O'Connor, 1993). These authors contend that the tensions between these realms are lived out in the moment of the nursing act (O'Connor, 1993).

 ## An Example: A Turning Point

Mr. Gray's body was swollen beyond recognition. He was septic following a bone marrow transplant and was critically unstable. I (Colleen) had been expecting his wife to return to the unit with their daughter who was flying in from California, not having seen her dad since he had become ill. Mr. Gray was semiconscious, and although I could not be sure he heard and understood me, I talked to him continuously as I suctioned his endotrachael tube, completed my routine vital sign checks, and titrated his drugs, trying to maintain some sort of blood pressure. At the same moment as his wife and daughter arrived, the senior resident came in the room (Mr. Gray was on reverse isolation), urgently told me to take a new set of cardiac output and hemodynamic parameters, and gave me several new drug orders. The resident was not the sort of physician who appreciated being contradicted, and my habit was to 'follow orders'. However, the look in his daughter's eyes as she took in the alien sight of her father amidst the multiple lines, monitors, tubes, lights, and sounds led me to say 'I think it is more important for his daughter to have some time right now'. I was shocked at myself (this marked a turning point for me in my practice), and at the resident's response. He nodded, and quietly left.

In this example, although technology and technological expertise are visible, and were obviously in the foreground of Mr. Gray's care, it is possible to see Colleen as the nurse move into the intersubjective space to 'be with' and attend 'all at once' to Mr. Gray, his family, and the resident. And, as Paterson and Zderad (1988) have described, it is possible to see the challenge of actualizing humanistic nursing in the face of the hectic demands of everyday nursing practice. In Colleen's case, it took a certain kind of strength and initiative to challenge the resident in order to 'presence with' Mr. Gray and his family. Although this type of presencing was not always at the center of her nursing care, responding as she did at that particular moment marked a turning point in her work as a nurse and the inspiration to persevere toward that way of being in future. Paterson and Zderad (1988) contend although no nurse may be able to live humanistic nursing in every moment of practice it is 'a goal worth striving for; an attitude that strengthens one's perseverance toward attaining the difficult goal; or fundamentally, a major value shaping one's nursing practice' (p. 15).

An Example: Through the Screen Door

The following story was told to me (Gweneth) by a public health nurse during a workshop I was conducting on health-promoting practice with families. As we discussed the intricacies of how we might join families in ways that were respectful and responsive, one of the more senior nurses spoke of the importance of honoring the family's choice and right to decide when and how we entered their lives. She offered the following story as an example. As I listened to the story I was reminded of Paterson and Zderad's (1988) humanistic nursing and how the description of this nurse's practice exemplified many of the concepts within their theory.

The nurse told us about a family she was working with who included a young, teenage mother and her children. The family met all of the criteria of a 'high-risk' family and therefore public health nursing had been notified by the hospital on discharge. The family had not requested a visit from the public health nurse and in fact was obviously very guarded and on edge about public health's involvement in their lives. This had been communicated indirectly, yet clearly, by the mother. However, because the family was deemed 'high risk' the public health nurse was compelled to visit them. The nurse described how during the first visit the mother watched her approach from behind a screen door. When she climbed the stairs the mother did not open the screen door and did not invite the nurse in. The nurse (paying close attention to unspoken information that was being communicated by the mother and to her own feeling of 'what was right') introduced herself through the screen door, explained that she had been asked to visit the family over the next several months to assist them in any way she could. Following this brief exchange, she departed. The nurse described to us how the visits had continued in this way for several months. She would inform the mother by telephone prior to her visit and they would conduct their visit through the screen door. Although she made frequent visits to the family, she was never 'allowed' into the house. However, although the screen door stayed between them for many months, over time they began to develop a fairly good relationship. The young mother began phoning the nurse to ask the occasional question or to find out when she would be coming again. One day when the nurse arrived the woman opened the screen door and invited the nurse in for tea.

Stop for a minute and consider how the nurse was living Paterson and Zderad's (1988) humanistic nursing theory. For example, how was the nurse present and with the mother? What were the forces within the situation that shaped the intersubjective connection between the mother and the nurse? How did each exercise their freedom and choice in the situation? How did the nurse promote well-being and more-being of both the mother and herself? Can you see the central processes of here and now, nursing as dialogue, all at once, and so forth being lived and practiced?

Newman's Theory of Health As Expanding Consciousness

In her book *Health as Expanding Consciousness*, Margaret Newman (1994) describes what she came to learn as she cared for her mother who lived with Amyotrophic Lateral Sclerosis.

> 66 *I learned that my mother, though physically incapacitated, was a whole person, just like anybody else. I came to know her and to love her in a way I probably never would have taken the time to experience had she not been physically dependent. The five years I spent with her before she died were difficult, tiring, restrictive in some ways, but intense, loving, and expanding in other ways. (p. xxii)* 99

This personal experience informed Newman's subsequent work as a nurse theorist. Her work focused on articulating an understanding of disease as a meaningful aspect of health. For Newman, health and illness are not at two different ends of a continuum, but rather are integrally related aspects of the unitary process of life. From this theoretical orientation, health is conceptualized as a process of expanding consciousness and the ultimate goal of nursing is to foster higher levels of consciousness. Consciousness in this sense is defined as information—how/what people know of themselves in the world. The theory proposes that as people gain more knowledge and information (expand their consciousness), life

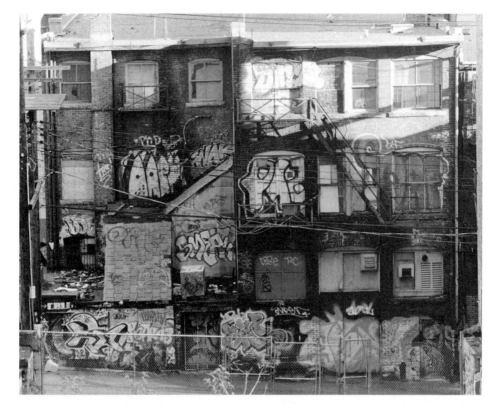

Patterns. (Photograph by Len Budiwski.)

patterns can be identified and transformed. Although Newman does not directly speak of families in her descriptions, the way she conceptualizes people and human being in terms of pattern and energy allows her to transcend the distinction of family as an entity. That is, she speaks about 'persons' in a way that has meaning for any grouping of people including individuals, families, communities, and so forth.

Identifying Patterns

Newman (1994) contends that the task of nursing is not to try to change another person's pattern but to recognize it as information that depicts the whole of their life. For Newman the understanding of pattern is basic to the understanding of health.

> *From the moment we are conceived to the moment we die, in spite of changes that accompany aging, we manifest a pattern that identifies us as a particular person: the genetic pattern that contains the information that directs our becoming; the voice pattern that is recognizable across distances and over time; the movement pattern that identifies a person known to us a long way off even though no other features can be seen. These patterns are among the many explicate manifestations of the underlying (whole) pattern. It is the pattern of our lives that identifies us. (p. 71)*

Because all people/families have their own unique patterns, this theory proposes that nursing action cannot be generalized but must be in response to people in particular situations (for example, we do not give the same information about asthma in the same way to all families). Borrowing from Vaill (1984–1985) Newman (1994) emphasizes the importance of *process wisdom* and *response-ability*—of nursing being open, relational, and in synchrony with people/families. A nurse practicing from this theoretical orientation requires the capacity to be conscious of his or her involvement with others and to act from a knowing that transcends the material and intellectual level. Knowledge must also include the moral/ethical knowing that 'what you are doing is somehow right' (Newman, 1994, p. 77). Notice how Newman's perspective resonates with the spiritual lens that we described in Chapter 2.

Shifting Nursing Practice

Based on this understanding of health as expanding consciousness, Newman emphasizes the following shifts in nursing practice:

1. The shift from treatment of symptoms and disease to a search for patterns
2. The shift from viewing pain and disease as wholly negative to a view that pain and disease are information about the life pattern and an opportunity for growth
3. The shift from seeing the body/family/community as a machine in good or bad repair to seeing the body as a dynamic field of energy
4. The shift from seeing disease as an entity to seeing it as a process

Nursing Intervention As a Relational Process

A central premise within Newman's theory is that intervention aimed at producing a particular result is problematic. 'To intervene with a particular solution in mind is to say we know what form the pattern of expanding consciousness will take, and we don't' (Newman, 1994, p. 97). Interestingly, if you stop and think about this quote you will likely be able to identify how what Newman is saying resonates with the principles of complexity theory discussed in Chapter 2. The theory of health as expanding consciousness articulates nursing intervention as a relational process where the nurse enters into partnership with the family, often at a time of chaos, with the mutual goal of participating in an authentic relationship through which the nurse and the family may emerge at a higher level of consciousness (for example, by developing more knowledge, evolving existing patterns).

Moving Beyond Problems

The theory of expanding consciousness also informs us that nursing practice must move beyond the deficit approach, which focuses on identifying what is wrong with a family, why it is wrong, and then takes steps to fix the problem. Newman emphasizes that often people are brought to the attention of a nurse when they are in a situation that is new, disruptive, and/or one that they do not know how to handle—they are at a place where their old rules and patterns don't work or are not relevant. Rather than viewing such a situation as a problem to be fixed, Newman emphasizes that such situations are opportunities for promoting health—for expanding consciousness and evolving new patterns. For example, illness can provide 'a kind of shock' that reorganizes the relationships and pattern of a person/family's life in more harmonious ways.

> 66 *Consider the function of a high fever, or an emotional crisis, or the accident that occurs at a particularly crucial time. These, and other critical incidents, may provide the shock that facilitates a jump from one pattern to another . . . if we view disease as something . . . to be avoided, diminished or eliminated altogether, we may be ruling out the very factor that can bring about the unfolding of the life process that the person is naturally seeking. (Newman, 1994, p. 11)* 99

In this way, disease and illness provide the opportunity for people/ families to expand their consciousness (gain information about their life patterns). Such experiences may lead them to 'transcend a situation that seems impossible, to find a new way of relating to things, and to discover the freedom that comes with transcending the old limitations' (Newman, 1994, p. 99).

Entering into the Difficulty
Because of the emphasis on *not* fixing and *not* reducing life situations/ experiences to problems, this theory highlights the importance of nurses entering into the difficulty of families' health and healing experiences and 'hanging in there' with families as they live and experience uncertainty and chaos in their lives. 'The task . . . is to stop trying to change the world in accordance with our own image of what is healthy . . . to give up the old agenda to fix things' (Newman, 1994, p. 103). According to Newman, focusing on change and doing to people leads nurses into a pattern of diminished sensitivity. She emphasizes that change is unpredictable and transformational. Therefore the intention guiding practice is for nurses to be in-relation with people as they are, view their behavior and experience as an indication of their current life pattern, and relate to that information (to their expanding consciousness) as it unfolds. As people expand their consciousness and gain information about their life patterns their power and choice of action is enhanced.

Responding to Patterns
Overall this theory informs us that nursing actions must be offered in appropriate response to the patterns of the people/families involved. Pattern extends to all bodily and contextual aspects including temporal patterns (such as natural body rhythms). Newman (1994) contends that such patterns have a profound bearing on how people respond to other people, to therapeutic interventions and so forth. She offers the example of a drug that may have a fatal effect at one point of the circadian cycle and a therapeutic effect at another point. In her theory, Newman emphasizes the importance of nurses orchestrating the timing of their interactions in response to people's readiness and need. Consequently, 'sensitivity to knowing when the need is there to connect with the client and when

TRY IT OUT 3.1. **Trying Out Humanistic Nursing**

Revisit the example of the public health nurse in 'Through the Screen Door'. Reread the story and consider the story in light of Newman's theory of expanding consciousness. How did the nurse demonstrate response-ability in this situation? How did she attend to this specific mother in this specific situation? What do you notice about the relational process that was experienced and lived between them? What new information (expanded consciousness) do you think each gained through the experience? In what ways did the mother and the nurse 'transcend a situation that seemed impossible'? What new way of relating did they find? How did the situation provide an opportunity for them to each 'discover the freedom that comes with transcending old limitation'? How did their expanded consciousness enhance their power and choice of action and foster new life patterns?

"There is enough," is an important skill for nurses to acquire' (Newman, 1994, p. 56). She calls this skill *interactional synchrony*. Use the questions in Try It Out 3.1 to think about the relevance of Newman's theory.

Parse's Theory of Human Becoming

Parse's theory of human becoming was created through a synthesis of ideas from Roger's (1970) science of unitary human beings and existential phenomenology. Some of the language and ideas within Parse's theory are quite abstract and complex and this abstractness poses a challenge to us as writers—how to relate the ideas in a way that is understandable in terms of your everyday practice while not losing the depth and complexity of Parse's theoretical concepts or changing the way she has chosen to language those concepts. Subsequently, we decided to use her original words and to offer descriptions of how *we* have found her theory to be relevant to our work in family nursing. Because it is only our interpretation, it might be quite helpful for you to explore Parse's ideas further with your classmates and instructor. We have also drawn on Cody's (1999) translation in an attempt to strengthen our interpretation.

Parse begins with nine philosophical assumptions (Parse, 1999, pp. 5–6). As you read the assumptions following, pay attention to the core themes that are running throughout the assumptions—meaning, rhythmicity, and transcendence. Also pay attention to the phenomenological (remember Chapter 2) underpinnings that are obviously embedded in the assumptions.

1. The human is coexisting while co-constituting rhythmical patterns with the universe.
2. The human is open, freely choosing meaning in situations, bearing responsibility for decisions.
3. The human is unitary continuously co-constituting patterns of relating.
4. The human is transcending multidimensionally with the possibles.
5. Becoming is unitary human living health.
6. Becoming is a rhythmically co-constituting human-universe process.
7. Becoming is the human's patterns of relating value priorities.
8. Becoming is an intersubjective process of transcendence with the possibles.
9. Becoming is unitary human evolving.

As can be gleaned from these assumptions, Parse views people and the world as inseparable. Throughout, we can hear the remnants of phenomenological thought and the relational view of human life that is central to complexity theory (remember Chapter 2). We can hear the phenomenological notions of constituted and situated that we discussed in Chapter 2 running through the assumptions. It also seems that there might be elements of liberal individualism discussed in Chapter 1, embedded within the ideas of free choice and responsibility for decisions. In addition it is possible to see a similarity between Newman's notion of 'pattern' and Parse's assumption of rhythmical patterns. For Parse, people are living patterns in the world. Within this theory, health is conceptualized as a process of human becoming. This human becoming is evolved in and through living experience. Health is the quality of life from the perspective of the person. Regardless of whether nurses are working with individuals or with families, the goal of nursing practice is to participate in co-creating quality of life. Parse believes that humans are free agents who bring the innate capacity to make intentional choices in situations and it is in this capacity for choice that possibilities for transcendence lie. Through this capacity people are able to change moment to moment as they are in relation with the world—to invent new ways to actualize their dreams.

Looking Beyond the Words

When I (Gweneth) first read Parse's theory several years ago I remember struggling greatly with the language and abstractness. Yet at the same time, the ideas within her theory resonated with what I 'knew' about nursing. In reading about 'health as a process of human becoming' I found myself thinking back to particular nursing moments that had affected me deeply and I could 'see' that at the center of those moments was the human becoming process that Parse was describing. I found myself remembering people/families for whom I had cared in the emergency department, in adult and neonatal ICU, in psychiatry, and in my community work as a nurse. Regardless of the context of my practice, even in the briefest of moments the lives of the people/families I worked with and my own life had changed and become something more. Whether it was a child with an acute otitis media who was brought to the ER by an exhausted mother or a family who was living with a diagnosis of schizophrenia, health as a process of human becoming was central. As I thought about the significance of those human-becoming moments, it highlighted the importance of my own nursing actions and in particular how I was 'with' people in those moments. I resonated with Parse's contention that nurses should take the role of 'nurturing gardeners' (as opposed to fix-it mechanics) and could see how that description was in keeping with how I had intuitively found myself responding. At the same time the distinctions she drew between biomedically based approaches and a human science approach to nursing echoed the limitations that I had experienced in the service-delivery model of health care that seemed to dominate and limit my nursing potential.

Looking Beneath the Words

When reading Parse's work I (Colleen) too struggled with the language. However, I was drawn to what I understood to be Parse's take on the stance of nursing. That is, according to Parse, nurses are not 'experts' engaged in doing to and for people. Rather, it seemed to me that Parse advocated more egalitarian relationships than what I regularly witnessed in my critical care practice. However, first I wondered how nursing and non-nursing knowledge was to be drawn on. Second, I saw the ability of people/families to freely choose meaning and bear responsibility for decisions as severely constrained by available resources and discourses. To me the constrained 'possibilities' often overwhelm the ability of families to 'freely choose' and I continue to question relative importance of the role of nurses in expanding the possibles and co-creating quality of life.

Parse's Theory of Family

Interestingly, Cody (1999) describes how Parse's theory was originally presented using family life situations. In Parse's theory the term 'human' is used to refer to all human phenomena including individuals, families, and communities. Parse (1981) defines family as 'the others with whom one is closely connected' (p. 81). Cody draws an important distinction between Parse's theory and other views of family. He contends that historically scientists have conceptualized 'family' in accordance with the prevailing norms. In contrast, Parse does not conceptualize family according to a particular structure or function. Rather, although family might be construed as a 'unit' in contrast to a configuration of people, Parse considers family as a unit of meaning (Cody, 1999). 'It is not a hypostatized structure or system with roles and functions but, rather, a flowing experiential process of interrelating' (Cody, 1999, p. 15).

Although each person's life is one's own, because people interface multidimensionally (for example, physically, energetically, rhythmically) with others and the world, their evolution and becoming is always in-relation with others and the world. For this reason, Parse contends that family is always with any person regardless of circumstance. This idea is exemplified by the experience of John, the man in Chapter 1 who worked at the shelter and described his experience of family while living on the street.

Practicing from True Presence

Nurses who practice from this theoretical perspective live and practice nursing in "true presence . . . [Nursing from this perspective] is an unconditional loving, non-routinized way of being with, in which the nurse bears witness to changing health patterns of persons and families" (Parse, 1997, p. 34). The nurse enters people's worlds as a not-knowing stranger (Parse, 1996), is open to what people are experiencing, and is willing to share in particular moments. Parse (1981) emphasizes that all nurse-person processes are led by the person. In this way, 'family health is co-created by persons as they live family process' (Cody, 1999, p. 14). Parse articulates particular ways of relating including face-to-face discussions (dialogue and conversation), silent immersion (a deep place of no words), and lingering presence (being still to reflect and abide with).

To Illustrate

Coby Tschanz is a nurse who works in palliative care and who, as part of her graduate-level studies, has come to choose Parse as the nursing theory that guides her practice. I (Gweneth) asked Coby if she would describe her practice to offer an illustration of how the theory might look in everyday nursing work. The following is Coby's description in her own words:

A poem by Rumi entitled 'Love for Certain Work' reads 'Each has been given a strong desire for certain work. A love for those motions, and all motion is love' (1991, p. 17). For me, most days, that 'certain work' is the practice of hospice palliative care nursing. Significantly, the theory of human becoming offers a language for me to speak about this work.

Recently, a nursing professor asked why, out of all possible theories of nursing, I was particularly interested in the theory of human becoming. Instead of offering my prepared response, I found myself claiming: 'The theory sounds, it *is* like poetry to me'. I think we were both surprised by that answer. After all, theory is science. The language of Parse's theory can seem difficult, and the concepts are not necessarily easy to understand. And, as with any other science, it takes a fair deal of study, reflection, and practice to become comfortable with using new words and conceptualizations until these things seem almost invisible.

Oddly enough, a few days after meeting with the professor I came across an article in which a nurse scholar referred to theory as 'the poetry of science' (Levine, 1995, p. 14). Interesting! Levine's words surfaced a new awareness of both theory and poetry as modes of representing and inviting innovative understandings of human experiences. In my case, the theory of human becoming provided me with a way to tell of my certain work and offered support for practicing in ways congruent with my beliefs about humans and health experiences.

For me, practice guided by the theory of human becoming means I am supported to work with respect for human experiences of mystery, diversity, and paradox. In some ways, it is a relief as a nurse and as a person to be guided in illuminating and co-creating meaning, plans, and hopes with others without necessarily seeking to construct, identify, or solve human experiences as problematic, and normal or abnormal. This way I seek to discover what quality of living and dying means to each person and what his or her own experiences and visions of health are. Still, it is sometimes a struggle to be clear about my ideas and beliefs, to live them out in practice with others, and to meet the demands of a complex health care system. In the midst of what seems a similar struggle, Kuhl (2002) shares insights from his research with persons who are dying. Significantly, he writes that the people he interviewed '*longed* [my italics] for others to know about them' (p. xxxvii–xxxviii). How, in nursing practice, can I honour such longing? Whatever theoretical perspective one chooses, it seems vital to continue to explore ways of discovering what it is each person values when he or she is with a nurse.

Think through Parse's theory for yourself by using the ideas in Try It Out 3.2.

> **TRY IT OUT 3.2.** **Trying Out Human Becoming**
>
> Revisit the example 'Through the Screen Door' one more time and consider it in light of Parse's theory of human becoming. For example, how did the nurse enter the family's world in a manner that is similar to Parse's not-knowing stranger? In what ways did the nurse bear witness to the mother's changing health pattern over time? How was the nurse-person process led by the mother? Are there other aspects that seem to reflect the human becoming process?

● What Makes a 'Good' Theory?

Through the earlier discussion it becomes evident that just as there is no 'right' answer to 'What is family?' there is no right answer to 'What is family nursing?' But this does not mean that all theory is of equal merit. Theorizing our practice is *not* merely a matter of deciding for ourselves how we will practice. Rather, theories are chosen for their pragmatic correspondence and responsiveness to families. This means that *any theory must be scrutinized according to how well it responds to experience—how useful it is in sensitizing us and enhancing our capacity to respond in ways that promote the health and well-being of families*. This may mean that you might choose one theoretical perspective as your central guiding perspective, or may choose a more eclectic approach, drawing on multiple theories that you judge to be congruent and/or complimentary.

● A Reflection

The nursing theories from the human science paradigm that we have described in this chapter draw attention to aspects of family in nursing that are not typically emphasized within a biomedical-only approach. As an intensive care nurse, I (Colleen) learned to devalue the aspects of my practice that had to do with emotion, comfort, relationships, caring—the 'soft', nontechnological, 'nonscience' aspects of my practice. I learned that my skill with technology, drugs, and equipment, and my knowledge of physiology, pathophysiology, and pharmacology were of value. My ability to use this knowledge in an 'efficient' manner was also of value. This primarily meant getting the tasks all done quickly, keeping up with q15 vital signs and hourly checks, having my unit look tidy, and moving my patient on quickly. Moving my patient on meant getting the patient stable enough so that my assignment could be doubled (so I could look after more than one patient), or getting patients discharged, or, in the case of dying patients, getting decisions regarding withdrawal of treatment made expeditiously.

   Without any particular nursing theory guiding me, I practiced predominantly from a biomedical perspective. However, I never quite let go of my belief that the essence and value of my practice was 'something more'. I hung on to the connections I made with patients and family members, the instances of knowing that I had made an important difference in someone's life or death. When I first encountered nursing theories, such as those we have described here, I thought they were a bit 'flakey' and 'soft', until I realized that I was playing into discourses and ideas that devalued what I truly believed in. Eventually such theories helped me to think and talk about and value openly that 'something more'.

As I (Gweneth) consider the nursing theories within the human science paradigm from a pragmatic perspective it becomes evident that these theories support nurses to attend to the larger life force of people/ families and their lives. In line with the hermeneutic and spiritual lenses we presented in Chapter 2, the theories can guide us as we attempt to be with people/families in ways that attend to what is meaningful and significant in their lives and the spirit, energy, and power that is at the center of their life force. Each of these theories deals with the sociopolitical context of health and health care differently and to a different extent. For example, I (Colleen) read these theories, and to some extent still do, as focused on *relationships* between and among people, but not necessarily taking into account people *in relation* to their contexts (cultural, economic, sociopolitical, language, and so on). However, in tandem with sociopolitical theories that help take context into account (what we are calling a *relational* approach), these theories can help us to push back at the taken-for-granted assumption that practice that is oriented to humans in-relation (as opposed to, for example, bodies on stretchers) is no longer possible in the world of health care reform. These theories can also help us see when families are overlooked and/or treated as a means to meet corporate objectives.

In subsequent chapters we provide opportunities for you to continue theorizing and retheorizing *your* family nursing practice. As you proceed, keep the notes you have made during this chapter so you can track the evolution of your living theory as you continue to reimagine your nursing practice with families.

THIS WEEK IN PRACTICE

What Are the Central Ingredients of Your Theory of Nursing?

If you are in practice, read over the following, and when in practice pay attention to the decisions you make. Find two classmates or colleagues to meet with. As a group go through the following steps, using your most recent day in practice to provide examples (if there are three of you, each might take responsibility for one part, or act as a proponent for one of the theories):

Part 1: Read over the description of Paterson and Zderad's (1976, 1988) theory once again and any notes you made in response and consider each of your own perspectives. For example, Paterson and Zderad theorize nursing as 'a happening between people'. What do you each believe nursing is? Reread the beliefs that underpin Paterson and Zderad's theory. How are your beliefs similar and/or different from theirs? For example, do you believe all people have an inherent capacity to choose how to respond to situations in life? Do you believe people have the capacity to envision possibilities? Do you believe that through the process of relating people 'become more' and learn more about their uniqueness? Do you believe that what happens between nurses and the people they care for is always inclusive of both the nurses' and the patients' history, meanings, hopes, fears, and possibilities? If so, how do these beliefs shape your nursing actions? If you did share these beliefs and wanted to retheorize your own practice in light of them, what changes would you make to how you went about your nursing work? What aspects of your theory are different from Patterson and Zderad's?

Part 2: Read back over the description of Newman's (1994) theory and the notes you made in response to it and begin to ask each other about your own views. For example, Newman views disease as a meaningful aspect of health. Her view is in contrast to a biomedical view that considers disease as the opposite of health. How do you each theorize health and disease and the connection between them? How are your theoretical views similar and/or different from Newman's? Newman contends that the task of nursing is to search for and recognize patterns. She theorizes that pain and disease are information about the life pattern and an opportunity for growth. As a result of this theoretical assumption she does not seek to 'fix' or 'cure' but rather to join families in their illness situations and promote their opportunity for growth rather than seek to change them or their situation. What do you theorize the goal and task of nursing to be? What beliefs and assumptions underpin this goal in your theory? If someone watched each of you in practice how would you look different as a result of the particular beliefs and assumptions you each hold? Based on her theoretical view, Newman identifies interactional synchrony as a skill that nurses need. What skills do you view as integral to practice given your theory of nursing? How do you think Newman's theory addresses contextual knowledge (as described in this chapter) or does it? What other aspects of Newman's theory resonated with your own? What differences between her theory and your own did you discover?

Part 3: Read over the description of Parse's (1981) theory once again and use the concepts within her theory to continue your own theorizing. For example, Parse identifies the goal of nursing practice as participating with people to co-create their quality of life. Believing that people are free agents who bring the innate capacity to make intentional choices in situations, Parse assumes that they can make the changes they need to actualize their dreams. What is your theoretical perspective on this? Do you each see this similarly or are there differences between you? Do you think people have the capacity to effect change in their own lives? How do you reconcile this belief with the knowledge that contextual elements can constrain choice? Given your answers to the preceding questions, what do you see as your role as a nurse? If you share the view that people have this innate capacity, how do you believe their history (e.g., remember postcolonial theory) might intersect with this capacity and the choices people make in their lives? Think about how each of you theorizes family. Parse theorizes family as a unit of meaning rather than as a unit of structure or function. What do you think family is?

CHAPTER HIGHLIGHTS

1. What are three ideas from the nursing theories in this chapter that resonated with you in regard to your own practice?
2. How do these human science nursing theories contribute to your own developing family nursing knowledge and practice?
3. How might the three theories described in this chapter work in concert with or in contrast to the lenses presented in Chapter 2?

REFERENCES

Banks-Wallace, J. (2000). Womanist Ways of Knowing: Theoretical Considerations for Research with African American Women. *Advances in Nursing Science, 22*(3), 33–47.

Belenky, M. F., Clinchy, B. M., Goldberger, N. R., & Tarule, J. M. (1986). *Women's ways of knowing: The development of self, voice and mind.* New York: Basic Books.

Benner, P., Tanner, C. A., & Chesla, C. A. (1996). *Expertise in nursing practice.* New York: Springer.

Browne, A. J. (2001). The influence of liberal political ideology on nursing practice. *Nursing Inquiry, 8*(2), 118–129.

Carper, B. A. (1978). Fundamental patterns of knowing in nursing. *Advances in Nursing Science, 1*(1), 13–23.

Chinn, P. L., & Jacobs-Kramer, M. (1988). Perspectives on knowing: A model of nursing knowledge. *Scholarly Inquiry for Nursing Practice: An International Journal, 2*(2), 129–139.

Cody, W. (1999). The view of family within the human becoming theory. In R. Parse (Ed.), *Illuminations: The human becoming theory in practice and research.* New York: National League for Nursing Press.

Grant, A. (2001). Knowing me knowing you: towards a new relational politics in 21st century mental health nursing. *Journal of Psychiatric & Mental Health Nursing, 8*(3), 269–276.

Hartrick, G. A. (1997). A critical pedagogy of family nursing. *Journal of Nursing Education, 37*(2), 80–84.

Hartrick, G. (2002). Transcending the limits of method: Cultivating creativity in nursing. Research and Theory for Nursing Practice. *An International Journal, 16*(1), 53–62.

Kleffel, D. (1996). Environmental paradigms: Moving toward an ecocentric perspective. *Advances in Nursing Science, 18*(4), 1–10.

Kuhl, D. (2002). *What dying people want: Practical wisdom for end of life.* Toronto: Doubleday Canada.

Levine, M. E. (1995). The rhetoric of nursing theory. *Image: Journal of Nursing Scholarhsip, 27*(1).

Liaschenko, J. (1997). Knowing the patient? In S. E. Thorne & V. E. Hayes (Eds.) *Nursing praxis: Knowledge and action* (pp. 23–53). Thousand Oaks: Sage.

Liaschenko, J., & Fisher, A. (1999). Theorizing the knowledge that nurses use in the conduct of their work. *Scholarly Inquiry for Nursing Practice: An International Journal, 13*(1), 29–41.

Newman, M. A. (1994). *Health as expanding consciousness* (NLN Publ. No. 14-2626, 2nd ed.). New York: National League for Nursing.

O'Connor, N. (1993). *Paterson and Zderad humanistic nursing theory. Notes on Nursing Theories.* Newbury Park, CA: Sage.

Parse, R. (1981). *Man-living-health: A theory of nursing.* New York: Wiley.

Parse, R. (1996). The human becoming theory: Challenges in practice and research. *Nursing Science Quarterly, 9*, 55–60.

Parse, R. (1997). The human becoming theory: The was, is, and will be. *Nursing Science Quarterly, 10*(1), 32–38.

Parse, R. (1999). *Illuminations: The human becoming theory in practice and research.* New York: National League for Nursing Press.

Paterson, J. G. (1978). The tortuous way toward nursing theory. In *Theory development: What, why, how?* (NLN Publ. No, 15-1708, pp. 49–65). New York: National League for Nursing.

Paterson, J. G., & Zderad, L. T. (1976). *Humanistic nursing.* New York: Wiley.

Paterson, J. G., & Zderad, L. T. (1988). *Humanistic nursing* (NLN Publ. No. 41-2218, 2nd ed.). New York: National League for Nursing.

Polanyi, M. (1962). Personal knowledge. Chicago, II: University of Chicago.

Rogers, M. E. (1970). *An introduction to the theoretical basis of nursing.* Philadelphia: F.A. Davis.

Rumi. (1991). *One handed basket weaving: Poems on the theme of work* (Coleman Barks, Trans.). Athens, GA: Maypop.

Schaefer, K. M. (2002). Reflections on caring narratives: Enhancing patterns of knowing. *Nursing Education Perspectives, 23*(6), 286–294.

Schultz, P. R., & Meleis, A. I. (1988). Nursing epistemology: Traditions, insights, questions, *IMAGE: Journal of Nursing Scholarship, 20*(4), 217–221.

Smith, M. C. (1992). Is all knowing personal knowing? *Nursing Science Quarterly, 5*(1), 2–3.

Sweeney, N. M. (1994). A concept analysis of personal knowledge: Application to nursing education. *Journal of Advanced Nursing, 20,* 917–924.

Vaill, P. G. (1984–1985). Process wisdom for a new age. *Revision, 7*(2), 39–49.

Wainwright, P. (2000). Towards an aesthetics of nursing. *Journal of Advanced Nursing, 32*(3), 750–756.

Watson, J. (1988). *Nursing: Human science and human care. A theory of nursing* (NLN Pub. No. 15-2236). New York: National League for Nursing.

White, J. (1995). Patterns of knowing: Review, critique, and update. *Advances in Nursing Science, 17*(4), 73–86.

Zderad, L. T. (1978). From here to now to theory: Reflections on 'how'. In *Theory development: What, why, how?* (NLN Publ. No. 15-1708, pp. 35–48). New York: National League for Nursing.

2

Relational
Practice in
Context

4 Family and Nursing in Context

OVERVIEW

In Chapter 4 we use the theoretical lenses presented in the previous chapters to highlight the significance of context to relational nursing practice and illuminate how families, nurses, and health care are contextually shaped.

> 66 *Blood ties are almost always a bad place to begin to understand the boundaries between private and public life, the nature of the marriage bond, or tensions and sentiments between parents and children . . . it is best to start with the particulars of time and place, economic needs, social priorities and the exercise of power, because these are the environments in which childhood and family are embedded and within which they change. (Parr, 1982, p. 8)* 99

As we take up a relational approach to family nursing practice and as we try on different lenses through which to view family, we begin to see that the context within which we practice is integral to that practice. Our experiences of family shape our personal understanding of 'family' and what is 'usual' or 'normal'. However, these experiences don't 'just happen'. Our experiences have been shaped by the circumstances of our lives, and those circumstances are shaped by larger sociopolitical and economic forces. Therefore, family nursing practice must attend to the living experience of family *in context*. The lives, health, and experiences of the families with whom we work can only be understood in context. At the same time, relational family nursing practice requires exploration of how our ideas have been shaped, not just by our experiences, but also by our life circumstances and the forces shaping those circumstances. Finally, families and nurses come together under particular conditions and circumstances that shape the possibilities for practice. To be responsive and health promoting, nursing practice must attend to these conditions and circumstances.

To continue the tour-guide analogy that we used in Chapter 2, we are asking you now to stop at a crossroads, to look at the many roads down which the families you encounter have traveled, to think about the road behind you (where you have already traveled), and to look around at the area surrounding the crossroads where you will meet these families. Some of the families you will meet arrive at the crossroads footsore and hungry, others arrive with full packs and helpers to carry them. Some of you will have traveled through rich, sun-drenched valleys, some through deserts and rocky plains. There might be an oasis at the crossroads where you and a family meet, or the well might be close to dry. We believe that if you are going to cultivate practice that is relational you need to take into account these contexts: that of the families you encounter, your own, and the contexts you experience together—the hospitals, clinics, homes, and streets where as a nurse you join with families.

● Family in Context

When you meet families, are you in the habit of looking to see their absent family members, their ancestors, or their current friends hanging around them like ghosts? Do you immediately imagine the family's home, community, or history as an invisible backdrop? Or, do you envision the 'roads' they and you have traveled to a given health care encounter? What of visualizing the family as linked by invisible connections to various branches of the government, to schools, and to cabinets and computers full of files of information? Although you may not 'look to see' all of those structures, experiences, and people, they are all in fact shaping the living experiences of the families you come in-relation with. Paying attention to family in context draws attention to these features.

Together, the hermeneutic phenomenological, critical, and spiritual lenses draw attention to these features in particular ways. As we outlined in Chapter 2, these lenses draw attention to the way in which knowledge and the conditions that create such knowledge are meaningfully experienced, socially produced, and spiritually significant. A hermeneutic lens draws attention to the living experience of families in particular moments and particular situations. A critical lens draws attention to the way power operates and to the ways in which structural conditions create unequal power relations. Each of the perspectives we have discussed within the critical lens draws attention to particular features of the

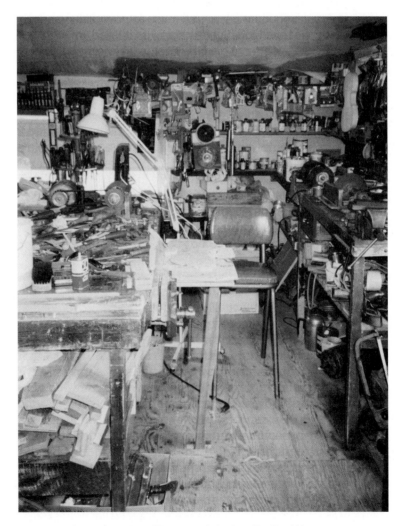

My father the violin maker. (Photograph by Len Budiwski.)

environment. A spiritual lens draws attention to the larger life force—to what is ultimately concerning and shaping people/families as spiritual beings in the world. Together the hermeneutic phenomenology, critical, and spirituality lenses turn attention to meaning, significance, power, oppression, gender, diversity, intersectionality, culture, history, racialization, language, faith, and spirit—to the ways families are situated, constituted, and inspired. In what follows, we illustrate how together these perspectives foster a relational inquiry that can enhance your ability to be responsive to particular families.

An Example: Seeing Red

Red was born in a rural Canadian community in 1954. As an Aboriginal child, she was sent to the Mission, a residential school, at age 6, where she remained until she was 12, and then off and on until she was 17. She described her life and experience of family as one of continuous rejection, not only because of being removed from her mother's care, but also because of how her mother and grandmother (who had both been in residential school) treated her.

▶ *My mom would come and get my other brothers and sisters and leave me and she did it twice. The first time . . . she said she didn't have enough money and kids came back and said she had lots of money. Another time she said she had no room and they came back and said she had lots of room. And then when I was 12, she took me and she said the only reason she took me was to baby sit . . . they used to drink a lot and [my mom] was always kicking me out.*

Red was released from residential school at age 17. Having neither access to further education nor employable skills, and unable to live with her mother, she 'ended up' living with a series of men. One of her longest relationships was with a man named Edward.

▶ *I ended up pregnant. I told him and he told me, 'pack your stuff, you're going back to town'. He dumped me off and said, 'Go have an abortion'. And he left me there. And I don't know how I got back, but I went back there and he said, 'As soon as that baby is born, you're giving it up for adoption'.*

She had several children, all of whom were either given up for adoption or apprehended by the state and placed in foster care. Despite not raising the children or having much contact with them, they remain a primary focus of Red's conversation.

Red has always been very poor, and as a young woman she spent time living on the street.

▶ *A lot of times we would just go to the dumpsters, you know, and dig around in there for, um, whatever. You know, bread, sometimes they'd throw bread out that was still in bags. Throw out fruit and all kinds of stuff you could just find in there. And other times, um, I went to a few people's places, you know, and they might give me something to eat. But, um, that's pretty much how I lived, you know, and in the end I started living with these two guys. They had a one-bedroom apartment . . . most of the time, we all three of us slept . . . in the living room, because a lot of times if you have a hangover, you're really depressed and so we would just watch TV. That was a spot where everybody came to drink and bring booze or Lysol.*

Today she has quit drinking, is struggling to get herself 'healthy', and hopes to have more contact with her children someday:

▶ *I thought, you know, I should write [my son] a letter for his birthday. I thought, no, not until I'm [pause] really to the point, you know, where more rejection isn't going to hurt me. I'm going to get myself healthy. Yeah. And, then I might try and find my [pause] daughter.*

Inquiry Into and About Context

As a nurse you may have cared for Red when she was a pregnant teen, or when she was giving birth to one of her children, or when she came to emergency, perhaps with an injury from abuse by her partner. More recently, you might have met Red as a family member when her older sister was admitted to psychiatry following a suicide attempt or when her mother was dying. In those encounters you might not have inquired in such a way as to learn her story. Yet her sociohistorical context is integral to who she is today and how you might best respond to promote her health and healing.

Take a minute and think about Red's story. What stands out for you about that story? What seems to be of concern and significance to Red? What is the meaning of family to her? What historical, political, economic, and social conditions shaped the experience of Red's family? How are these conditions shaping what is of concern and significance to Red?

To Illustrate

To understand Red and her family in context, the story must be understood against the background of colonialism and racism. However, such understanding must be developed thoughtfully and cautiously, because as Razak (1998) shows, understanding people in their cultural contexts can be a double-edged sword—in seeking to understand people's oppression, sometimes people are painted only as victims (and their strengths overlooked), or worse, painted as somehow inferior and responsible for their social circumstances. The history of Aboriginal people in Canada, the background to Red's life, is one of the clearest examples of how families are shaped by social, political, and economic contexts. In concert with policies and practices that stripped Aboriginal people of their lands and means of survival, the place where Red grew up was home to one of the most notorious residential schools in Canada, St. Joseph's Mission (Furniss, 1995, 1999). The state's intended project was the assimilation of Aboriginal people into 'white' society. A premise central to this project was that 'Aboriginal children would have to be removed for a lengthy period from the "destructive" influences of their families and communities' (Furniss, 1999, p. 42). For six decades, from 1891 to the 1960s, children of the Secwepemc, southern Carrier, and Tsilhqot'in people were sent to the Mission, where they were allowed little or no contact with their families and were 'subjected to a strict regime of discipline in which public humiliation, beatings and physical punishments were used to maintain their submission' (p. 43). Today the Aboriginal people of that area often speak of themselves as survivors of generations of residential school as they strive to heal the destruction of family ties, loss of culture and language, loss of parenting skills, and destruction of sense of self that is their legacy.

Red and her family are some of those 'survivors'. Red was not the first generation of Aboriginal children taken by the state. Rather, her mother, her grandmother, and children of earlier generations were taken from their families. These practices wrecked family ties, and entire communities of children grew up in successive generations not knowing their parents, their language, or their customs. Furthermore, the children were subjected to abuse and were taught that they were inferior. These practices were implemented along with other Indian Act policies that forced Aboriginal peoples into economic dependence and confined them to reserves without means of economic support other than state dependence. Despite amazing strength, resilience, and efforts to heal, the

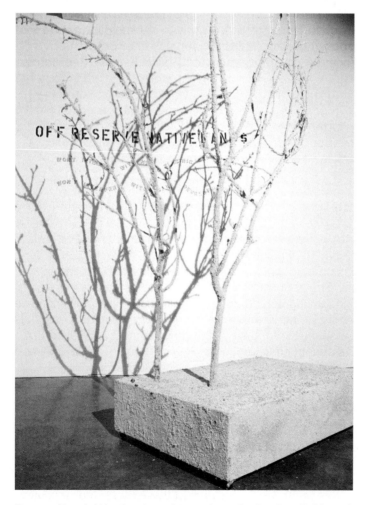

Reserved Land. (Wood and sawdust sculpture by Jocelyne Robinson.)

despair and destruction wrought continues to pervade many communities. With this background in mind, Red's mother's 'rejection' of her can be seen not as 'bad mothering' but as a direct consequence of state practices over many generations. In turn, Red's loss of her children to the state can be seen as a continuation of state practices in relation to Aboriginal people and at least in part as a failure of the state to take measures to attempt to remedy generations of abuse. Indeed it is only recently that lawsuits by Aboriginal people in Canada have drawn attention to these abuses and resulted in some attempts to implement measures such as treatment programs for residential school survivors. Still, despite years of bargaining, few treaty negotiations have been concluded in Canada, with the result that the enforced poverty and dependence of Aboriginal people continues. Had such remedies and treaties been in place, might Red have raised her own children?

For Aboriginal people in Canada, racism is a daily feature of life. In my work on a project in the rural area where Red grew up, I (Colleen) have been overwhelmed by the extent to which the Aboriginal people have been taught that they are inadequate, dysfunctional, and inferior and how deeply these messages have been absorbed. One woman, Rita (a very well-educated, accomplished woman), said to me 'When you are told by your family that you are a drunken Indian, that you will never be anything but a drunken Indian . . . then, you are unlikely to be anything but a drunken Indian'. Against the backdrop of widespread racism, enforced poverty, and her family's history, Red's life on the street and struggle with alcohol are more comprehensible. And her capacity— her effort to get healthy, to quit drinking, to hope for contact with her children— seems remarkable.

The this example illustrates that the knowledge that is required for relational family nursing practice is broad and includes knowledge of political, economic, social, and historical events. It is our contention that if family nurses are to practice in ways that are health promoting, they need to use different knowledge and use knowledge differently. In particular, nurses need to continually expand their knowledge of the sociohistorical context and its influences on families, health, and health care, and shift the ways they employ such knowledge. These changes start with fundamental shifts in thinking about nursing knowledge, health, and health promotion, shifts we began to suggest in Chapter 1.

● Building Contextual Knowledge of Family Health

As families can only be understood in their specific historic, geographic, and social contexts, family health can only be understood similarly. In addition to empirical knowledge about health issues and knowledge of the meaning of those health issues, contextual knowledge is required. For example, without analysis of context, high infant mortality rates among Aboriginal people might be seen as symptomatic of poor prenatal choices. However, once living conditions, poverty, and restricted access to health care because of rural geography and racism are taken into account, infant mortality can be understood differently, and thus more effective actions can be taken. Understanding family health in context requires seeking contextual knowledge regarding the health issues facing families.

To Illustrate

Childhood asthma may not be a health problem that you automatically think of as a social problem. Yet studies from countries as diverse as Canada, the United States, South Africa, and Britain (for example, see Akinbami, LaFleur, & Schoendorf, 2002; Klinnert, Price, Liu, & Robinson, 2002; Ng Man Kwong, Das, Proctor, Whyte, & Primhak, 2002; Poyser et al., 2002; Sin, Svenson, Cowie, & Man, 2003) show that prevalence and severity of asthma in children is linked to socioeconomic status, which in turn is linked to racial disparity. Researchers think that socioeconomic deprivation affects the physical environment (for example, poor ventilation and heating, cockroaches, mould), the quality of asthma management and access to asthma treatment, and/or symptom reporting. If we draw only on medically based empirical knowledge (which is also important) regarding the pathophysiology of asthma, medications, and clinical management, or if we draw only on the meaning of the experiences of asthma to children and their families, as nurses we may participate in 'downstream' asthma management while the homes and conditions in which children live remain unchanged. For example, health cannot be promoted solely by providing information regarding improving household ventilation to a family who will never be able to afford such improvements. Thus, nursing approaches to families of children with asthma must take into account the social, economic, and historical context of families' lives and include strategies to address the problem 'upstream' (remember the example of drowning victims from Chapter 1?).

In order to promote health, contextual (or sociopolitical) knowledge is required to complement other forms of knowledge. Indeed, as we discussed in Chapter 3, we believe that sociopolitical knowing is a frame within which to understand other ways of knowing. You will have acquired certain empirical knowledge from other sources. Much of the health-related knowledge you will have acquired likely is congruent with the biomedical model. For example, you will have learned about the etiology and pathophysiology of childhood asthma and the pharmacology of drugs used in the treatment of asthma. Some of you also may have learned about what asthma means in the lives of certain families, by working with families, from personal experience, or by reading research about the experiences of families. For example, Peterson, Sterling, Stout (2002) conducted interviews with 20 African American adult primary caregivers of children with asthma to understand asthma from their perspective. They found that the families' lived experience contrasted greatly with health care provider explanations of asthma. The families had their own explanatory models of asthma. They drew on

---

TRY IT OUT 4.1. **Family Health in Context**

1. Pick any family health issue in which you are interested.
2. Identify the structural conditions that might influence that health issue.
3. Do an Internet or library search to identify research that would help you better understand those structural conditions. If you have access to the Internet, an easy way to do this is to go to http://www.ncbi.nlm.nih.gov/PubMed/ This is a free resource, and you can quickly do a search on your health issue and combine it with another term to narrow your search. For example, the references in the example about asthma will be retrieved by entering 'childhood asthma' and 'poverty' or 'socioeconomic status'.
4. Get and read at least one research article that expands your knowledge 'contextually'.

---

their cultural context to understand asthma and drew much of their information about asthma from other family members and from personal experience.

Although these forms of knowledge are important, what we want to emphasize here is the importance of also understanding health from a contextual perspective. That is, how does the environment (social, political, economic, physical, and so on) shape health? Using the lenses we have offered helps build contextual knowledge of health and points to understanding health by considering economics, gender, colonization, racism, and language in relation to health. In the example of asthma, it is easy to see how economics and racial discrimination shape health. But what about gender? Is it possible that boys and girls are treated differently in their homes in ways that would affect asthma? Are boys and girls assigned better or worse sleeping accommodations, do they perform different chores, and so on? Again, our intent here is not that you acquire particular knowledge, but rather that you expand your ways of thinking to approach family health contextually. You might want to consider Try It Out 4.1 at this point.

● Building Contextual Knowledge of Families

> *Your car stereo is state of the art*
> *My ghetto blaster is fallin' apart*
> *But hey man, you're all show*
> *You only listen to techno*
>
> *Your ride goes from zero to sixty*
> *Well my ride's gone, ya, it must have missed me*
> *Cause i'm still standing here watching you drive by*
>
> *I am sick and you are healthy*
> *You are rich and i am filthy*
> *Congratulations on all your success . . .*
> *Bif Naked, 2003*

As we encounter families, the way that history, policy, and economics lives on in their lives serves to shape their health and health care experiences. The socioenvironmental perspective of health promotion (discussed in Chapter 1) directs us to attend to the context within which families live and experience health. One approach to understanding the environmental conditions that compromise health promotion and the interrelationships between social, political, and economic structures and the origins of health and illnesses is to begin with particular health issues. We suggested this in Try It Out 4.1.

Another way to expand your understanding is to begin with the environmental conditions and consider how they shape families and thus, their health. Again, the lenses we have offered point us to the economic, historical, political, and social circumstances of families' lives. The goal here is to widen our understanding of the range of influences that might be shaping families' experiences.

Influence of Economics on Families

Begin by thinking about how economics shape families. It might not be your habit to think of families as economic units. However, local and global economics are highly influential on the forms and functions that families serve. Indeed, every family you encounter is shaped by access to material resources. Do you know families whose adult children continue to live with their parents in order to afford to attend school? Or in order to afford to raise their own children? Every family you meet is also shaped by not just immediate, but also historical economic influences. For example, in the Southern United States, postabolition labour dynamics meant that African American people migrated into cities for jobs that subsequently disappeared, largely through automation, leaving many unemployed and thus unable to support families (Sharpe, 2001; Wilson, 2002). Thus the 'extended family' dwelling became an economic necessity, not merely a 'cultural preference'. Today, the intersecting influences of racism and economics continue to shape the family experiences of African Americans, particularly, for example, through the disproportionate incarceration of black men (Browning, Miller & Spruance, 2001; Miller, Browning & Spruance, 2001).

Influence of Colonization on Families

Integrally related to economics, colonization has also shaped and continues to influence families around the globe. Indeed, every family you encounter has been shaped by and is continuing to be shaped by, colonizing practices, whether the family is descended from early colonizers, those who have been colonized, or both, or whether the family has immigrated under neocolonial conditions. Colonial rule has shaped family forms and norms throughout the Western world, and indeed the globe. Because of the dominance of European colonial powers over the past centuries, and because of continued Western dominance through neocolonialist practices, many cultures have had to cope with the imposition of Christian-European family norms and with the values of their colonizers (Potthast-Jutkeit, 1997). However, despite such imposition, a wide variety of family forms have persisted, and former colonial powers in turn have been exposed to this greater variety of family forms, particularly through immigration from their former colonies.

In Canada, for example, the nuclear family began to emerge as an institution in the late 18th century and did so as a consequence of the complex social and economic influences of colonialism (Parr, 1982). However, these influences did not impact all people or all families in the same way. The impact of colonization on Aboriginal women and immigrant women of colour was quite different than for white women (Das Gupta, 1995; Dua, 1999). Aboriginal women and immigrant women of colour were governed by different policies (specifically the Indian Act for Aboriginal women and race-specific immigration policies for immigrant women). Various immigration policies have prevented marriage by certain immigrants, denied immigration to women, and allowed only temporary visas to workers in attempts to recruit domestic workers and labourers without providing citizenship (Arat-Koc, 1999; Das Gupta, 1995; Dua, 1999). Thus, colonial and state policies repeatedly denied immigrant people of colour and Aboriginal people the right to live in a family context and the right to have the family form of their choice. For example, early Canadian policies ensured that for Chinese and South Asian people, only male labourers could immigrate and their wives and children could not follow. Caribbean and black women were allowed to immigrate primarily as domestic labourers and their male partners and children could not follow. Despite these racist policies, and sometimes in response to them, various forms of family have endured. Indeed Das Gupta (1995) says that "Same-sex, communal and quasi-extended families have been formed as a bulwark against genocide and racism. These alternative families create a sense of support and solace from the harsh realities of life" (p. 169). Thus the idea of family as a 'safe haven' has particular meaning among some communities. Such historical and current restrictions must be considered if various family forms and experiences are to be understood rather than dismissed as deviations from the way in which the nuclear family operates in Canada, or indeed other Western countries.

Similar dynamics have shaped families in most Western countries. In the case of Aboriginal peoples in countries colonized by Europeans, such as Australia, New Zealand, and the Americas, policies of assimilation, subjugation, removal from traditional lands, and systems of reserves have had impacts similar to those in Canada. In the case of immigrant people, immigration policies have systematically discriminated against immigrants of color, particularly limiting the forms of family that are possible. Today's immigration policies, which are becoming progressively harsher in the post–September 11 era (see, for example, Kerwin, 2003), continue to discriminate in similar ways (Arat-Koc, 1999; Das Gupta, 1995).

Consideration of the impact of colonization on families must include consideration of religious practices and religious persecution. People have emigrated to escape religious persecution and paradoxically have imposed their religion on others through emigration. Religious beliefs and practices are deeply entwined with other aspects of the social, political, and economic context, with religious symbols often being the focal point

---

TRY IT OUT 4.2.   **Families in Context**

1. Get a big piece of paper and some crayons or coloured pens.
2. Consider your own community. Undoubtedly there will be a great diversity of people within that community, so take a few minutes to just think about the range of economic, historical, racial, social, and political experiences represented in your community.
3. Using different colours, first represent the different economic circumstances families in your community experience, then overlay the historical circumstances, political circumstances, and so on. You might use overlapping circles, pie-shapes, lines, or pictures.
4. Note the gaps in your knowledge. For example, if a particular religious group is part of your community, what do you know of their history?
5. Finally, see if you can locate actual families you know on your 'map'. Are there families located in particular areas of your map?
6. Compare your representation with a colleague or classmate's version.

---

for conflict. For example, in late 2003 and early 2004, a debate arose in France over the wearing of *hijab*, head scarves, in school by devout Muslim girls, with legislation being developed to ban such practices. The debate officially was framed as an issue of keeping religious symbols separate from secular schools, but many critics saw these moves as directed against Muslims in an atmosphere of intolerance and fear characterizing the post–September 11 era.

Understanding the Context of Families

Understanding the context of families' lives is essential to relational practice and a socioenvironmental approach to health promotion. Try It Out 4.2 suggest an activity to start. However, such understanding is not a matter of making assumptions about particular families based on a broad contextual understanding. For example, if you recall the example of Fatima in Chapter 2, assuming that Fatima's husband or brother-in-law was disadvantaged by immigration policies would have been inaccurate. Being very wealthy, they had immigrated as entrepreneurs, which gave them considerable advantages. Rather, understanding families in context involves looking and listening relationally to hear what is contextually significant to people/families' health and healing. This means holding your own experience in critical regard (an idea we explore in Chapter 5) and exploring the relationship between family narratives and the context.

● Bridging the Gap: Narratives to Context

Striving to understand families in context is not a simple matter. Families are not necessarily conscious of all the ways in which their lives are structured and influenced by the environments in which they live, so making such connections between family narratives and larger contexts requires a careful sort of listening.

We meet families in a 'discursive world'. That is, as we explained in Chapter 2, people and families are literally spoken into existence as they participate in the everyday language and discourse of their culture (Davies, 1990; Weedon, 1987). Nurses and the families we meet have access to similar discourses. But, as people participate in the discursive practices of their communities, to a great extent they do so unconsciously and eventually take them up, forgetting that the discourses are separate from who they are. Here we are not drawing on the idea of 'false consciousness', suggesting that people are 'cultural dopes'. Rather, we are acknowledging that as we all participate in our worlds in taken-for-granted ways, we have different levels of awareness of our own participation in various discourses. So, for example, in the health care world we are so accustomed to the discourse of the diabetic regime that when Artur told Rosa (the story we told in Chapter 1) that he was 'eating better', their mutual use of a discourse of diabetic nutritional compliance may not have been conscious. Artur shares with Rosa a common understanding of the expectations of health care providers regarding diabetic behaviour, and thus speaks to Rosa using that language and those ideas.

Listening for Narratives

These discursive practices mean that listening to families requires paying attention to the ways that families are telling their stories and how their stories are being shaped by dominant stereotypes and taken-for-granted norms. It means listening carefully to the language families use and the discourses they are taking up, perhaps unknowingly. For example, having lived within the service-oriented, biomedically dominated health care system, many families have taken up the discourse and practice of being 'patients'. As a result, they have learned how to turn to expert practitioners with their health problems. If one listens carefully it is often possible to hear how their health and healing stories are languaged in accordance with biomedical discourse. Although they may not do so consciously they script themselves as unknowing patients turning to the all-knowing professional. Similarly, many people attempt to shape themselves to fit into the discourses and narratives that depict family as a close-knit and loving group of people. Although this narrative may in fact depict a family's actual experience, the way the narrative is at times taken up may hinder health and healing. In my work with people/families who are experiencing the life-changing event of illness or death, I (Gweneth) have found that based on family narratives people sometimes believe that they 'should' feel certain things and act in certain ways because they are family. For example, in line with dominant narratives, people often act from the belief that as children they should feel love toward their parents or as wives they should be devoted to their husbands. When their experience does not reflect that narrative they become quite distressed, feel guilty, and so forth. It is important to listen for the narratives that are shaping particular people/families not for the purpose of challenging those narratives but rather to inquire into how they are shaping health and healing. For example, for some people and families, filial obligation is paramount. Thus, it is important to understand how particular people are shaping their choices and actions in concert with that particular contextual narrative. Such understanding offers the opportunity for people to affirm the choices they are making and/or consider options in light of their beliefs and customs and in light of their health and healing experience.

Understanding the Narrative

Hardin (2001) tells us that in trying to understand the connections between individual accounts and the cultural, historical, and social worlds from which those accounts emerge, it is useful to think of the environment as 'language'. Imagining that the environment is not just social, political, and economic draws attention to the 'available discourses'. Hardin uses the example of anorexia nervosa, explaining that psychological discourses (about individual and family pathology), feminist discourses (about women, society, and issues of control), and medical discourses (about brain chemistry and starvation) are all available in the language environment. People talking and thinking about anorexia can draw on these different discourses, each of which gives a different slant or interpretation. For those of you who have played Scrabble, it is comparable to having to form words out of the available letters and words that are in the dictionary—given that language environment your options for creating your own words are limited.

It is not that one discourse is 'bad' and another 'good'. Rather, it is important to pay attention to how any given discourse limits and expands what is understood. Introducing multiple and alternative discourses can then help us think differently, and ultimately be more responsive to families. Think back, for example, to the interaction between Fran and Erica regarding baby Lorraine in Chapter 2 (Purkis, 1997). Both Fran and Erica were limited by the discourse of growth and development. Even though Fran was focused on promoting health, what she saw and discussed was limited by her theoretical discourse. Similarly, following the lead of the nurse, Erica's choices about how to talk about her child were limited. As you think back to the example, can you identify other alternatives to the 'developmental discourse' that were available? What, for example, would a feminist discourse highlight? Think about the health issue you used as an example earlier in this chapter. What are the common discourses related to that issue?

Hardin (2001) describes how thinking about the environment-as-language draws attention to narratives as performance. That is, when stories are told, they are told for a particular audience, and in a particular context. A family's story is not an immutable truth. Rather a story is told in a particular way drawing on particular discourses for particular audiences and contexts. For example, Fran's position as a nurse invoked a developmental discourse to the extent that Erica required little prompting to participate. This means that as nurses listening to family we need to consider what discourses are being drawn on, how the story is being told, and how we, as nurses, are shaping that particular performance.

● Nurses in Context

> *Genocide has been done by people who thought they were 'doing good.' Just because actions are well-intended does not mean they are not harmful. (Blackstock, 2003)*

Nurses' own specific historical and social locations strongly shape and determine how they respond in the moments of everyday nursing practice. Therefore, an essential part of relational practice is being aware of your sociohistorical location or situatedness and how that location is shaping how you look at people/families, what you see, what you listen for, what you hear, and how you respond—including what you do and do not do. Although I (Gweneth) have for many years understood the importance of my sociohistorical location to my nursing work, I have found that as the years go on I continue to discover depths of contextual knowing I have within me that I have not previously accessed.

To Illustrate

A good example of this ongoing learning was the first time I took a postcolonial lens to myself and my practice and began to see how my thinking and ways of knowing families had been 'colonized'. Having grown up in a family where my grandparents immigrated from Scotland/England, and living in Saskatchewan, which was a land of indigenous peoples that had been colonized, my world was strongly shaped by colonial values, beliefs, and assumptions. These values and beliefs included taken-for-granted norms that were communicated to me both explicitly and implicitly, about what was 'right' and 'proper' conduct. I grew up with the privilege of being white, English speaking, and British descended in a country where British dominance was living out in the societal and institutional structures that shaped my everyday life. However, I did not see myself as privileged and in fact would probably not have been seen by others in my white world as privileged. As a single parent in the 1960s with a grade-8 education and four children to support, my mother struggled to even provide food and shelter for her family. As she worked hard in the face of those challenges, the 'story' that dominated my childhood was one that said that, although a person/family could know great struggle, through their own volition and work they could create a life where they could realize their aspirations. This liberal individualist story (remember Chapter 1) that portrays the autonomous individual as separate from and able to rise above contextual/situational adversity was the dominant value lens through which I was shaped and through which I learned to observe others.

Being in this white, English-speaking privileged position and assuming this liberal individualist ideology meant that the colonial values, structures, and ways of being that dominated my world were taken up by everyone around me, and by myself, as 'normal'. And as they were taken up as normal, they became invisible to me. That is, I was colonized. Perhaps one of the most detrimental effects of this normalizing/colonizing process was that I thought the values, beliefs, and norms were 'truth'. In phenomenological terms, I became constituted by them and did not see that I had embodied norms that I had not consciously chosen and in fact (thanks to postcolonial theory) would later realize I did not actually believe. For example, although I consciously would have said that to know someone you had to know them in their context, living in my colonial world I was subtly instructed to look at the surfaces of people. I heard people around me distinguishing between good and not good people by using criteria such as how people dressed, how well they kept their houses or yards, and how they followed the proper conduct and adhered to Eurocentric norms. Anyone or any group of people who was different from the norm was subtly and at times not so subtly deemed 'less than'. What is important to emphasize is that the people, including myself, who were making these distinctions were most often well-intentioned people who would not purposefully harm another person. However, having (through the process of colonization) taken up a Eurocentric view of people and the world, we were operating from the assumption that each person (regardless of their sociocultural context) had the same opportunities and choices.

When I first read postcolonial theory I could see how my view of people around me had been limited by my white, colonialist glasses. I had not seen or understood how the privilege I had as member of the dominant white society had shaped my personal story, how this privilege had served as a foundation from which I acted, and how in many ways it had enabled me to make the choices I had made and to pursue my life goals. As I thought about people who had not shared that privilege, even though they had grown up in the same city during the same era, I found myself thinking back to experiences I had had as a young nurse. The racist discourse I had heard throughout my nursing education echoed through me. I remembered my nursing school rotation on pediatrics where the nurses continually talked about 'those (referring to a particular racialized group) women who don't look after their kids properly and then when the kids get sick they dump them at the hospital' and how these nurses, who were serving as my mentors, had informed me in frustrated voices that 'you can never get a hold of the mothers to come and get their kids because they're off drinking somewhere'. As I listened to these voices of the past, the impact that colonialism had had on me and on those around me became increasingly clear. I began to realize how my colonialist upbringing had not only planted seeds of racism but also clouded my ability to step out of my privileged position and be able to see people/families from within their own contextual location. For example, in the case of the racialized families on pediatrics, I saw them through my privileged lens and did not see the backdrop of colonialism and the profound impact that backdrop had on their lives.

Interestingly, it was probably the confusion that I felt in hearing contradictory messages that led me to question the status quo colonialist knowledge that was being offered. That is, on one hand I was being told that as a nurse I should treat all people with respect and dignity, and on the other I was seeing particular people being treated very disrespectfully. This disjuncture and confusion led me to feel very uncertain about how to 'be a good nurse'. And it was that uncertainty that served as the inspiration to want to learn and develop more knowledge. Since my first reading of postcolonial theory I have been compelled to continually scrutinize my current practice and ask myself how my own contextual location is constraining my ability to know and be with families in ways that are respectful and relationally appropriate to them.

You might now want to try the activities suggested in Try It Out 4.3.

TRY IT OUT 4.3.   **Understanding Your Living Contextual Location**

1. Take a minute and think about the historical context of your life. Draw your family's history on a time line as far back as you can go, and then insert what you consider to be major historical, social, and economic features—what are the key features of the historical context of your life story? (For example, what events shaped your life, the lives of your parents or grandparents?)
2. If possible, compare your time line to someone else's. What features did you particularly note on your time line and how are they similar and/or different from the other person's? Examine your time line in light of colonialism—in terms of the colonized/colonizer relationship, how was your family affected?
3. Think back to Red's experience and consider how the social, economic, and political elements shaping your life compare with those underlying Red's.
4. How do your 'life chances' (opportunities, material wealth, positive influences) compare with Red's?
5. How do you think your ideas about family might compare with Red's and how much of the similarity or difference could be explained by the context of your different lives? How might these similarities or differences play out if you were caring for Red or say, for example, her dying mother?

Knowing Our Own Location So We Can See Beyond It

We might think that knowing and responding to people in ways that are relevant and respectful might be easier and more likely when responding to those who have had similar experiences to ourselves. However, that is not always the case. As hermeneutic phenomenology tells us, although we may have similar experiences we are unique beings who make our own particular meaning of experience. Because we make our own meaning of experiences it may well be that when we have shared similar experiences with people we might actually have more difficulty seeing beyond our own 'knowing' of what a particular experience is like. For example, when I (Colleen) was first doing research on how nurses respond to violence against women, I thought that people who had experienced violence would be more understanding and empathic than those who had not had such an experience. Therefore, I was surprised by a nurse who described how she had left home where her father had been very abusive, saying 'if I could get out, anyone could'. She said this to express disapproval of women who did not leave abusive situations, but she did not seem to consider how her situation might differ in terms of such things as economics, responsibilities, or relationships. Next, I was surprised by a nurse whose mother had been battered by her father. She told me that she did not understand women who 'chose' to stay with abusive partners, and that her job was to 'teach women how not to push men's buttons'. What I eventually realized was that these nurses were interpreting violence and the women they met through their own personal history as well as the dominant societal discourses that tell us people are autonomous agents who have 'free choice'. These discourses, grounded in liberal ideals (remember Chapter 1), led these nurses to see their own relative advantages (say, being middle class, for example, or having a sense of self agency) as a matter of personal strength and achievement rather than as a matter of privilege and/or chance at birth and/or life experience.

These examples once again exemplify the power of the concerns and selective interests we bring as people/nurses. Although we may be expected to be neutral as nurses, not to have any biases or prejudices, hermeneutic phenomenology informs us that no person is neutral—that as living human beings we are always 'concerned' in particular ways; we are always 'selectively interested'. What is important is to be as aware of our concerns as possible so that we can strive to ensure that our concerns and prejudices do not hinder our ability to know and respond to the families with whom we work. We will be exploring other ways to help us see beyond our own values, concerns and prejudices in Chapter 5.

● Families and Nurses in the Health Care Context

The lenses and perspectives we have described in Chapter 2 draw attention to the fact that health care organizations are part of the structural conditions that shape families' experiences of health and health care. Further, these lenses and perspectives draw attention to the way power operates in the health care context and how dominant values shape the experiences of families. Health care contexts and the structure of nursing practice in Western countries are largely shaped by economics and gender and in accordance with heterosexual and Eurocentric values.

Economics of Health Care: Consequences for Families and Nurses

Families have become economically important to health care in the new millennia. In most Western countries 'the state is withdrawing from its previously defined responsibility for the health and well-being of the nation' (Björnsdóttir, 2001, p. 3). Families are expected to fill in the space created by this withdrawing. The widespread withdrawal of health care services has been accomplished largely in the name of cost cutting and economic 'efficiency', although the withdrawal has been accompanied by ideals about home as the place to be, especially when ill or infirm (Björnsdóttir, 2001). Families are expected to take up the caregiving activities previously provided by the state. These dynamics have had a number of impacts. Despite expectations, there may be no suitable family member to provide care to any given person, leaving that person in limbo and creating strain on those who cannot provide the care. Families are not necessarily equipped to provide care. The shift has occurred at the same time as other trends in families have occurred. Women, who do most of the caregiving, increasingly work outside the home and various configurations of families may mean that any given person may not have a family member who is a suitable candidate as caregiver. Those who do take up caregiving have been shown to suffer depression, ill health, financial problems, and other social burdens (e.g., see Cousins, Davies, Turnbull, & Playfer, 2002; Langa

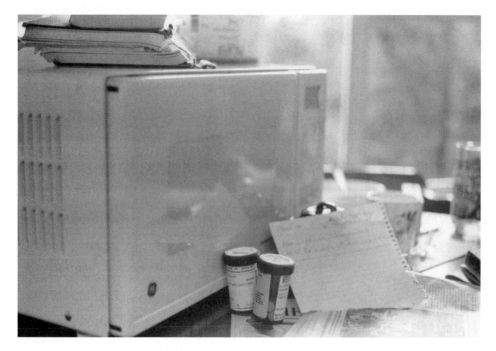

Homecare. (Photograph by Gayle Allison.)

et al., 2001; Pinquart & Sörensen, 2003; Rossi Ferrario, Zotti, Ippoliti, & Zotti, 2003; Williams, Forbes, Mitchell, & Corbett, 2003). The shift in state expectations and responsibilities has rippled down to shift the relationship between health care providers and family members. Nurses are increasingly working under the mandate of business practice with the goal of discharge taking primacy over the goals of care (Rankin, 2004; Varcoe, 2001; Varcoe, Rodney, & McCormick, 2003). Increasingly health care providers, particularly nurses, are the managers of care provided by family members.

An Example: Bundle Them Out the Door

In her dissertation, Janet Rankin (2004) shows how nurses subvert their clinical concerns to concerns with short-term economic efficiency. She illustrates with the story of a nurse discharging an elderly male patient. The patient had undergone a radical retropubic prostatectomy for cancer. The man was mildly confused and combative. On day 7 of his hospitalization—the planned discharge date—the priority was teaching the man's wife about his prescriptions and his bowel medications, explaining about his incontinence, and telling her where she could buy Attends (adult diapers). The woman, however, became upset, telling the nurse that she could hardly manage her husband *before* the surgery. The nurse, operating under managerial interests and pressure to empty the bed, 'bundles them out the door'.

▶ *So you talk to the Team Leader to see if you can get more home follow-up on this guy, but he's got to go, its day 7. . . . I mean there's just no way. . . .*

I can't hang on to him because his wife got teary. So I mean . . . you just kinda kindly bundle them out the door and keep your fingers crossed that home care will catch up with them and then you start looking after the next one. And let's face it, it might feel like hell, but that's not our job, I mean, it might not look like it's very caring, but it's just not efficient use of resources to hang onto this patient for another night just because his wife is having trouble coping. There are all those other patients waiting for surgeries to think about. (p. x)

If you think back to Bulbir's experience with Lena and her mother (Chapter 2) you can imagine some possible consequences of the practices described in this example. Business and economic models increasingly dominate health care. The emphasis is on 'efficient' use of resources, meaning that the greatest number of patients should be provided a particular service. For example, some health care settings discharge women on the same day following a radical mastectomy, paring down the care provided to physical preparation, the surgery, and immediate postoperative physical care. Discharge teaching, emotional support, and monitoring for complications and adverse affects are eliminated or replaced with brochures of instructions for the patient and family. Cost savings are at least partly to be achieved by shifting the caregiving to family members. And nurses are instrumental in achieving this shift.

Economics of Health Care: Consequences for Nurses

In off-loading caring work to family members, first, the acuity of the patients who remain in health care institutions increases. This in turn contributes to the compression of nurses' caring work or emotional labour into ever-smaller spaces—the same number of nurses looking after more acute patients moving more quickly through care systems leaves less space for work that is not readily counted in workload measurements. Second, as the example of the elderly male patient and his wife illustrates, the nurse's role shifts from a provider of care to a manager of family caregiving. Third, as nurses manage greater numbers of more acute patients, the number of nurses is reduced under continuing efforts to reduce labour costs and increase profitability and certain efficiencies. As the workloads continue to mount, nurses are less able to provide 'good' care and become more distressed. For example, when we and a team of colleagues (Varcoe et al., 2003) studied nurses' ethical practice in a wide range of clinical settings, we found that nurses experienced serious moral distress. However, this distress was not simply a consequence of their victimization by circumstances beyond their control but was created partially by their own participation in coercive practices to bring patients and families into line with organizational and managerial business goals.

It does not seem that these dynamics are working very well for nurses, so why do nurses participate in the ways that they do? Part of the answer to this question is that, as previously discussed, ideas of individualism and the 'new efficiency' are congruent with traditional nursing knowledge. The ideals of pursuing 'concrete' and predetermined goals dominate traditional nursing knowledge. These ideas are congruent with the 'outcomes', 'deliverables', 'benchmarks', and 'evidence base' that characterize the 'efficiency' approach to health care. Nurses in the studies that we have conducted (e.g., Varcoe, Rodney, & McCormick, 2003) took the idea of scarce resources for granted and wove it through their practices, rationing care and resources without explicit managerial direction, even when clinical concerns suggested otherwise.

A Business Approach: Consequences for Families and Nurses

Another part of the answer is that business ideas and language are being integrated with nursing language to make it seem as though business interests and nurses' interests are the same. Rankin (2004) shows how nurses do the work of implementing managerial efficiencies, even though it does not seem to be in the interests of nurses or their patients, partly because this mingling of types of language cover up differences in interests. She shows how, for example, the term "patient centered" (her analysis would apply just as well to "family centered") seems to be a commonsense idea that nurses believe in. However, used in a 'business' way, it means getting the patient (or family) to take as much responsibility for care (financially and otherwise) as is possible. Rankin points out that a concrete example of this 'taking up of business language' is offered in Wright and Leahey's (1999) description of beliefs that constrain nurses from engaging with families. These authors offer examples of beliefs they have heard nurses express such as 'If I talk to family members, I won't have time to complete my other nursing responsibilities' or 'If I talk to family members I may open up a can of worms and I will have no time to deal with it' (p. 260). This discourse of time and efficiency echoes business language and interests, and as Wright and Leahey describe, is highly constraining to responsive nursing practice. What is interesting is that rather than challenging the business approach to health care and the subsequent busy-ness nurses live in their practice, the response has been to find ways to help nurses 'do better' within that business and busy-ness. For example, Rankin argues that 'the 15-minute (or less) family interview' (Wright & Leahey, 1999) that is meant to inspire nurses to be more responsive to families ends up instructing them on how to better conform to managerial efficiencies. Rankin argues that theorizing nurses' time constraints with families as arising from nurses' 'constraining beliefs' and nurses' lack of knowledge about 'efficient ways to conduct brief family interviews' (Wright & Leahey, p. 260) glosses over the ways managerial reforms organize nursing work with families. Nurses take up the call to 'minimize suffering' without realizing that nursing language and interests are being used to further business interests. Challenging Wright and Leahy's contention that in the face of 'budgetary constraints and staff cutbacks' nurses need to find 'more efficient ways . . . to conduct brief family interviews' (Wright & Leahey, 1999, p. 259), Rankin argues that instead of joining in with this business model of efficiency we need to address the pressures (increased acuity, increased workload, deskilling of the workforce, and so on) that require 'brief interviews'. This is not to say that the beliefs Wright and Leahey identify and challenge are not problematic but rather that we need to more critically consider what leads nurses to form those beliefs. By challenging the beliefs *and* challenging the underlying business value structure, there is more potential to achieve the goal that Wright and Leahey are calling for—that of supporting nurses to be more responsive to families.

Gendered Expectations

Nurses and other health care providers may unconsciously (and to their own detriment) 'buy in', not only to the ideas of individual responsibility and scarcity, but also to the gendered expectations that accompany and support the move to family caregiving. Wuest (1994) argues that 'familism' (the taken-for-granted ideology of the nuclear family in which women provide domestic labor and altruistic caregiving) is a gendered pattern that is also evident in the gendered hierarchy of the health care system. The economics of health care fit comfortably with and take advantage of traditional gendered roles. This similarity between the health care system and dominant ideas about family may assist in rendering the ideas, practices, and shifts in health care invisible and unproblematic.

Heterosexism

Health care contexts and practices are both gendered and largely shaped by assumptions of heterosexuality. Although there has been some attention to the relationships between gender, sexism, health, and health care, policy makers and health care professionals have paid limited attention to sexual identity and heterosexism in health and health care (Wilton, 1998, 2000). 'Heterosexism is the system of institutions that supports heterosexuality as the norm and treats any other sexual identity as either nonexistent or abnormal' (Livingston, 1996, p. 253). Heterosexism is also linked to homophobia—the irrational fear of, aversion to, or discrimination against homosexuals (O'Hanlan et al., 2001). However, Braun (2000) explains that the term heterosexism refers both to the assumption of heterosexuality as 'normal' and to discrimination based on sexual orientation.

'Heterosexism is intimately linked with sexism—they are two systems of oppression that rely on one another' (Livingston, 1996, p. 253). Livingston goes on to explain that sexism is the belief system that supports patriarchy, that is, the rule of men over women and the assumed superiority of men over women. She explains that sexism and patriarchy depend on compulsory heterosexuality and enforces rigid role expectations for both males and females, regardless of their sexual orientation. For example, remember the experiences of male nurses that we described briefly in Chapter 2? If you are a man, what was your experience with your family when you decided on a career in nursing? What has been the experience of your male nursing colleagues with their families or with other people?

In the health care setting, assumptions of heterosexuality can lead to misrepresentation by patients and misunderstanding by health care providers with negative consequences for health care, including alienation from the health care system, reduced response to health problems, and avoidance of health care situations (O'Hanlan et al., 2001; Simkin, 1998).

An Example: I Never Had Intercourse

A young woman visits a family physician for the first time. During the course of a physical examination, the physician asks, 'When was the last time you had sexual intercourse?'

'I've never had sexual intercourse,' she replies.

'Never?'

'No'.

'Do you have a boyfriend?'

'No'.

'Well, don't worry. You will soon. Let's talk about birth control'.

The physician finishes the discussion about contraception and writes in the chart 'Not yet sexually active. Not in relationship. Contraception counselling given'.

The patient never returns, but the next year goes to see another family physician for her physical. During the course of the examination, the physician asks, 'Are you sexually active with men, women, or both?'

'Yes', she replies, 'with a woman. I'm a lesbian'.

'Are you in a relationship?'

'Yes—for 8 years now. In fact, I wonder if my partner could come to see you, too? We're thinking about having children.'

'Of course, I'd be delighted to meet her'.

And so begins a long, healthy physician–patient relationship.

(Simkin, 1998, p. 370)

As the example above illustrates, assuming heterosexuality can render invisible those people who do not conform to this dominant norm. Worse, discrimination based on sexual orientation negatively affects health and health care. Research has documented that lesbians and gay men have higher lifetime rates of depression, attempted suicide, and substance use as a consequence of living with the societal stress of heterosexism (e.g., Cochran & Mays, 2000; Cochran, Sullivan & Mays 2003; O'Hanlan et al., 2001). Furthermore, health care providers may deny care or provide reduced or inferior care based on sexual orientation (O'Hanlan et al., 2001; Simkin, 1998).

The assumption of heterosexuality as normal is so pervasive that it is almost invisible. Wilton (1998, 2000) explains that from the mid-19th century on, European biomedicine claimed jurisdiction over understanding sexuality. In this process of 'medicalizing' sexuality, those behaviours, desires, and experiences that deviated from what medical science (dominated by middle-class European men) thought was normal were seen as pathological. The 'pathologization' of same-sex relationships continues to influence ideas about family and health care providers' attitudes and practices and the structures and delivery of health care.

The taken-for-granted assumption about family is that the normal family is the heterosexual family. For example, the term 'family values' is used in the United States as though it does not refer to *particular* family values, but there is no doubt that this refers to value for heterosexual married couples with children and the assumption that this configuration is normal. A quick glance at most forms of media will confirm this message of the heterosexual family as normal. Such a powerful taken-for-granted assumption means that it is very difficult for us to experience other forms of family without seeing them as other or less than. For example, those of you who have been 'single' may have experienced pressure to be in a couple relationship. Friends and family may be anxious to help you 'meet someone', or may ask questions such as 'when are you getting married?', implying that your single status is just a less-than-satisfactory state of waiting to be in the preferable situation of not-single. For those of you who do not have children (think of the difference between labelling this as 'childless' or 'childfree'), you may have experienced pressure to have children, and particularly to have them within a heterosexual relationship, whether you want children or not.

The assumption of heterosexuality as normal and the pathologization of other experiences and forms can lead health care providers to overlook and misunderstand the experiences of the families with whom they interact, as the earlier example from Simkin illustrates. Such misunderstanding can have unintended negative consequences for families.

An Example: A Psychiatric Consult

Recently, a friend told me (Colleen) about taking her 11-year-old daughter to the hospital for severe stomach pains. My friend and her partner had adopted their daughter from overseas when she was an infant. Because their daughter had been severely malnourished prior to the adoption, she had experienced various gastrointestinal problems throughout childhood. Once in the emergency, the staff focused on the fact that the child had 'two moms'. The 'treatment' this family received consisted of a psychiatric consult for the child, presumably to deal with the 'problem' of living with two women who are partners. The stomach pains persisted until their daughter began menstruating.

Heterosexism can be conveyed in health care by subtle and not-so-subtle means. Inquiring about someone's 'husband' or 'wife' can convey an assumption of heterosexuality. Excluding a same-sex partner from the privileges of 'family' (e.g., visiting privileges, giving information) can similarly convey a heterosexist assumption and limit family support. Or, as the example about the child with two mothers illustrates, heterosexism can be conveyed by pathologizing families who do not fit with heterosexual expectations. What if my friend's daughter had been experiencing a life-threatening problem such as a ruptured appendix or a bowel obstruction?

Nurses often have little or no education regarding sexuality and sexual identity (Gray et al., 1996). Further, the theories nurses use (as we discussed in Chapter 2) are often based on heterosexist assumptions. For example, Gray and colleagues (1996) point out that nurses are often taught growth and development using Erickson's theory, which specifies (among other heterosexist ideas) that the developmental task of adolescence is to resolve bisexual conflicts. As an example of how heterosexist role expectations can affect nursing practice, Gray and colleagues describe how a male nurse explained that he was reluctant to show caring behaviour toward patients for fear that he would be seen as feminine or assumed to be gay. The research by Evans (discussed in Chapter 2) shows that his experience is commonplace among male nurses. As Gray and her colleagues say, heterosexism diminishes and hurts us all. It is a form of oppression that pervades health care and intersects (remember the concept 'intersectionality'?) with other forms of oppression.

Eurocentrism

A final set of values that dominate health care and thus influence nursing practice is Eurocentrism—that is, seeing values associated with European-descended (primarily Caucasian) people as central and preeminent. In most Western countries, Eurocentric values dominate health care contexts and practices, regardless of the ethnic diversity of the population. For example, hospital visiting policies may be developed based on what might work for a 'nuclear' family (mother, father, children) that is sometimes assumed to be the family form typical of European-descended (primarily Caucasian) people. Because Eurocentrism inherently values some people over others on the basis of ethnicity and race, racism accompanies Eurocentrism. Although racial discrimination is widespread, nursing has paid little attention to racism, discrimination, and social inequities in health care (Browne, Johnson, Bottorff, Grewal, & Hilton, 2002; Condliffe, 2001; Shaha, 1998). Like heterosexism, racism extends beyond individual expressions of discrimination to the structure and delivery of health care. Whether unintentional or intentional, racism can result in alienation from the health care system, the withholding of care, and the provision of inferior care. We return to these ideas later in the book and consider racism, sexism, heterosexism, and other forms of discrimination in relation to health promotion and relational family nursing practice.

● A Suggestion

In order for family nursing practice to be health promoting and responsive, nurses need to understand the living experience of family *in context*. The lives, health, and experiences of the families with whom we work can only be understood in context. Similarly, our practice as nurses can only be understood within the contexts of practice, such as health care organizations and the wider culture that shapes the possibilities for practice. We have suggested in this chapter that relational family nursing practice requires exploration of how our ideas have been shaped, not just by our experiences, but also by our life circumstances and the forces shaping those circumstances. In the next chapter, in theorizing family nursing practice further, we turn your attention in more detail to this exploration, particularly emphasizing the skill of reflexivity. In order to pull together the ideas in this current chapter, and set the stage for this deeper development of the reflexivity, consider your own cultural context by following the suggestions outlined for This Week In Practice.

THIS WEEK IN PRACTICE

Your Culture

The exercise suggested for This Week In Practice is an observational exercise that can be completed individually or in pairs. The purpose is to increase your sensitivity to context and culture, so that you can better analyze how context affects family health and health care. Here is how to proceed.

Choose

Choose a public location (a mall, a coffee bar, a street corner, a bus, a train or subway station, a hospital lobby, and so on) where you might observe your culture in action. Choose a location in a public setting where you can observe a variety of people. You might want to think of some of the concepts discussed in this chapter (context, culture, economics, heterosexism) or some of the ideas from previous chapters (racialization) when making a choice. You might wish to pick a location that is already familiar to you (your favourite coffee place?) or one that is unfamiliar (e.g., a street corner 'notorious' for illegal activity).

Observe

Spend half an hour in the location of your choice. Observe the world around in you careful detail, and record your observations. What are you seeing, hearing, smelling, feeling? (Try dividing your paper in half lengthwise, writing your observations on one half of the paper, and saving the other half for your paper for your analysis.)

Analyze

Analyze your observations. To what did you pay attention, and why? How do you identify people and families? Did you use labels, categories, terms that you were surprised that you used? What does this tell you about your 'culture', and what does this tell you about how you are seeing your culture? What does this tell you about how you see family? What do your observations tell you about your attitudes and values, particularly about family, gender, sexuality, ethnicity, class?

Summarize

Create a brief written summary of your analysis. In one paragraph identify one important insight you have had from this experience.

Compare

Share your notes, analysis, and summary paragraphs with someone else. What can you learn?

CHAPTER HIGHLIGHTS

1. Given your contextual background, in what ways do you think you have been shaped by colonialism?
2. How would you begin to alter your practice to attend to families in context?
3. What is one way that the health care context in which you are currently practicing or studying limits people/families experiences of health and healing and your own ability to practice relationally?

REFERENCES

Akinbami, L. J., LaFleur, B. J., & Schoendorf, K. C. (2002). Racial and income disparities in childhood asthma in the United States. *Ambulatory Pediatrics, 2*(5), 382–387.

Anderson, J., Perry, J., Blue, C., Browne, A. J., Henderson, A., Khan, K. B., Reimer-Kirkham, S., Lynam, J., Semeniuk, P., & Smye, V. (2003). "Rewriting" cultural safety within the postcolonial and postnational feminist project: Toward new epistemologies of healing. *Advances in Nursing Science, 26*(3), 196–214.

Arat-Koc, S. (1999). Gender and race in "non-discriminatory" immigration policies in Canada. In E. Dua & A. Robertson (Eds.), *Scratching the surface: Canadian anti-racist thought* (pp. 207–233). Toronto, ON: Women's Press.

Ballou, K. A. (2000). A historical-philosophical analysis of the professional nurse obligation to participate in sociopolitical activities. *Policy Politics and Nursing Practice, 1*(3), 172–184.

Björnsdóttir, K. (2001). From the state to the family: Reconfiguring the responsibility for long-term nursing care at home. *Nursing Inquiry, 9*(1), 3–11.

Blackstock, C. (2003). Keynote presentation. International Child and Youth Care Conference, Victoria, Canada, August 2003.

Braun, V. (2000). Heterosexism in focus group research: Collusion and challenge. *Feminism & Psychology, 10*(1), 133–140.

Browne, A. J. (2000). The potential contributions of critical social theory to nursing science. *Canadian Journal of Nursing Research, 32*(2), 35–55.

Browne, A. J. (2001). The influence of liberal political ideology on nursing practice. *Nursing Inquiry, 8*(2), 118–129.

Browne, A. J., Johnson, J. L., Bottorff, J., L., Grewal, S., & Hilton, B. A. (2002). Recognizing discrimination in nursing practice. *Canadian Nurse, 98*(5), 24–27.

Browning, S. L., Miller, R. R., & Spruance, L. M. (2001). Criminal incarceration dividing the ties that bind: Black men and their families. *Journal of African American Men, 6*(1), 87–102.

Burt, S. (1995). The several worlds of policy analysis: Traditional approaches and feminist critiques. In S. Burt & L. Code (Eds.), *Changing methods: Feminist transforming practice.* Peterborough: Broadview.

Canadian Nurses Association. (2002). Code of ethics. Ottawa: Canadian Nurses Association.

Cochran, S. D., & Mays, V. M. (2000). Lifetime prevalence of suicide symptoms and affective disorders among men reporting same-sex sexual partners: Results from NHANES III. *American Journal of Public Health, 90*(4), 573.

Cochran, S. D., Sullivan, J. G., & Mays, V. M. (2003). Prevalence of mental disorders, psychological distress, and mental health services use among lesbian, gay, and bisexual adults in the United States. *Journal of Consulting & Clinical Psychology, 71*(1), 53–61.

Condliffe, B. (2001). Racism in nursing: A critical realist approach. *Nursing Times, 97*(32), 40–41.

Cousins, R., Davies, A. D. M., Turnbull, C. J., & Playfer, J. R. (2002). Assessing caregiving distress: A conceptual analysis and a brief scale. *British Journal of Clinical Psychology, 41*(4), 387–404.

Das Gupta, T. (1995). Families of native peoples, immigrants, and people of colour. In N. Mandell & A. Duffy (Eds.), *Canadian families: Diversity, conflict and change* (pp. 141–174). Toronto: Harcourt Brace.

Davies, B. (1990). Positioning: The discursive production of selves. *Journal for the Theory of Social Behavior, 20*(1), 43–63.

Drevdahl, D. (1995). Coming to voice: The power of emancipatory community interventions. *Advances in Nursing Science, 18*(2), 13–24.

Drevdahl, D., Kneipp, S. M., Canales, M. K., & Dorcy, K. S. (2001). Reinvesting in social justice: A capital idea for public health nursing. *Advances in Nursing Science, 24*(2), 19–31.

Dua, E. (1999). Beyond diversity: Exploring the ways in which the discourse of race has shaped the institution of the nuclear family. In E. Dua & A. Robertson (Eds.), *Scratching the surface: Canadian anti-racist thought.* Toronto, ON: Women's Press.

Furniss, E. M. (1995). *Victims of benevolence: The dark legacy of the Williams Lake residential school.* Vancouver: Arsenal Pulp Press.

Furniss, E. M. (1999). *The burden of history: Colonialism and the frontier myth in a rural Canadian community.* Vancouver: UBC Press.

Gray, P., Kramer, M., Minick, P., McGehee, L., Thomas, D., & Greiner, D. (1996). Heterosexism in nursing education. *Journal of Nursing Education, 35,* 204–210.

Hardin, P. K. (2001). Theory and language: Locating agency between free will and discursive marionettes. *Nursing Inquiry, 8*(1), 11–18.

Kendall, J. (1992). Fighting back: Promoting emancipatory nursing actions. *Advances in Nursing Science, 15*(2), 1–15.

Kerwin, D. (2003, June 23–30). Undermining antiterrorism: When national security and immigration policy collide. *America,* 11–14.

Kleffel, D. (1996). Environmental paradigms: Moving toward an ecocentric perspective. *Advances in Nursing Science, 18*(4), 1–10.

Klinnert, M. D., Price, M. R., Liu, A. H., & Robinson, J. L. (2002). Unraveling the ecology of risks for early childhood asthma among ethnically diverse families in the southwest. *American Journal of Public Health, 92*(5), 792–798.

Kneipp, S. M. (2000). The consequences of welfare reform for women's health: Issues of concern for community health nursing. *Journal of Community Health Nursing, 17*(2), 65–73.

Langa, K. M., Chernew, M. E., Kabeto, M. U., Regula Herzog, A., Beth Ofstedal, M., Willis, R. J., et al. (2001). National estimates of the quantity and cost of informal caregiving for the elderly with dementia. *Journal of General Internal Medicine, 16*(11), 770–779.

Livingston, J. A. (1996). Individual action and political strategies: Creating a future free of heterosexism. In E. D. Rothblum & L. A. Bond (Eds.), *Preventing heterosexism and homophobia* (pp. 253–265). Thousand Oaks, CA: Sage.

Marck, P. (2000). Nursing in a technological world: Searching for healing communities. *Advances in Nursing Science, 23*(2), 62–81.

Mill, J. E., Allen, M. N., & Morrow, R. A. (2001). Critical theory: Critical methodology to disciplinary foundations in nursing. *Canadian Journal of Nursing Research, 33*(2), 109–127.

Miller, R. R., Browning, S. L., & Spruance, L. M. (2001). An introduction and brief review of the impacts of incarceration on the African American family. *Journal of African American Men, 6*(1), 3–12.

Ng Man Kwong, G., Das, C., Proctor, A. R., Whyte, M. K., & Primhak, R. A. (2002). Diagnostic and treatment behaviour in children with chronic respiratory symptoms: Relationship with socioeconomic factors. *Thorax, 57*(8), 701–704.

O'Hanlan, K. A., Lock, J., Robertson, P., Cabaj, R. P., Schatz, B., & Nemrow, P. (2001). *Homophobia as a health hazard: Report of the Gay and Lesbian Medical Association.* Portola Valley, CA: Gay and Lesbian Medical Association.

Papps, E., & Ramsden, I. (1996). Cultural safety in nursing: The New Zealand experience. *International Journal for Quality in Health Care, 8*(5), 491–497.

Parr, J. (1982). Introduction. In J. Parr (Ed.), *Childhood and family in Canadian history* (pp. 7–16). Toronto, ON: McLelleand & Stewart.

Peterson, J. W., Sterling, Y. M., & Stout, J. W. (2002). Explanatory models of asthma from African-American caregivers of children with asthma. *Journal of Asthma, 39*(7), 577–590.

Pinquart, M., & Sörensen, S. (2003). Associations of stressors and uplifts of caregiving with caregiver burden and depressive mood: A meta-analysis. *Journals of Gerontology Series B: Psychological Sciences & Social Sciences, 58B*(2), 112–129.

Potthast-Jutkeit, B. (1997). The history of the family and colonialism. *History of the Family, 2*(2), 115–121.

Poyser, M. A., Nelson, H., Ehrlich, R. I., Bateman, E. D., Parnell, S., Puterman, A., & Weinberg, E. (2002). Socioeconomic deprivation and asthma prevalence and severity in young adolescents. *European Respiratory Journal, 19*(5), 892–898.

Purkis, M. E. (1997). The "social determinants" of practice? A critical analysis of the discourse of health promotion. *Canadian Journal of Nursing Research, 29*(1), 47–62.

Ramsey, J., Richardson, J., Carter, Y. H., Davidson, L. L., & Feder, G. (2002). Should health professionals screen women for domestic violence? Systematic review. *British Medical Journal, 325*(7359), 314–318.

Rankin, J. (2004). *Fundamentals of health management technology.* Unpublished doctoral dissertation, University of Victoria, Victoria.

Razak, S. (1998). *Looking white people in the eye: Gender, race and culture in courtrooms and classrooms.* Toronto: University of Toronto Press.

Ribeiro, M. C. S., & Bertolozzi, M. R. (1999). Nursing and the environmental matter: A proposal for a theoretical model for the professional practice. *Revista Brasileira De Enfermagem, 52*(3), 365–374.

Rossi Ferrario, S., Zotti, A. M., Ippoliti, M., & Zotti, P. (2003). Caregiving-related needs analysis: A proposed model reflecting current research and socio-political developments. *Health & Social Care in the Community, 11*(2), 103–111.

Shaha, M. (1998). Racism and its implications in ethical-moral reasoning in nursing practice: A tentative approach to a largely unexplored topic. *Nursing Ethics, 5*(2), 139–146.

Sharpe, T. T. (2001). Sex for crack cocaine exchange, poor black women, and pregnancy. *Qualitative Health Research, 11*(5), 612–630.

Simkin, R. (1998). Not all your patients are straight. *Canadian Medical Association Journal, 159*(4), 370–375.

Sin, D. D., Svenson, L. W., Cowie, R. L., & Man, S. F. (2003). Can universal access to health care eliminate health inequities between children of poor and nonpoor families?: A case study of childhood asthma in Alberta. *Chest, 124*(1), 51–56.

Smye, V., & Browne, A. J. (2002). Cultural safety and the analysis of health policy affecting Aboriginal people. *Nurse Researcher, 9*(3), 42–56.

Stevens, P. E. (1989). A critical social reconceptualization of the environment in nursing: Implications for methodology. *Advances in Nursing Science, 11*(4), 56–68.

Stevens, P. E. (1992). Who gets care? Access to health care as an arena for nursing action. *Scholarly Inquiry in Nursing Practice, 6*(3), 185–200.

Stevens, P. E., & Hall, J. M. (1992). Applying critical theories to nursing in communities. *Public Health Nursing, 9*(1), 2–9.

Varcoe, C. (2001). Abuse obscured: An ethnographic account of emergency nursing in relation to violence against women. *Canadian Journal of Nursing Research, 32*(4), 95–115.

Varcoe, C. (2004). Violence, women and ethics. In J. Storch, P. Rodney, & R. Starzomski (Eds.), *Toward a moral horizon: Nursing ethics for leadership and practice* (pp. 414–432). Toronto, ON: Pearson.

Varcoe, C., Doane, G., Pauly, B., Rodney, P., Storch, J. L., Mahoney, K., McPherson, G., Brown, H., & Starzomski, R. (2004). Ethical practice in nursing—Working the in-betweens. *Journal of Advanced Nursing, 45*(3), 316–325.

Varcoe, C., Rodney, P., & McCormick, J. (2003). Health care relationships in context: An analysis of three ethnographies. *Qualitative Health Research, 13*(6), 957–973.

Weedon, C. (1987). *Feminist practice and post structural theory.* New York: Basil Blackwell.

Wilber, C. K. (Ed.). (1998). *Economics, ethics and public policy.* Lanham, MD.: Rowman & Littlefield.

Williams, A., Forbes, D., Mitchell, J., & Corbett, B. (2003). The influence of income on the experience of informal caregiving: Policy implications. *Health Care for Women International, 24*(4), 280–292.

Wilson, J. Q. (2002). Slavery and the black family. *The Public Interest, 147,* 3–23.

Wilton, T. (1998). Gender, sexuality and health care: Improving services. In L. Doyal (Ed.), *Women and health services: An agenda for change* (pp. 147–162). Buckingham: Open University Press.

Wilton, T. (2000). *Sexualities in health and social care.* Buckingham; Open University Press.

Wright, L. M., & Leahey, M. (1999). Maximizing time, minimizing suffering: The 15 minute (or less) family interview. *Journal of Family Nursing, 5*(3), 259–273.

Wuest, J. (1994). Institutionalizing women's oppression: The inherent risk in health policy fostering community participation. In A. J. Dan (Ed.), *Reframing women's health: Multi-disciplinary research and practice* (pp. 118–128). Thousand Oaks, CA: Sage.

5 The Skill of Reflexivity

OVERVIEW

In this chapter we ask you to look inward, to cultivate the skills of reflexivity and self-knowing. You will be particularly aware, having read the preceding chapters, how important your own social location and experience of family are to your knowing of family. We invite you to consider these influences, to hone your self-knowing, particularly drawing on 'bodily' knowing.

n Chapter 3, we invited you to begin explicating the theories that are guiding your practice by offering you some example theories and suggesting a careful look at your own values, beliefs and assumptions—at your own theory of family nursing practice. In Chapter 4, we asked you to consider how your contextual location shapes the way you approach families and take up your nursing role. You might have found this process of trying to articulate your theory and contextual location challenging. As you observed yourself in your practice you might have also found that what you thought and said you believed is not always reflected in the way you practice. For example, many nurses with whom we have worked have said that they share the assumptions of the human science paradigm of nursing, including the belief that nursing practice is people focused rather than disease-treatment focused. Yet as they observe themselves in practice, they see how their actions are focused on fixing or treating disease conditions and how at times they may practice in a way that gives precedence to the disease process over the person living with the disease condition. Their espoused values and theories are not congruent with their theories in action. This incongruence between our espoused theories and our theories in action is most often because of having taken up values, beliefs, and habitual ways of being (remember Chapter 1's discussion about habits of conduct) of which we may not be aware. For example, as discussed earlier, the contexts in which we grow up strongly shape how we view the world and how we act. Dominant norms and discourses are taken up unwittingly and may be living out in our actions. Similarly, the contexts in which we practice may profoundly shape how we take up our nursing work. Therefore, to be able to more consciously choose the ways you will theoretically practice—ensuring that the theories you consciously believe in and choose are lived in your everyday actions requires that you develop the *skill of reflexivity*. Reflexivity involves a combination of self-observation, critical scrutiny, and conscious participation. It involves paying attention to who, how, and what you are being/doing in the moment as you work with families, observing your own living experience of that being/doing and critically scrutinizing your experience, knowledge, and actions. In this chapter we discuss the skill of reflexivity and provide an opportunity for you to explore how reflexivity is central to competent, theoretical nursing practice.

● The Skill of Conscious Participation: Paying Attention to What Concerns Us in the Here and Now

Paterson and Zderad (1988) describe that a central form of nursing knowledge is 'authenticity with the self' (p. 57). To practice in a knowledgeable way involves striving for awareness of one's self—of how one is living one's history, present, and future within the multiple and at times conflicting values and demands of everyday practice. This awareness includes paying attention and tuning into how one's past experiences and anticipated future is shaping the perceptions and responses to people in the 'here and now'. One of our intents in this chapter is to offer an opportunity for you to become more aware of how your past, present, and future are shaping your here-and-now nursing practice and an opportunity for you to begin cultivating and/or to further cultivate conscious participation.

As we described in Chapter 2, from a phenomenological perspective people do not merely exist in the world but are involved in their world. Heidegger (1962) calls this phenomenological (human) way of being involved 'concern'. In essence phenomenological concern highlights how people experience the world and each other in terms of meaning. Basically our concerns signal or attune us to what is important and meaningful to us at any particular time. Remember back to the story in Chapter 2 about the student nurse who was concerned about the food the mother was buying at the grocery store. Because she was situated in a health-promotion course, as a nurse she felt a sense of responsibility to promote health in the family. Her nursing knowledge informed her that good nutrition was essential to growth and development of children and therefore the food that the mother put in the cart (which the student thought held little nutritional value) was meaningful to her as a nurse. This offers an example of how as people, our lives are ordered by our own networks of concerns. Being aware of the concerns that are guiding our thoughts, feelings, and actions is crucial if we are to enhance the effectiveness of our nursing practice.

Nursing concerns (what matters to nurses) clearly differ from nurse to nurse and from situation to situation, because each nurse is situated and constituted differently (remember the discussion about phenomenology in Chapter 2?). For example, as Colleen described in Chapter 1, when she was a nurse working in cardiac surgery, based on her own understanding of family and of health, initially her overriding concern was ensuring that her patients had stable vital signs and monitor readings. Based on her perspective of health and her beliefs about family and about her nursing role, family held little meaning in terms of the patient's vital signs, and was therefore of little concern to her (unless the family members got in the way of the activities she did to keep the patient stable). However, as she had experiences that challenged her own personal (and theoretical) ideas of what family was and what health was, she began to realize that she needed to change her nursing practice. As her personal/theoretical understanding changed so did her nursing concerns. Each nurse who worked with Colleen would have had a unique approach to the care of people in the unit based on his or her own personal values, beliefs, and assumptions. Although as nurses who worked in cardiac care they had shared understandings (for example, what 'normal' vital signs were) and practices (for example, the frequency with which to monitor vital signs), their unique person shaped how they went about their practice and what they deemed to be significant to good cardiac care at any moment (for example, to what they paid attention in assessing the person/family, whether family was even acknowledged, the priorities they set for intervention, and so forth).

Identifying Our Ultimate Concern: An Examination of Faith

In attempting to identify the nursing concerns that are dominating our work it can be helpful to revisit the notion of faith that we explored in Chapter 2. As we described, faith is central to every person's life regardless of whether they are religious and/or adhere to any formal religious doctrine. Tillich (1958) describes faith as the state of being ultimately concerned. Faith is not a matter of mind in isolation or of the soul in contrast to mind and body. Rather, faith is the centered movement of the whole personality toward something of ultimate meaning and significance (Tillich, 1958, p. 106). Tillich contends that our faith as ultimate concern is analogous to our 'god values'. One commits to these values and is shaped by them (Fowler, 1981). Tillich (1958) provides the example of the ultimate concern for success, social standing, and economic power as god values that have dominated the post–World War II era. According to Tillich, this ultimate concern is the god of many people, demanding 'unconditional surrender to its laws even if the price is the sacrifice of genuine human relations, personal conviction, and creative eros' (p. 3). Because our ultimate concerns are so central to our lives, they strongly shape how we act and respond as we go about our nursing work. Identifying the ultimate concerns that are central to our work—that is, engaging in a process of faith clarification offers an opportunity for us to consciously and intentionally choose which god values we will adhere to as nurses (Hartrick, 2002).

To begin identifying the god values or ultimate concerns that shape your practice as a family nurse, begin by asking yourself the following questions: What commands and receives my best time, my best energy? What power or powers do I adhere to, do I fear, do I dread? What powers do I rely on and trust? What are the most compelling goals and purposes in my nursing life? (Fowler, 1981; Hartrick, 2002). As you reflect on these questions it is important to be mindful of Street's (1992) contention that one's espoused values may be incongruent with one's values in use. That is, what you say you value—your spoken responses to those questions—may be contradicted by your actions in practice. Consequently, this reflexive process requires careful examination of your work with people/families to see what values are reflected in your practice.

When I (Gweneth) first engaged in a process of faith clarification like the one cited earlier, I began to notice patterns in my practices and simultaneously tried to identify the values that seemed to underlie them. I also contemplated how these values were related to, and shaped by, the values that dominated the nursing profession and the larger health care arena. Following I describe one god value that was particularly influential in my work when I first entered nursing. My intent in providing this example is to highlight the significance of faith (ultimate concern) in the daily practice of family nursing and to spark your own reflexive inquiry into the god values that currently dominate your practice.

An Example: A Faith of Certainty

As a new nurse the god value of certainty had a profound impact on my practice. Fueled by successes of medical science, and the desire to be a scientific practice, the nursing profession had developed a tradition of looking for foundations (nursing theories, techniques) that could offer clear and certain direction for practice. Certainly as a new nurse I remember being soundly indoctrinated and schooled in nursing as a knowledgeable practice. I was taught 'a competent nurse knows'. Within this mantra was the assumption that knowledge provided certainty. If one had knowledge, one could be certain she or he was practicing in a safe, competent, and scientific manner. I am still not sure whether I personally made this assumption, whether the assumption was one that my nursing instructors held and communicated to me, or if it arose through a combination of the two. However, as a new member of the nursing community it seemed there was a strong tradition of 'certain practice', and as a member of the community I began living out and practicing that tradition. In essence, I began to put my faith in the 'god value' of *certain* knowledge and practice. Being knowledgeable and therefore certain would provide a safe and solid foundation from which to practice nursing.

My faith in certainty shaped the way I approached my work as a nurse, how I engaged with people/families, and how I used nursing knowledge. Basically, I 'set my heart on' being certain. I hoped for *certain* knowledge that could lead to *certain* practices that would find *certain* solutions to the problems people/families presented. As a result, *my* knowledge and practice became the overriding focus. Guided by a faith of certainty I put an enormous amount of time and energy into becoming and being an expert. When approaching a family, I concentrated on being certain—saying and doing the *right* thing in the *right* way so the *right* reality would be discovered (by me). When at times I felt uncertain (e.g., about what was happening for a person/family or about how I should approach a family), I interpreted that uncertainty as a lack of knowledge or skill. Guided by my ultimate concern for certainty I subsequently would seek ways of gaining more knowledge, more technical expertise, and so forth.

Although my faith in certainty served to ensure I had a scientific and knowledgeable foundation from which to practice, it simultaneously directed my attention away from families. As I set my heart on being certain, the theories and frameworks that had been developed from nursing knowledge took primacy. For example, to assess a family's health status, I followed the established assessment tools and asked the series of questions that made up those tools. I rarely stopped to determine whether the questions were relevant and/or reflected the priorities and needs of the particular family I was working with. I 'had faith' that the tool would illuminate any thing of importance and would ensure I made a full and accurate assessment. Overall, my ultimate concern for certainty directed my attention toward expert knowledge and away from families and their experiences. Moreover, it contributed to a proscriptive form of practice and led me to assume the overriding responsibility for the family's health and healing process.

Gradually, I experienced a growing doubt within my faith. Although I did not doubt the value and importance of practicing in a knowledgeable way, I began to question the god value of certainty. As Fowler (1981) describes, images of faith are not static—there are times when faith images undergo profound changes. The doubt I experienced grew from my gradual realization that no matter how thorough my knowledge or how scientific I was in the pursuit of knowledge, nursing was essentially an uncertain practice. As this conviction grew, I began to doubt the god of certainty. Yet I was unsure how to honour the uncertainty and also meet the creed of competent, knowing nurse. How could I be uncertain and be a competent nurse? How could I honour my own expertise if I was uncertain? Similar to Mason's (1993) contention that many practitioners find themselves caught between the duality of either being certain in their work with families or acting as if they don't have any expertise, I struggled to reconcile certainty and uncertainty. It was this collapse of my faith in certainty, and the doubt and questions it evoked, that opened up the possibility for me to reimage my faith—to consciously and intentionally choose new god values to put my faith in. This faith-clarification process also served to highlight the importance of reflexively paying attention to how I 'am' and how responsive I am being to people/families.

Paying attention to the concerns that are shaping our practice offers the opportunity to ensure our 'ultimate' nursing concerns are relevant and responsive to the people/families with whom we are working. Learning to pay attention involves developing awareness of who and what we are bringing to our practice and the ability to reflexively shape our practice to ensure that we do not inadvertently privilege our own concerns over families. This skill continually guides us to inquire into ourselves, into what is meaningful and significant to the particular families with whom we are working, into the contextual forces that are shaping our health care encounters and to consciously and intentionally decide how to proceed most responsively in each particular situation.

● Cultivating the Skill of Reflexivity

> *When you get into the ward, there are constraints. You've got the pressures of the other nurses, your colleagues, administration, clients and clients' families, I found myself and what I believe, can get lost. (fourth-year nursing student)*

> *I'm focused now on graduating and passing the requirements to graduate, so my focus is not being present with the patient because I am worried about . . . all those medications that Oh, my goodness, I have to give these to my patient. (fourth-year nursing student)*

The above words spoken by two nursing students who participated in an ethics research project (Storch, Hartrick, Rodney, Starzomski, & Varcoe, 2000) highlight how the practice of individual nurses is profoundly shaped by both internal and external processes. The expectations of others, institutional factors, personal history and beliefs, and present and future goals all factor in to how a nurse is in any moment of

---

TRY IT OUT 5.1. **Whose Concerns? What Concerns?**

1. *Think* back to your last day in practice.
2. *Try visually representing* your 'concerns' (perhaps draw a target or 'bull's-eye' with your concerns at the center, a mountain with your concerns at the top, a schematic with arrows). Where were you working? Who and what was at the center of your nursing practice? What were the pressing concerns of the day? How did you feel as you went about your work? What contextual elements were pressing in on you? What concerns did you as a person/nurse bring to the day? How did those concerns guide your work? Were you consciously aware of those concerns at the time? Did you inquire into what was of meaning and particular concern to the people you cared for? Whose concerns took precedence? As you reflect back on your practice that day, can you see how your own concerns shaped your responsiveness to the people/families with whom you were working?
3. *Compare* your picture to someone else's. Are there similarities? Differences? Themes?

---

practice. For the student in the second quote, her concern for her future goal of graduating was one of the most dominant factors determining how she was going about her nursing work. However, because this student practiced the skill of reflexivity she was able to recognize how her own anxiety about meeting the requirements to successfully graduate was dominating her 'here-and-now' practice and constraining her ability to be present with her patients. That reflexive self-awareness offered her the opportunity to not only critically consider this knowledge and understand its significance in regard to her nursing practice, but also offered her the opportunity to make conscious and intentional choices as she went about her work.

This example demonstrates that who you are and what you are particularly concerned about at any moment shapes your being/knowing/doing as a nurse. Your self and your concerns penetrate any nursing activity that you undertake. Try your own concerns out with the activities suggested in Try It Out 5.1.

The skill of reflexivity is vital to family nursing practice. To be able to acknowledge and honour the complexity of family and of families' health and healing experiences we must be aware of who and what we bring to the here and now of any nursing moment. This includes being aware of and reflexively scrutinizing our emotional and embodied knowing in our everyday nursing work.

● Emotions As Integral to the Reflexive Process

66 *Each one of us has a resource within ourselves. It again needs to be named. It's that voice that comes from our heart, discovering it, defining it, and learning how to communicate with it. And I am starting to find that that's a major resource for me . . . when I look*

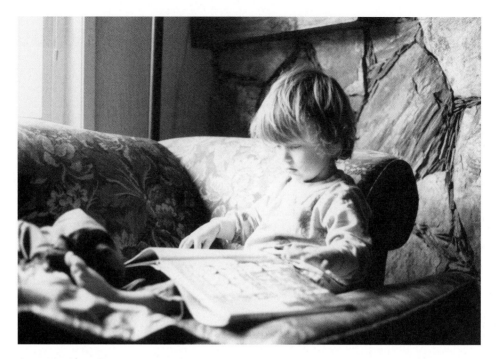

Quiet Moments (Photograph by Gayle Allison.)

> *at things from that point of view, it lets me know who I am in partic-*
> *ular instances. And it lets me know what I need to do, if I need to*
> *do anything. (fourth-year nursing student)* **99**

It was long believed that the personal emotions of nurses were a barrier
to professional nursing practice. It was assumed that by becoming emotionally involved with the people for whom they cared, nurses ran the
risk of not only losing the ability to carry out their professional responsibility but also experiencing burnout. Recent research, however, has
shown just the opposite. Acknowledging emotions and attending to them
can both serve to help nurses meet their professional responsibility to
people/families and may well prevent burnout (Benner & Wrubel, 1989;
Storch et al, 2000). The phenomenological understanding that human
beings are 'involved in their world' highlights that nurses have little
choice about being involved or not. As human beings our very presence
with people and in situations means we are always involved experientially.
The question is, *how* do we involve ourselves? Do we consciously
distance ourselves from the emotion that is being expressed and that we
are feeling or do we acknowledge and respond to others' and our own
emotional experience? The importance of this choice was highlighted in
our research into nurses' experience of ethical practice (Varcoe et al.,
2004). Our findings revealed that when nurses took up an objective,
rational stance in their practice and pushed aside their own personal
emotions and experiences, those emotions and experiences stayed with
them. Although not necessarily conscious, the emotions and experiences
were imprinted bodily and did not subside over time (Doane, 2002). For

example, during the focus groups we conducted, many nurses told stories of previous experiences that had been particularly concerning or distressing. Interestingly many of the stories the nurses chose to tell had occurred some years prior (for some, up to 20 years earlier). In the telling they became quite emotional and impassioned as they described their experience. A central theme in the stories was how at the time of their experience the nurses had pushed aside their 'personal' thoughts and emotions in order to be 'professional' and carry on with their nursing duties. For many the focus group was the first time they had actually voiced their experience and it was the first time they had expressed the emotion they had carried with them. Although the emotions had gone underground and were not readily accessible, they continued to live inside. By choosing to not attend to their emotions, the nurses missed the opportunity to understand and meaningfully integrate the experiences and emotions into their lives. In addition, this stance meant that they did not experience support and nurturance by others. Some had not even told their life partners about the experiences, despite continued distress. Seeking to manage by distancing from their emotions mirrors Benner and Wrubel's (1989) description of how burnout occurs when nurses detach from their person to avoid an emotional situation or relationship. These authors contend that burnout actually results from a loss of caring.

Nurses are not always able to act in a way that they would like. Recently, rather than describing nurses as simply 'burned out', some authors in health care (e.g., Bell, 2003; Hamric, 2000) have related these dynamics to moral distress, that is, the negative feelings that result from situations in which moral choices cannot be turned into moral actions (Storch, 2004). Webster and Baylis (2000) call the long-term impact of such situations 'moral residue'.

When nurses engage as people and intentionally involve themselves with families, they have the opportunity to acknowledge the emotions and vulnerabilities they experience in working with families. Moreover, they have the opportunity to express their experience and be supportive in it, and to thus optimize their potential to influence the situations in which they are working. At the same time they can experience what Montgomery (1993) describes as the alchemical quality of human caring. For many nurses, such involvement is 'the spark'. Without it, nurses' work would be 'bleak' (Montgomery, 1993, p. 99). As Moccia (1988) describes 'When we get past our science and theories, our technical prowess, our titles and positions of influence, it is this shared moment of authenticity—between patient and nurse—that makes us smile and allows us to move forward in our own life projects' (p. iv).

Overall, the conscious and intentional emotional involvement of nurses promotes ethically responsive practice with families (Doane, 2004). Emotions are our value feelings—they mark what matters to us— 'we experience emotion only in regard to that which matters' (Donaldson, 1991, p. 2). Emotions, as value feelings, are a precondition of moral perception (Thompson, 2001). It is through emotion that people actually experience the objects of moral judgments (Nussbaum, 2001; Vetlesen, 1994). As Vetlesen explains 'emotions anchor *us* to particular moral circumstance, to the aspect of a situation that addresses *us* immediately, to the *here* and *now* . . . (emotion is required) to identify a situation as carrying moral significance in the first place' (p. 4).

It is our emotions that make us experientially aware of ourselves (Thompson, 2001), of others, and of the situation. By paying attention to and acknowledging our emotions, we have the opportunity to learn from them (Doane, 2004). Our emotions can help us gain clarity about our own values and concerns and also cue us to what might be meaningful and significant to the families with whom we are working. Indeed, Jaeger (1989) claims that emotions are vital to systematic knowledge and necessary to developing a critical perspective on the world.

An Example: A Crazy Day

The following is a story told to us by a fourth-year nursing student during our ethics research project. The story exemplifies how listening to oneself and one's emotions is central to ethical nursing practice. The story also depicts how by listening to the different emotions, the opportunity to make more conscious and intentional clinical decisions is created.

It was a crazy day on the ward, my preceptor was busy with other things going on . . . this woman was going for ECT because psychotic depression. And she did not want that at all. She was in severe pain and she was upset that they weren't looking into what the pain was because of. They were telling her it was in her head. And I was looking at the situation . . . there was something going on . . . it was not just pain, she did need psychiatric help. But the way they were planning on going about it, I didn't like. So I just tried to make a change for her . . . I was feeling powerless because I didn't know, like that was my own constraint on myself, because I'm thinking 'I'm just a student, really, what can I do?' But I just kept phoning the doctor.

TRY IT OUT 5.2.   A Meaningful Experience

1. *Think* back to an experience you have had in your nursing work that has stayed with you. It might have been a particularly rewarding experience or one that was in some way distressing.
2. *Write* in a descriptive paragraph, poetry, a word picture, or a flow-of-consciousness free-writing (put your pen on paper, and don't lift it for 10 minutes—writing whatever comes to mind, including road blocks!). Describe the situation including who was involved, what happened, and what you personally experienced. As you write, try to remember the emotions you felt during that experience. Did you feel unease, frustration, distress, despair, anger, joy, excitement, peacefulness or. . .? After you have finished writing, reread your description and consider the knowing that the emotions were offering you. For example, did they point to contextual aspects or procedural aspects that were problematic as in the story above? Did they inform you about what might be meaningful to other people in the situation? Did they highlight and offer insight into particular values that guide you as a nurse? If you listened and responded to the emotions, at the time consider how they enhanced your nursing practice. If you did not pay attention to them at the time consider now how, had you listened, they might have affected your action and response during the situation.

Within the story it is possible to hear the student's own emotional response to the way the woman was being treated. Although she understood the need for psychiatric treatment, the way the woman was being approached and not being listened to in the process of the provision of that treatment was ethically problematic. By listening to her emotions (e.g., 'I didn't like (it)' and 'I was feeling powerless'), the student nurse was able to identify what really mattered to her, step beyond her feeling of powerlessness, and live her value of responsive ethical nursing care. Try It Out 5.2 suggests that you review an experience of concern of your own.

● The Body As Integral to Reflexivity

The skill of reflexivity also involves learning to tune into and pay attention to our bodily sensations. Body sensation (bodily knowing) offers a rich source of knowledge and a guiding foundation for nursing practice (Doane, 2004, 2003a). Merleau-Ponty (1962) describes that our bodies are our first opening to the world. Our bodies do our living—they sense themselves in our physical, cultural, social, human situations, and environments.

   Take a minute and tune into your body. Try taking some slow deep breaths to help you begin to feel your bodily sensations. Pay attention to the air going into your lungs and to how it feels when you breathe out. As you breathe out what bodily sensations do you feel? Sitting at my computer, and having done so for the past few hours I (Gweneth) am aware of how tight my shoulders are from sitting over my computer so long. This simple example shows how, if we listen and pay attention we can physically sense our bodies implying the situation and the next steps we should take (Gendlin, 1992a). For example, my tight shoulders serve as cues to remind me that I should take a break and replenish myself if I want to continue thinking clearly and be able to carry on working. In this way our bodies sense the intricacy of a situation and implicitly shape our next action (Gendlin, 1992a). Our bodies are the *site* of knowledge and decision making as well as the *medium* for action and knowledge development.

   Although we may not tune into or be aware of it, this implicit, intricate body-sense functions in every situation and according to Gendlin (1992b) we would be quite lost without it. Gendlin (1992b) offers the example of walking home at night

> ❝ [Y]ou sense a group of men following you. You don't merely perceive them. You don't merely hear them there, in the space back of you. Your body-sense instantly includes also your hope that perhaps they aren't following you, also your alarm, and many past experiences—too many to separate out, and surely also the need to do something—walk faster, change your course, escape into a house, get ready to fight, run, shout. (p. 346) ❞

The example reveals how body sense includes more than conscious awareness. Gendlin contends that body sense is not merely perception or feeling but involves an intricate interaction of conscious and unconscious 'knowing' that offers more than you can see, feel, or think. Our bodies are a site where many forms of knowing come together, are present simultaneously, and are weighed and interrelated as possible next moves (Gendlin, 1992c). It is this understanding of how knowledge comes together in the body that highlights the significance of bodily knowing for nursing practice. The body allows one to navigate and flourish in the ambiguity of everyday nursing practice (Benner, 2000) by offering a site where multiple knowledges (for example, personal, experiential, theoretical, contextual, cultural) come together and imply direction. A simple example of bodily knowing in a nursing context is when I (Gweneth) worked as an emergency room nurse. Often my more experienced nursing colleagues would describe 'having a gut feeling' that a particular patient was going to code. As a new nurse I quickly learned that, more often than not, bodily sense—that gut feeling—was accurate. I also learned to rely on my bodily sensing during tasks such as starting an intravenous line. Once I started listening to my bodily sense and let my fingers *sense* the way, I became much more adept at successfully finding and entering a vein.

Bodily knowing is determined by sensory organs, the detailed structure of our living body, contextual forces and structures, and our interactions. What we know and take to be true, therefore, is shaped by all of these factors. Subsequently embodied knowledge is not objective knowledge nor is it merely subjective. Embodiment keeps it from being purely either (Lakoff & Johnson, 1999). Our bodily sense is shaped by our cultural, social, and corporeal world. As Merleau-Ponty purported the flesh of our bodies is inseparable from the 'flesh of the world' (cited in Gendlin, 1992c). Our bodies are intimately shaped by and shape what we touch, taste, smell, see, breathe, and move within. It is through sentient bodily interaction that we take up language, history, and culture and also exceed them (Gendlin, 1992). In this way, the body conveys knowledge and information about ourselves, others, and the sociopolitical context that we may not yet be capable of languaging. For example, think about how both men and women often attempt to shape their bodies to reflect (or less often refute) gendered expectations.

Overall, our bodily sense offers a window into the complex and multifaceted aspects of nursing situations including knowledge about the personal, professional, and political elements. At the same time, bodily sense implies a step in the right direction without defining the right direction (Gendlin, 1992). For example, although my body is implying that I best get up from my computer and take a break, it is not defining how exactly I should move—whether I should go to the gym, lie down for a rest, and so forth. As we consciously access our bodily sense and also tap the knowledge that may be gleaned through a more explicit process of thinking and analyzing (for example, critically considering what our bodies might be implying: to what we need to pay attention and act on in the situation, what knowledge of the sociopolitical context our bodies convey, what would be the best action, and so forth), our family nursing practice can be profoundly enhanced. Attending to bodily sense offers the opportunity to step out of and possibly challenge habitual ways of practicing and/or the dominant sociocontextual norms that may be constraining us.

An Example: A Gun To Your Head

Perhaps one of the most striking examples of bodily sensing was described spontaneously by an operating room nurse during the ethics research project (Varcoe et al., 2004) we mentioned earlier. To understand the meaning of ethics in everyday nursing practice, we conducted a series of focus groups with nurses from a broad range of clinical areas. During a focus group with OR nurses, the nurses began discussing how their work environment was making it difficult for them to practice ethically. As they attempted to put the challenges they faced in their work environment into words, the following interaction occurred between them:

Nurse 1: The pressure is relentless. It is relentless . . . it's one of the most demoralizing environments you can ever imagine being in.

Nurse 2: I can speak of having to do 10 cataract extractions every day and feeling as though you're working with a gun at your head. Literally, that is the emotional feeling that I have.

Nurse3: That's it, that describes the feeling perfectly. A very real and present revolver at your temples.

This interaction offers an excellent example of how our bodies sense, take up, and help us express knowing that we may not yet have put into thoughts or language. By becoming aware of the knowing living in our bodies at any moment we are offered the opportunity to expand not only our understanding of ourselves and our reactions but also what might be happening for others in the situation and what contextual factors are pressing on us. This bodily sensing can also enhance our ability to articulate aspects of our experience more clearly and serve as a compass to help us navigate through the complexities and ambiguities of any nursing situation.

The example cited earlier shows how emotions are a form of bodily knowing. However bodily sense is more than emotion and feelings. Bodily sense is wider and at first may be unclear and murky. Although a feeling such as anger is felt bodily, as Gendlin (1992c) describes, if one waits a few moments one often finds that the anger is part of something wider—a larger felt sense. For example, for the OR nurses their bodily sense of practicing with a revolver at their temple conveyed numerous emotions and at the same time reflected their overall experience. In this way bodily sense may be less clear than naming particular emotions. One might experience a slight unease, a tightness, or a jumpy feeling (Gendlin, 1992c). What is important is that we develop the reflexive ability to tune in and listen to the knowing our body is communicating. In the case of the OR nurses, their bodies were informing them about particular things that needed to be addressed in their workplace (for example, workload, support, power dynamics, and so forth). Try It Out 5.3 invites you to pay attention to your own bodily knowing by reflecting on your nursing work.

> **TRY IT OUT 5.3.**   **Thinking Back to Yesterday's Concerns**
>
> As you cultivate the skill of self-knowing you may find it feels somewhat cumbersome at first, especially if you try to enact it in the moment of your experience. A good way to start is by going through the process retrospectively. Begin by thinking about a person/family you worked with during your last clinical day. Try to recollect the emotions, bodily sensations, and thoughts that you experienced. Consider what beliefs, assumptions, aspirations, and concerns you were bringing to the situation. Ask yourself: What *in me* led to this response? What habits of practice were constraining me? Consider what your self-experience reveals about *you*. What values, beliefs, assumptions, concerns, and habits of practice can you see? Next, take the opportunity to scrutinize this self-knowing in light of the theories and ideas presented in the first four chapters and in light of your espoused values. For example, do you see how some of the values or concerns that were guiding you were incongruent with responsive health-promoting practice? Try and name what concerns you would *like* to have guiding you in practice. During your next clinical day, try keeping those newly identified concerns at the forefront of your mind as you go about your day.
>
> As with any skill or behaviour, you will find that as you play the What Can I Learn About Me? game and practice the skill of self-knowing it will become second nature to you. You will find that you automatically begin living that skill in your moment-to-moment practice with families.

● Reflexivity As Integral to Conscious Participation and Self-Knowing

As we have emphasized, reflexivity involves conscious participation and self-knowing in the moment. We have purposefully languaged 'self-knowing' as a verb rather than a noun (e.g., self-knowledge) to emphasize the living, ongoing nature of the skill. Self-knowing as a verb highlights how reflexivity is a living process that is integral to any nursing moment. The skill of reflexivity offers important knowledge and also enhances your ability to use your self and your knowledge in more intentional ways.

As you cultivate the skill of reflexivity, it is important to understand that it does not merely involve paying attention to one's feeling and thoughts and responding based on those feelings and thoughts. Rather, reflexivity involves learning to pay attention to the thoughts and emotions and bodily responses one is having at any moment and reflexively considering those responses in order to more consciously and intentionally choose how to act and respond (Doane, 2004, 2003a). Reflexivity involves critically questioning the meanings, concerns, and values that are shaping one's experience. Reflexively attending to one's experience and scrutinizing the knowledge gleaned through it can enhance our power and choice in practice in two ways. First, it allows us to more thoughtfully bring ourselves to our work and make conscious choices about how to respond and use the capacities we have at our disposal. Second, because our bodily sensations, emotions, and thoughts are often sparked in response to what is happening externally, self-experience offers a window to the world and directs our attention to certain aspects of that world. Paying attention to and critically reflecting on our bodily and emotional experiences can inform us about institutional practices and structures that might be problematic and/or in need of revision.

 To Illustrate

Reflexivity is one of the central skills of relational practice. The nurses to whom I (Gweneth) have taught relational practice have found this skill of reflexivity to be very empowering. For example, as I have worked with students and encouraged them to tune into their own experience (rather than distancing from it or pretending it isn't happening), they begin to see the meanings and concerns that are guiding them as they engage with others. By paying attention to how they are acting and what they are feeling in a situation they often begin to see how their behaviours and responses flow out of their own concerns and how their own concerns are at times overriding those of the people with whom they are working. One typical discovery nurses often make about themselves is that they begin to feel anxious when they are with people who are upset and in emotional pain. Just as they would ease physical pain they begin to recognize that they have an overriding concern and sense of responsibility to 'make it better' or 'fix' the emotional pain and suffering. As they become aware of this overriding concern, they are able to observe this concern in action. That is, they can track how this concern leads them to act. They are often surprised to see how it immediately moves them away from the person. They get so focused on trying to fix the pain that they end up in-relation with the pain (which they most often turn into some form of concrete problem) rather than the person. Once in-relation with the problem, they set about trying to fix it. However, more often than not, the emotional pain is not really fixable and this leads to further emotions such as frustration, fear, powerlessness, and so forth. Although we discuss this relational practice process in much more depth in Chapters 6 and 7, what is important to highlight at this point is how, by reflexively naming their concerns (and their subsequent actions), they are often able to see how they are practicing from a service model of health care (discussed on Chapter 3) where the expert health care provider is expected to treat and cure the health problems of the people being serviced. By coming to understand how this concern is dominating their practice, they have the opportunity to retheorize their practice. They can, for example, scrutinize their assumption of responsibility and concern to fix the problem in light of the socioenvironmental approach to health promotion (that emphasizes the role of people in promoting their own health). Or they can consider the assumption in light of Newman's theory of health as expanding consciousness or Parse's theory of human becoming that emphasize how a fixing approach diminishes nurses' sensitivity to people and contravenes the health-promoting process. Paying attention to their self-experience and actions and engaging in a thought-full reflexive examination of their experience and action enhances their ability to retheorize their practice and intentionally choose actions that are responsive, ethical, and congruent with their theoretical intent.

Overall the nurses with whom I have worked have told me that when they begin to see how their self-experience and knowing is central to their nursing practice and more intentionally tap that knowing, they find they are able to be much more responsive to the families with whom they work. They can participate more fully and humanly with families in an intentional way. They do not become consumed by their own concerns. For example, nurses who work with families who have been deemed 'high priority' or 'high risk' have told us how difficult they find it to work with families who are engaged in behaviours they view as potentially harmful. Recognizing and naming their own experience allows nurses to see beyond their concerns—to not give precedence and/or get lost in their own concerns (e.g., trying to get the family to stop the high-risk behaviours) and to listen and involve themselves in what is meaningful to the family. As nurses get clear about what their concerns are and also clear about the concerns of the family with whom they are working, the opportunity to look for common ground arises. We explore the process of looking for common ground to connect across difference in more depth in subsequent chapters, however, we wish to highlight that connecting across difference is enabled through the skill of reflexivity.

● Intentionally Living Our Knowledge

As I (Gweneth) worked with families and practiced the skill of reflexivity, it became clear to me that none of the existing theories I had studied in family nursing addressed the experiential/relational aspect of family— what Moore (1994) describes as the 'soul' of family that I had come to know. As I considered the theories that informed family nursing practice and thought about the 'deeper stirrings and intuitions' (Mumford, 1957, p. 179) within my experiences of family that were not reflected in existing theoretical perspectives, I began to look beyond the extant theories in an attempt to stretch my way of thinking and seeing family. That is, I began retheorizing my practice. My retheorizing has been supported through an ongoing reflexive process that has included actively paying attention to my own self-knowing (to my own experiences and responses), listening carefully to learn from families, scrutinizing existing theories in terms of their adequacy, and donning different theoretical lenses such as the ones described in previous chapters (Doane, 2003b). As part of my reflexive process, I have paid attention to my bodily knowing, what I am feeling, what I am sensing, what I am thinking, the questions I am asking myself and/or want to ask others, what I feel clear about and what is confusing me, what I want to know more about, and so forth. I have found this reflexive process and the information it affords has served as an important compass alerting me to when I need to stop and reflect, question, or seek more knowledge as well as helping me know the direction in which to move to continue my knowledge development process.

 An Example: "I Only Know of Unlove"

One important reflexive experience that depicts the value of bodily knowing occurred during a conference I (Gweneth) attended where one of the keynote speakers was Ryan, a young man about 19 years of age. As part of his presentation Ryan told his story of growing up in foster care, of eventually living on the street, and of what 'made the difference' and helped him 'get on with his life'. At the time of his presentation, Ryan was working with a grassroots initiative with children who were

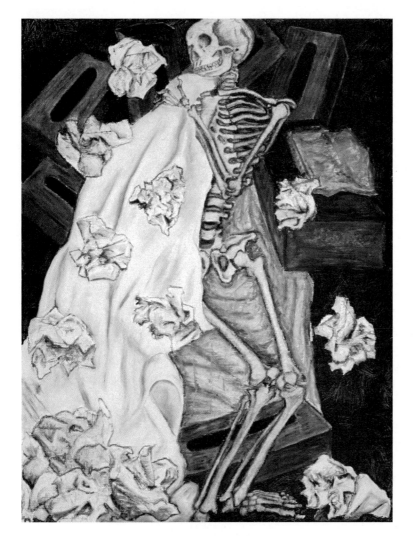

Unlove. (Oil Bar on Rag Paper Danaca Ackerson.)

currently living on the street to help them reconnect with mainstream society. Although Ryan had many important insights to offer the professionals sitting in the audience, he particularly emphasized how vital each moment of connection was to a child who had never known deep connection. I was so struck by his words that I actually wrote them down:

▶ *What do I know of love. I only know of unlove, being bought on a street corner, being given a cigarette by a guard to beat up another kid . . . remember that connection with you might be the only experience of love that kid has ever had. Although a 5-minute connection may not seem important to you, it has a different meaning to a kid who has never had anyone care. It can make a big difference.[1]*

---

[1] This story, which has previously been published in *Nursing Philosophy*, has been reprinted with permission from Blackwell Publishing.

As I listened to Ryan's words, I knew that the reason they were having such an impact on me was because they were echoing the deeper stirrings I had experienced about family (Doane, 2003b). Although Ryan had never had or known family in the literal sense, he was speaking of what I had come to know about family both as a person and in my work as a nurse. He was speaking of the deeper intent that guided me when I intervened with literal families in instrumental ways. As he spoke, I heard echoes of what I had heard embedded in the stories of other nurses as they described 'improving family function' 'making a home visit to a new mom' 'doing discharge planning for a man who has just had a stroke'. What Ryan was speaking of was *deep connection*—of deeply touching another and of being deeply touched. I was struck by how in many ways Ryan's story highlighted what it is that makes actual families so vital. We want to improve family structure and function and family communication, promote healthy family systems, and so forth because more than any other place, families are where people have the greatest chance of experiencing deep connection. Family is supposedly the societal medium through which people:

- are seen as individuals and experience that they matter and that other people matter,
- experience being loved and loving others,
- experience being valued and how to value others,
- experience a sense of belonging and connection to something more than themselves.

In essence, our society bequeaths to family the responsibility for peoples' relational growth and experience.

Moving Beyond the Literal View of Family

My awareness of the harsh reality that not all families are mediums for nurturing deep connection and relational experience emphasized more than ever the importance of moving beyond thinking of family in its literal sense. That is, Ryan described that although he had never lived or experienced deep connection in an actual family, he could still experience deep, loving connection with others. He could still have relational experiences where he had the opportunity to come to know that feeling of being seen and cared about, to learn how to care toward and for others, to experience being part of the human family—to belong and be a part of something bigger. It was this relational experience that was significant to his health and healing, not necessarily a literal family.

Certainly what Ryan had to say was not 'new'. We have known for years that relational experiences of deep connection promote health. However, as I listened carefully to Ryan's story and to my own bodily resonance with what he was saying, I was able to articulate my deeper stirrings and knowing of family. In particular, I was able to more fully articulate my dis-ease at the limitations of my own practice and the limitations of existing conceptual understandings of family. Although I had known for a long time that there was more to family than was reflected in conceptualizations I had studied, I found that by reflexively scrutinizing existing conceptualizations and theories in light of my self-knowing and in light of what Ryan was saying I could more clearly see how my current practice was limited. For example, I could see how thinking of family as a configuration of people was incongruent in many ways with my ultimate nursing goal of promoting human flourishing. At the same time I began to see that my work as a family nurse was about creating opportunities for nurturing, relational experiences. And that this may or may not happen in a literal family.

Nurturing Relational Experiences

Through this experience I (Gweneth) revised the image of family that was guiding my practice. Imaging family as a relational, living experience, I began to scrutinize my practice and ask myself how I might enhance my ability to nurture relational experiences in my everyday work. For example, although I had always focused on promoting relational experiences in the 'actual' families with whom I worked, viewing family as an entity had limited the depth and breadth of that focus. As my field of vision expanded and I began paying more attention to each moment as a potential experience of deep connection in a very pragmatic way, I began to understand that family nursing was not just about actual families. Rather, I could see that promoting family health was about enhancing the opportunity for people to experience being deeply touched and deeply touching others in ways that are nurturing and growth producing for them. Aided by the different lenses and theories we present in the first four chapters, I began, in my everyday practice, to pay close attention to how I was (and at times, was not) fostering the experiences we hope people can have in actual families, including the experience of being seen, being valued, and feeling of value; the experience of learning about themselves in all of their complexity; the experience of being part of something that is more than oneself; experiencing the capacity, strength, and also vulnerability that lies within them; and developing their own relational capacity to nurture growth and wellness in others. This process involved paying close attention to the societal and health care norms and structures that were shaping my practice and the practice of colleagues around me.

Overall, the inquiry into my practice enabled me to understand the importance of promoting relational experiences regardless of the existence of a literal family and regardless of the health, abilities, or resources of any actual family. That is, I intentionally began fostering relational experiences in every moment of my practice. As in Ryan's experience, I realized that I might do that in a 5-minute connection with an individual I met only once or I might work with a family for several months. I came to see that family transcended the literal, taken-for-granted conceptualization that had previously governed my practice and I also began to see how I might more effectively promote family experience and health in my everyday nursing practice.

● What Can I Learn About Me?

One powerful way we have found to learn more about ourselves and cultivate reflexive self-knowing is to play the What Can I Learn About Me? game.

Try It Out 5.3 offers a learning activity to help you cultivate your self-knowing through reflection and This Week in Practice suggests a general way for you to bring this 'game' into practice and set the stage for tuning into particular situations. When we are with a family and find ourselves having a strong response or wanting to take charge and fix the family or situation, we purposefully turn our attention to ourselves and tune into our sociohistorical location, bodily sensation, emotions, and thoughts. To get a clearer sense of our own part in these responses, we reflexively consider what *in us* is sparking those sensations, emotions, and thoughts. We might ask ourselves what beliefs, assumptions, aspirations, and concerns we are bringing. We ask ourselves the question: What *in me* is leading to this response? This turning of attention serves two purposes. It allows us to move beyond the assumption that it is the family who is being or doing something problematic (for example, 'if only that mother would stop smoking around her child with asthma!'). In addition, it allows us to learn more about ourselves and move beyond habits of practice that might be constraining us (for example, how we tend to look at the half-empty part of families and problematize them rather than look for the half-full and enhancing existing capacities). Identifying the concerns that are shaping our responses and the habits of practice that are getting in our way of developing a responsive working relationship with the family creates the opportunity for us to:

- better recognize the complexity of the situation, the influences shaping us, shaping families, and shaping how we are practicing in between all of these forces;
- explore what really matters to the family, to see beyond our own concerns and seek to understand the concerns of the family (for example, what the mother sees as important, the meaning smoking has for her in her life, what it is like to have a child with asthma and still want to smoke);
- act and respond in ways that address our nursing responsibility while simultaneously honoring the power and choice of families.

 To Illustrate

One example of reflexive self-knowing in which I (Colleen) have recently engaged is related to the role of spirituality and religion in my nursing practice. Having been educated in a strictly secular manner, I was taught to distance religion (like emotions) from nursing practice. Over the years I have set my heart on nonoppressive and empowering nursing practice and saw this as including not imposing personal religious beliefs and practices on others. Recently in my work with women who have experienced violence, the women with whom I was working decided to make a video. The video was intended to convey to women living with abusive partners 'women's wisdoms' about how to deal with intimate partner violence. In concert with my philosophy and the project we were doing, the women had control over making the video. However, when I saw the video, I was quite uncomfortable about the extent to which they included segments of women talking about faith and finding strength in God (variously referred to, as the video included women of many religions, including Muslim, Christian, Buddist, Seik, and Hindu). I was uncomfortable because I worried that the video would convey the message that with faith, women could better put up with, tolerate, and endure violence, a message that is contrary to my commitment to reducing violence. I resisted the urge to wrest away control of the video and tried to sort out my discomfort. I realized that to some extent, I wanted my version of empowerment to dominate. My commitments and the way I saw those commitments led me to overlook or discount what was of meaning and significance to the women. Many of the women's values regarding the importance of family were related to their particular religions and had led them to find it very difficult to leave their violent partners, and I feared those values. Further, my secular nursing education, and my training in splitting body/mind/spirit led me to see spiritual issues as separable from other concerns in life. Although I have not resolved how to reconcile my belief that women should not have to endure violence with some women's beliefs that faith will help them do so, I am a little more open to recognizing the importance of other's commitments.

Overall, the skill of reflexivity enables us to be in-relation with people in ways that are meaningful and responsive. It helps us to more consciously and intentionally bring ourselves to relationships. In the next chapter, we continue the exploration of being in-relation by examining other skills and capacities that support responsive, relational practice.

THIS WEEK IN PRACTICE

Explicating Assumptions About Family Health

Your bodily sense can inform you not only about your own personal concerns and values but also about the world in which you are practicing. This week in practice, take the opportunity to play with this idea of bodily knowing. Just as you might do vital signs on a patient you are caring for, take readings of your bodily sensing several times throughout each day. Begin your reading by noticing the first sensation of which you become aware. For example, as you stop and tune into your body at that moment, do you immediately become aware of knots in your stomach, of tension in your shoulders, of a lightness in your step, or . . . ? As you begin to notice the sensations in your body, move your gaze to the context you are in. What in the context might be contributing to your bodily sensations? Do you have a heavy workload pressing in on you? Do you notice that you are working with particularly supportive colleagues today? Are you finding it challenging to communicate with a person/family you are working with? What is happening around you that you are sensing and perhaps taking up and wearing/living bodily? Next, shift your gaze to your thoughts. What has been dominating your thoughts over the past hour? How has what you have been thinking about perhaps been contributing to your bodily sense? It can be interesting to record these vital signs. Similar to charting on a patient, by recording your self-observations you might begin to identify patterns that can provide further insight into what is supporting and/or constraining you as you go about your nursing work and the changes you might need to effect in order to be more effective in your nursing work.

CHAPTER HIGHLIGHTS

1. What self-knowing have you discovered as you have worked your way through this book so far?
2. When you are in a challenging situation, where do you first know that in your body (e.g., knots in your stomach, tight shoulders, etc.)?
3. How might *you* enlist bodily knowing more intentionally to inform your practice?

REFERENCES

Bell, S. E. (2003). Ethical climate in managed care organizations. *Nursing Administration Quaterly, 27*(2), 133–139.

Benner, P. (2000). The roles of embodiment, emotion and lifeworld for rationality and agency in nursing practice. *Nursing Philosophy, 1,* 1–14.

Benner, P., & Wrubel, J. (1989). *The primacy of caring.* Menlo Park, CA: Addison-Wesley.

Bergum, V. (1994). Knowledge for ethical care. *Nursing Ethics: An International Journal for Health Care Professionals, 1*(2), 72–79.

Buber, M. (1958). *I and thou.* New York: Scribner.

Doane, G. (2004). Being an ethical practitioner: The embodiment of mind, emotion and action. In J. Storch, P. Rodney, & R. Starzomski (Eds.), *Toward a moral horizon: Nursing ethics for leadership and practice* (pp. 433–444). New York: Pearson.

Doane, G. (2003a). Reflexivity as presence: A journey of self-inquiry. In L. Finlay & B. Gough (Eds.), *Reflexivity. A practical guide for researchers in health and social sciences* (pp. 93–102). Oxford: Blackwell Publishing Company.

Doane, G. (2003b). Through pragmatic eyes: Philosophy and the re-sourcing of family nursing. *Nursing Philosophy, 4*(1), 25–32.

Donaldson, M. (1991). *Human minds: An exploration.* London: Penguin.

Fowler, J. (1981). *Stages of faith.* New York: Harper & Row.

Freire, P. (1989). *Pedagogy of the oppressed.* New York: Continuum.

Gendlin, E. T. (1992a). The primacy of the body, not the primacy of perception. *Man and World, 25*(3–4), 341–353.

Gendlin, E. T. (1992b). Thinking beyond patterns: Body, language, and situations. In B. den Ouden & M. Moen (Eds.), *The presence of feeling in thought* (pp. 21–151). New York: Peter Lang.

Gendlin, E. T. (1992c). The wider role of bodily sense in thought and language. In M. Sheets-Johnstone (Ed.), *Giving the body its due* (pp. 192–207). Albany: State University of New York Press.

Hamric, A. B. (2000). Moral distress in everyday ethics. *Nursing Outlook, 48,* 199–201.

Hartrick Doane, G. A. (2002). Am I still ethical? The socially mediated process of nurses' moral identity. *Nursing Ethics, 9*(6), 623–635.

Hartrick, G. (1997). Relational capacity: The foundation for interpersonal nursing practice. *Journal of Advanced Nursing, 26,* 523–528.

Hartrick, G. (2002). Beyond polarities of knowledge: The pragmatics of faith. *Nursing Philosophy, 3*(1), 27–34.

Heidegger, M. (1962). *Being and time* (J. MacQuarrie & E. Robinson, Trans.). New York: Harper & Row.

Jaeger, A. (1989). Love and knowledge: Emotion in feminist epistemology. In A. M. Jaeger & S. R. Bordo (Eds.), *Gender/body/knowledge: Feminist reconstructions of being and knowing* (pp. 145–171). New Brunswick, NJ: Rutgers.

Lakoff, G., & Johnson, M. (1999). *Philosophy in the flesh: The embodied mind and its challenge to Western thought.* New York: Basic Books.

Mason, B. (1993). Towards positions of safe uncertainty. *Human Systems: The Journal of Systemic Consultation and Management, 4,* 189–200.

Merleau-Ponty, M. (1962). *Phenomenology of perception.* (C. Smith, Trans.). London: Routledge and Kegan Paul.

Milton, C. L. (2001). Articulating nursing's moral residue. *Nursing Science Quarterly, 14*(2), 109.

Mitchell, G. J. (2001). Policy, procedure and routine: Matters of moral influence. *Nursing Science Quarterly, 14*(2), 109–114.

Moccia, P. (1988). Preface. In J. Paterson & L. Zderad, (Eds.), *Humanistic nursing* (NLN Publ. No. 41-2218, 2nd ed., pp. i–iv). New York: National League for Nursing.

Montgomery, C. L. (1993). *Healing through communication. The practice of caring.* Newbury Park, CA: Sage.

Moore, T. (1994). *Soulmates, honoring the mysteries of love and relationship.* New York: Harper Collins.

Mumford, L. (1957). *The transformations of man.* London: Allen & Unwin.

Nussbaum, M. (2001). *Upheavals of thought.* New York: Cambridge University Press.

Paterson, J. G. & Zderad, L. T. (1988). *Humanistic nursing* (NLN Publ. No. 41-2218, 2nd ed.). New York: National League for Nursing.

Storch, J. (2004). Nursing ethics: A developing moral terrain. In J. Storch, P. Rodney, & R. Starzomski (Eds.), *Toward a moral horizon: Nursing ethics for leadership and practice* (pp. 1–16). Toronto: Pearson.

Street, A. (1992). *Inside nursing: A critical ethnography of clinical nursing practice.* Albany: State University of New York Press.

Thompson, E. (2001) Empathy and consciousness. In E. Thompson (Ed.), *Between ourselves, second person issues in the study of consciousness* (pp. 1–32). Charlotte, VA: Imprint Academic.

Tillich, P. (1958). *Dynamics of faith.* New York: Harper & Brothers.

Varcoe, C., Doane, G., Pauly, B., Rodney, P., Storch, J. L., Mahoney, K. et al. (2004). Ethical practice in nursing—Working the in-betweens. *Journal of Advanced Nursing, 45*(3), 316–325.

Vetlesen, J. (1994). *Perception, empathy and judgment: An inquiry into the preconditions of moral performance.* University Park: Pennsylvania State Univesity Press.

Webster, G. C., & Baylis, F. (2000). Moral residue. In S. B. Rubin & L. Zoloth (Eds.), *Margin of error: The ethics of mistakes in the practice of medicine.* Hagerstown, MD: University Publishing Company.

6 Being In-Relation

OVERVIEW

In this chapter we discuss the significance of relationships in family nursing. This discussion includes a description of the types of relationships and the capacities and skills that support relational family nursing practice.

n the preceding five chapters we focused on philosophical and theoretical perspectives that are helpful in promoting a relational approach to family nursing. At this point we now shift the focus of discussion to the practical being/doing of relational family nursing practice. It is important to emphasize, however, that although we are shifting the focus we are not ceasing to speak of knowledge and theory. How we are and what we do as nurses is integrally shaped by the knowledge and theory that inform us—thus knowledge and theory are always part of any discussion of practice. The analogy of looking through a camera can be helpful in understanding the synergy of theory and action. As you look through the camera, depending on how you adjust the lens, the picture will foreground certain things and background others. However, even as you focus the lens on a particular aspect, everything else still remains in the picture. In this chapter we are continuing to look at the 'whole' picture of relational family nursing practice; however, we are adjusting the lens to bring one aspect—ways of being in-relation—to the foreground of the discussion. In Chapter 7, we shift the lens once more to foreground processes and strategies that support relational practice.

● How Is Being In-Relation at the Center of Family Nursing Practice?

Whether we are aware of our relational connection or not, relationship is central to every moment of family nursing practice. Thayer-Bacon (2003) describes how we 'use' relations throughout our daily lives in a number of ways. We use relations to draw comparisons—how big or small something is in comparison to something else. We use relations to make associations. For example, we may associate a certain song with someone we have known or with a past experience—we 'relate' the song to that experience (Thayer-Bacon, 2003). We also use relations to understand functional interactions. For example, Thayer-Bacon (2003) offers the example of relating the sound of an ambulance siren to an emergency rescue. Another way we relate is when we relate or tell others about ourselves or what happened to us in a particular experience. We also relate when we describe how one idea is relevant and related to what we are saying. By relating ideas in this way, we are able to create new ideas—to see and know things in new ways.

Similarly, relationships are a site where knowledge is developed and acted on. For example, in stopping to think about it you will probably be able to identify ways in which your knowledge has been altered as you have engaged in relationships with other people/families. It is through relationships that

- knowledge is exchanged between you and the people/families with whom you work,
- you have the opportunity to learn from families and become better informed by them,
- knowledge (both yours and families') is enacted, developed, and expanded.

It is through relationships with people/families that you are able to expand your 'knowing' and at the same time figure out what knowledge might be significant to the particular people with whom you are working and/or how you might offer that knowledge in relevant ways. Overall, relationships are the medium through which you and the families with whom you work come to 'know more' and the site where the knowledge you all have is used to promote health and healing.

● We Are Always In-Relation and Affecting Others

In all of the different ways of relating, there is a common theme of connection to someone or something else (Thayer-Bacon, 2003). And in each of these circumstances relations are *transactional* (Thayer-Bacon, 2003). That is, each element (for example, each person, idea, experience) is affected and in some way altered through the relational transaction. Because relating and relationships are so central to our lives, to assume that we function independently (that is, that we function separately from each other and from our world) is to miss all of the ways we are connected and relating. And, assuming this separateness in our nursing practice results in a failure to see all of the ways we are affecting everyone and everything else with whom we are in contact in our everyday nursing work. To exemplify this relational aspect of practice, we offer the following story of an experience I (Gweneth) had while in a hospital a number of years ago following the birth of my daughter Teresa. The story illustrates that whether nurses intentionally engage or disengage with people, they are always in-relation and those relational moments are always affecting and shaping the health and healing process.

 ### An Example: Two Relational Moments

    The nurse knocked gently on my door and, thinking I was asleep, came quietly into my room. As I opened my eyes, she smiled, said hello, and began to check my IV. Silence seemed to fill the room. As I lay there in the silence I could feel the nurse's discomfort. I watched her busily checking tubes and dressings. Throughout her tasks she did not look at my face—she seemed to be carefully avoiding my eyes. I was puzzled by the gentleness and concern I could sense she felt toward me and yet her seeming desire to not engage with me. I asked if it would be possible for me to go and see my baby. (My baby daughter had been born by C-section the day before. She had stopped breathing in the delivery room, was on a ventilator, and was progressively becoming worse. No one could figure out what was causing her distress.) As I began to get myself up, I could feel the emotion rising within me and found myself swallowing hard to keep the tears in. The nurse busily got the wheelchair and helped me into it, all the while avoiding my eyes. Just as we were about to head out of the door, an old (medical) friend stepped into the room with a big smile on his face. He had seen my name on the patient list and had wanted to stop in to congratulate me. As I tried to speak, the emotion welled up. Looking into his eyes that showed such care and warmth, it was like the dam broke and the tears began to pour out. Without saying a word, my friend took two steps across the room and reached out to hug me. It felt so good to express the emotion I felt! As the tears slowed and I reached for some Kleenex, I looked around for the nurse and realized she had left.

I have often thought about that nurse and wondered what her experience was that day. What led her to be in-relation by maintaining such a distance between us? I remember that the ward was very quiet, so time did not stop her from engaging. Also, I could sense her caring and compassion, and yet she was giving a very clear message that she was not willing to 'be with' me in my pain. In response, I found myself desperately trying to keep my pain within me. She had clearly communicated that this was not a place where it was OK to open up to my vulnerability and *be* what I was experiencing.

The response of that particular nurse is not unique. Many nurses choose such distance in their relationships. It is not uncommon to hear nurses say things like 'I didn't know what to say' or 'I didn't want to open that can of worms'. Often nurses believe they have to know how to 'handle' a patient's discomfort—they have to 'do' something with it. As a result of that belief, they offer advice or choose not to speak with people about difficult things. Their own discomfort with not being able to 'make things better' and/or at the uncertainty of what might happen (for example, 'what if the person gets more upset or starts to cry?' or 'what if I don't have a response or answer?') sometimes leads nurses to pull back. At times nurses may also pull back because they themselves (as people) do not want to feel such deep emotion and pain.

Nurses may also distance themselves at least in part because of the messages they get about what is and is not of importance and value within the practice context and in order to deal with the way they are expected to practice within the business-driven context of health care. In my research on emergency nursing, I (Colleen) found that nurses devalued one another for being 'too emotional' or 'too involved' (Varcoe, 2001, 2002). They called nurses who spent time with patients 'PR nurses', 'bleeding hearts', and so on. Nurses modeled and promoted emotional distance, and although they talked about wanting 'more time to talk with patients', emotional engagement did not fit with the overall work pattern that was focused on 'emptying the stretchers'. Even when they had ample time, many nurses often chose to sit at the desk engaging with colleagues rather than with patients and families. With other colleagues who noted similar practices in other clinical settings, I concluded that nurses disengaged relationally to some extent in order to make the organization 'work' (Varcoe, Rodney, & McCormick, 2003). They disengaged and kept emotional distance in order to be ready for the next stretcher, in order to 'bundle' a family 'out the door' (Chapter 4) or in order to survive 'practicing with a gun to your head' (Chapter 5).

Whatever the underlying reasons, as nurses distance themselves (and thereby distance others) their capacity to respect, honour, and promote people's health and healing process is hindered. Not only does this distancing lessen their ability to ensure they are fully informed and knowledgeable about the people they are caring for, we believe that as nurses pull back they lose their greatest source of satisfaction. As cited in Chapter 5, it is the 'shared moment of authenticity—between patient and nurse—that makes us smile and allows us to move forward in our own life projects' (Moccia, 1988, p. iv). Therefore, in this chapter we focus on the personal, professional, and political skills and capacities that we believe will create more health-promoting practice environments and ultimately more responsive ways of being in-relation. We begin by considering some constraining myths and problematic assumptions nurses often hold. However, in doing so we want to emphasize that practicing in-relation is not just a matter of individual nurses examining and changing their practice toward families. Rather, nurses need to work with their colleagues and leaders to create practice environments that foster and support relational practice.

● Some Constraining Myths

As discussed in previous chapters, many nurses approach their practice believing they are responsible to 'make things better, quickly'. Given the dominance of the biomedical model in health care and the rise of the business model in the delivery of that care, it is not difficult to understand how they have formed that belief. Situated in a health care system that is completely structured according to a disease-treatment, service-oriented, business model of care, nurses can't help but be shaped by the values and assumptions that underpin biomedical and corporate approaches.

Take a look back at the discussion in Chapter 1 that distinguished the medical approach to health promotion from the socioenvironmental approach. As you re-read that discussion, think about how the different definitions of health (such as the medical definition and the socioenvironmental definition) would each give rise to different kinds of relationships. For example, if health is defined as the absence of disease, it makes sense that nurses would want to engage in such a way as to 'make people better' (for example, by getting rid of whatever is bothering them). The dominance of this disease-treatment approach in health care has shaped health care relationships to the point that many family-nurse relationships reflect the underlying assumptions of the biomedical model. These biomedical, disease-treatment assumptions often are evidenced in how relationships are conceptualized in nursing literature and how nurses engage relationally in their everyday practice.

Also think back to the discussion in Chapter 4 that outlines how business and managerial interests have come to dominate health care delivery. The business emphasis on 'efficiency' and reducing costs has reinforced the biomedical model resulting in disease treatment being prioritized over more long-term prevention and health-promotion efforts. Profit-generating activities (for example, pharmaceutical or information technology or biotechnology production) of biomedicine also support the business model of health care. These profit-generating activities and the corporate and business assumptions that underpin them give rise to different kinds of relationships than does an emphasis on health promotion.

If one looks carefully at how relationships are conceptualized in nursing literature and how nurses engage relationally in their everyday practice, it is possible to see the biomedical and corporate underpinnings at work. In particular, there are three assumptions that arise from a biomedical model of care and are reinforced and shaped within a corporate model of health care delivery that profoundly hinder nurses' relational practice (Hartrick, 2002):

1. Relationships are simply a means to an end.
2. It is possible to provide health care without a relational connection.
3. Communication skills are the foundation of relational practice.

Problematic Assumption 1: Relationships Are a "Means to an End"

If you pay close attention to how relationships are talked about and how they are described in the nursing literature, you will notice that relationships are assumed to be tools or media that can be used in the daily work of nursing to effect certain outcomes. For example, students are often taught that relationships and good communication can foster good family assessment, intervention, and treatment outcomes. Relationships and communication skills are valued for what they produce (for example, more accurate information for diagnosis, faster discharge, less psychological distress, more rapid assessment of families' caregiving potential). Although good relationships may well enhance care and treatment, conceptualizing relationships as merely a means to an end is problematic in three interrelated ways:

1. It assumes that nurses are in control of relationships.
2. It suggests that nurses' concerns and commitments drive the relationship.
3. It obscures the worth of relationships in and of themselves.

First, thinking of relationships as a means to an end further assumes that relationships are under the control of the nurse—it is the nurse who determines and uses the relationship. Scrutinizing this assumption against the values and beliefs underpinning a socioenvironmental approach to health promotion not only shows the incongruity, but also highlights the disease-care and business underpinnings. For example, in disease care the health practitioner is the chief actor doing the assessment, diagnosing, and treating and might therefore strategically 'use' good communication to support expert intervention. However, from a socioenvironmental perspective of health promotion, people/families are the chief actors and decision makers. This means that relationship is no longer under the control of the nurse. Rather, in health-promoting relationships, families and nurses collaborate and work together.

The second problem that arises out of this means to an end assumption is that if the 'ends' are controlled by the nurse, rather than the family, they arise from the nurses' concerns and commitments. As we described in Chapter 4, corporate objectives increasingly steer nurses and their work. Increasingly, efficient use and conservation of resources dominates over the promotion of health in nursing practice. In health promotion, the people whose health is being promoted need to have a voice in determining the ends as opposed to having the ends determined by corporate objectives.

The third problem with the means to an end assumption is that it serves to conceal the inherent experiential worth of relationship. That is, the relational experience of deeply connecting is, in and of itself, health and healing promoting. People who involve themselves in meaningful caring relationships appear to experience an increased sense of integrity and personhood (McMillan, 2003; Montgomery, 1993). This heightened sense is manifested in courage, endurance, and aliveness within their health and healing experiences (Montgomery, 1993). Through caring relationships, people have the opportunity to experience the power of human connection in the healing process. Subsequently, they are often inspired to more intentionally care for themselves (Montgomery, 1993).

My (Gweneth) work with families who are grieving has exemplified this health-promoting quality of relational connection. When I am with families in their grief and we enter into the realm of deep relational connection, it is common for one or more of the family members to afterward question how it is possible to feel so out of control and in such incredible pain and yet simultaneously feel they are 'OK'. I have come to understand that, at least in part, what promotes this feeling of being OK is the deep connection we are living as we honour and live their grief together. Although our togetherness does not lessen their grief or pain, it provides the space and opportunity for them to live what they are experiencing—to open up to their grief and express it. Our relational connection promotes their reconnection with themselves and promotes a feeling of choice and centeredness amidst their grief. As Jordan (1997) describes, the deepest sense of one's self is formed in-relation with others. Therefore, "although relationships may well promote certain outcomes, their most significant value is the intrinsic capacity and connectedness people experience when they are in-relation" (Hartrick, 2002, p. 51).

Problematic Assumption 2: It Is Possible to Provide Health Care Without a Relational Connection

If you listen to the way that many nurses speak, you can often hear the underlying assumption that it is possible to provide care and promote health without relationally engaging with a person. This assumption is exemplified by such statements as 'I'm too busy' or 'I have no time' (to form relationships with patients/families). Similarly, it is evident in the everyday practice of the busy surgical nurse who goes to do postop care on the 'appendectomy in room 4', or the community health nurse with a heavy caseload who completes a well-baby visit by following a postnatal checklist and never stops to determine whether the checklist is relevant or significant to the family with whom she is working.

What is being obscured is that whether nurses are aware of it or not and whether they attend to it or not, there is a relational flow happening in every human encounter. Relationships are not formed they are lived.

Just as there was a powerful relational flow happening between myself (Gweneth) and the nurse who cared for me in the hospital when my daughter was born, relational connection is operating in all situations, is always present and influential. As such, the relational flow/connection can have an empowering or disempowering influence on health. The question, therefore, is not *whether* one engages but rather *how* one engages in-relation. Do you engage by distancing yourself or by objectifying people/families (for example, rushing them out the door in the name of efficiency), or do you open yourself up and invite connection? Relational practice is not just a matter of whether you have time to form relationships but rather *how* you live the relational time you have (even if that relational time is a minute or two as you take vital signs, dispense a medication, or complete a home care evaluation). Relationally connecting does not simply require more time, rather it requires that you intentionally choose how you spend the time you have.

This intentionality of relational engagement involves not only how we talk to people and what we say verbally, but also how we communicate in other more subtle ways. For example, the nurse who cared for me (Gweneth) when my daughter Teresa was born communicated to me through her actions, through her body language, and also 'energetically'. That is, in the quietness of the relational moment I could 'hear' her discomfort and trepidation at being with me in my pain—she communicated this to me in the way she moved around the room and avoided any kind of physical connection with me. At the same time, energetically I could sense (e.g., remember bodily sensing in Chapter 5) the warmth and caring that was also living through her in that moment. All of this was communicated to me without her speaking a word and without her necessarily realizing what and how she was communicating.

An Example: Communicating Energetically

The power and subtleness of communication has been highlighted for me through a research project that I (Gweneth) am involved in on a medical oncology unit. As with many current health care milieus, the nurses on the unit often face overwhelming workloads, lack of resources, and difficulty in providing the quality of care they wish to provide. At the same time, being on an oncology unit, the nurses are continually in-relation with people who are living through some of life's most intense and significant moments, including end of life. Many of the nurses who work on the unit have described how the hectic pace and demands combined with the emotional intensity of their work take its toll on them personally. They have described that while at work they are so focused on 'keeping everything going' that they often don't realize what and how they are being effected until afterward. It is like they take up the ward milieu and carry it home bodily where it profoundly affects their personal life. They describe this 'taking up' as similar to an ink blotter—without their conscious awareness they are soaking up the energetic intensity of the ward and they find it difficult to 'purge' themselves at the end of a 'stressful' day. As an outsider going onto the unit, I find myself acutely aware of this wall of energy when I walk on to the ward. If I pay attention to my bodily sensing I am often 'hit' with this energetic force and 'know' the emotional and physical state of the ward before listening to any kind of verbal report. One of the nurses recently described to me how, understanding the significance and intensity of this energetic force, she has begun to consciously pay attention to it and more intentionally choose how she herself is going to 'relate' energetically—both in what she communicates and in what she takes up. For example, when coming on duty she has begun to stop for a moment as she walks onto the unit at the beginning of her shift and center herself to connect with her own inner compass. Similar to the processes we described in Chapter 5, she pays attention to her bodily sensing so that she is able to maintain her energetic compass and be aware of what she herself is communicating energetically and what she is receiving from others. In contrast to the past where she found herself profoundly affected by colleagues who were subtly and not so subtly communicating negative emotions and attitudes, she now reflexively buffers herself so she does not take that negative energy up. At the same time she is more purposeful in her own communication with others including paying attention to what and how she is relating to the patients/families she cares for as well as the colleagues with whom she works.

Understanding the power of this energetic form of communication highlights the profound influence that the context of practice has on your ability to practice relationally. Indeed, we have come to believe that a commitment to practice relationally requires both paying attention to oneself as well as joining with others to take action to optimize the practice environment. Not only is it vital to pay attention to the subtle (yet powerful) ways the context is shaping your own personal way of relating, but it is also necessary to scrutinize more concrete and systemic forms of communication that shape relational practice. For example, policies and tools in practice settings that outline a clinical pathway that proscribes a mastectomy that is done through an admission and discharge on the same day implies that a relational connection between health care providers and women who are undergoing radical breast surgery is expendable. The pursuit of a 15-minute family interview (Wright & Leahey, 1999) or a 5-minute screening tool for woman abuse (Greenberg, McFarlane, & Watson, 1997) reflects the pressure for nursing practice to control relationships in the interests of spending as little time as possible with any given patient or family. No matter how committed a nurse may be to practicing relationally, it becomes increasingly challenging to do so under these directives and in the absence of support for relational practice. Thus, to move beyond the problematic assumption that 'it is possible to *not* form and/or be in relationship when "doing" health care' involves not just changing one's understanding of relationality at the individual level. It also involves collectively joining with other nurses to effect change at the larger systemic levels.

Problematic Assumption 3: Communication Skills Are the Foundation of Relational Practice

Another assumption that has dominated nursing is that good behavioural communication skills are the foundation for relational practice. Again, this arises out of the disease-treatment model where the health professional is the one with the power and expertise to intervene and is augmented by a business model in which the dispensing of service (outputs) must be limited. However, if one pays close attention to a nurse who is in deep relation with a family, it quickly becomes apparent that the attributes of human relating extend far deeper into human 'being' than behavioural skills (Arndt, 1992; Gadow, 1985; Hartrick, 1997; Hartrick Doane, 2002; Montgomery, 1993; Watson, 1988). Human relating is a caring process that involves values, intent, knowledge, commitment, and actions (Watson, 1988). Although communication skills may be a helpful resource, to enter into deep relation, a nurse must move beyond thinking of relating as being comprised of using expert communication skills where one 'knows the right thing to say' or knows the right thing to 'do'. To deeply connect with another requires that we move beyond our trusty tools and techniques and open ourselves up to be in the uncertain waters of human relating.

● Transcending the Fear of Uncertainty

Perhaps one of the main reasons that we turn to communication skills and other tools or methods of practice is to try and control the health care encounter in order to reduce the uncertainty (Hartrick, 1997; Hartrick Doane, 2002b). Gadow (1999) maintains that nurses often bring a concern for certainty to their practice that leads them to adopt a reductionist perspective (that is, reducing things down). Wanting to be certain leads them to want to nail things down—to know what is 'really' going on. As a result nurses rely on a single, objectively identifiable element in a client's situation—searching for the 'real thing' (for example, the diagnosis; the real problem) underlying their client's symptoms and experiences. This search for certainty erodes the possibility of tuning into the meaningful experience of the family and ultimately leads all involved to reduce complex experiences to a singular explanation.

The following is a story told to me by a former nursing student who had previously been enrolled in a relational practice course I (Gweneth) taught. The story depicts how as nurses we are with families in their most vulnerable moments—moments of intense sorrow, fear, joy, and uncertainty. Yet we often fear those moments and feel inadequate—not knowing what to say or do. We share the story because it is one where the nurse was able to transcend her own fears and make a profound difference in the life of a family.

An Example: Night Shift In-Relation

I came on night shift and the charge nurse asked me if I *would special* a baby boy who had been born that day with a number of congenital anomalies. The parents had been told that their baby would likely die sometime during the night. I experienced a moment of panic. 'Can I actually do this? How will I do it? What will I say? I don't have the skill to do this!' The charge nurse told me that there was no one else and the parents really needed some support. I began to think back on the relationship course I had taken, 'What did I learn that would help me with this?' I remembered our class discussions about the importance of joining in-relation and that there was never a right thing to say or do. I reminded myself that what was important was my desire to connect and to care and my willingness to bring myself to that caring relationship. Those thoughts served as my guide throughout the night I spent with the family.

I went into the room and introduced myself to the parents. I explained that I would be with them during the night. In a very quiet voice the father told me the doctor had said their son would likely die soon and they wanted to have as much time with him as they could so they would have memories of him after he was gone. As he spoke, his wife began to cry. Without really being aware of what I was doing, I bent down next to the mother and baby and reached out to stroke the baby's face. Through a cracking voice and watering eyes I asked what they had already come to know about their son through their time together. They began to describe the little movements and gestures they had noticed, the family likenesses they could see, and other important things about their son. Throughout the night, we cried, laughed, talked, and were silent together as we watched and came to know their baby. At about 5:00 in the morning their son died in his mother's arms.

Weeks later, I received a 'Thank You' card from the parents. In the card the parents told me that although I had been with them in their son's death, their memories of that night were more about the short life I had helped them to have and to share with their son. They thanked me for my caring and for my compassion, and wrote it was one of the treasured memories from that night they would always carry with them (Hartrick, 1997).[1]

Perhaps the thing that stood out most for me (Gweneth) when the nurse in the story phoned to tell me of her experience was how she had opened up to, and honoured, the family's experience. She did not 'do' anything with their tears. Rather she intentionally chose to *be with* the family as they lived the joy as well as the sorrow they were experiencing being with their son. In joining the family, the nurse did not have to take responsibility to make it better or do anything to comfort them. Rather, following the lead of the family, she took the opportunity to learn from them about how she could be in-relation. That is, what she did was just follow the family's lead—they had told her that the most *significant* and *meaningful* thing to them was their desire to know and experience their son's short life. The nurse *listened* and *honoured that meaningful health and healing experience* by joining in with it. In order to do this, she needed to move beyond her own fears and angst—beyond what was meaningful to her in that moment—to attend to the family's experience. Once she shifted her attention to the family (and away from what was concerning her—for example, what *she* as the nurse should say or do for parents of a dying child), she spontaneously and intuitively knew how to join the family and *be in-relation with* them. In recounting the story to me, the nurse described that while she had perhaps helped the family, the experience had also served to transform her own vision of herself as a nurse. She learned from the family that she did know how to be in-relation—that deep within her she had the innate, human capacity and knowledge. Moreover she learned that she just needed to look beyond her own fears

---

[1] This story has been previously published in Hartrick, G. A. (1997). Relational capacity: The foundation for interpersonal nursing practice. *Journal of Advanced Nursing, 26,* 523–528 and is reprinted with permission from Blackwell Publishing.

and concerns, learn to trust herself and believe in the strength and capacities of families to be in and live through difficulty. This story illustrates how, as discussed in Chapter 5, consciously and intentionally paying attention to what we are finding of meaning and of concern enables us to transcend the fear of uncertainty, to join families and be informed by them and thus be more responsive to the people/families with whom we work.

As I (Gweneth) described in Chapter 5, one place where I have frequently observed concern for certainty is when I am teaching relational practice to nurses. Their feeling of responsibility and their desire to make things better for people who are experiencing difficulty often leads them to look for a problem to solve. Rather than joining families in their difficulty (remember Newman's theory of Health as Expanding Consciousness in Chapter 4) to open and learn about a person/family's experience in all of its complexity, many nurses immediately reduce families' situations and experiences to 'a problem' and focus the discussion on what can be done to address or fix the problem. When, in the case of death, for example, there is no action that can fix things they are ultimately left feeling helpless and inadequate—not knowing what they might do.

Stepping out of this habit of fixing is not easy. For example, when I work with students we videotape or audiotape the simulations and practices so we can relisten to the conversations. As we relisten, the students are often surprised and dismayed at how they have and/or have not responded. Although their intent is to listen and be responsive, they can hear how their own concern with fixing the problem was dominating to the point that they did not even hear what the person/family was trying to say. As they relisten to the tapes and observe themselves, they have the opportunity to hear their habits and concerns in action and begin to acknowledge how their fix-it habits are shaping what they focus on and how they respond when in-relation with families. This reflexive recognition is the first step in moving beyond the habit of fixing and toward more relational practice.

As nurses we are never *not* involved with the people for whom we care. Although we may believe that we can be objective, as Gadow (1999) purports, objectivity is merely a formula that gives precedence to nursing concerns rather than the concerns of the people with whom we work. To be aware of the personal/nursing concerns we bring, we must first acknowledge our own meaningful participation and involvement as a person/nurse. Through such acknowledgment we have the potential to move away from objectifying people and begin to respond to families in ways that are of meaning and significance to them.

As we described earlier, the nurse in the story was a student in our baccalaureate program. Subsequently she had read theory and ideas that informed and potentially enhanced her relational practice. However, what was crucial to her being able to join the family was relationally opening herself up to the fear and uncertainty she felt. As she acknowledged her own fears and addressed them (by listening to them, recalling knowledge that could guide her and refocusing her attention on being with the family), she came to know her own human capacity to be in caring relation. Therefore, as you continue to read, reflect, and 'try on' some of the ideas in this book, we hope you will take the opportunity to come to know yourself as a relational being—and that you will open up and experience the relational capacity that is already living within you.

● Beyond Objectification of Families

A distinguishing feature of relational family nursing practice is that *people* (as opposed to objects) are at the center. That is, families are not perceived and/or treated as objects to be observed and assessed and nurses do not detach from their person to don the role of professional (and objective) nurse. Family nursing that is relational does not reduce families to the moral status of objects.

Buber's (1958) distinction between I-It and I-Thou relationships is helpful in understanding the difference between objectified relational connections with families and humanly involved ones. An I-It relationship involves a relationship between a person and an object. Yalom (1980) describes that when relating to 'It' people hold back a part of themselves. From this detached stance they inspect, categorize, analyze, and make judgments about the 'other'. In this way I-It relationships are functional relationships that lack mutuality. Within the scientific, biomedical world of health care such functional relationships have tended to be the norm. As Parse (1998) describes, within the biomedical view practice focuses on diagnosing, treating, and/or preventing disease. For this reason the relationships formed are often very functional ones where the health professional inspects, categorizes, makes judgments about, and treats the "disease."

In contrast, the I-Thou relationship is a mutual relationship involving a full experiencing of the other (Yalom, 1980). Within the I-Thou relationship, one's whole being is involved. According to Buber (1958), whenever one person relates to another with less than her or his whole being—that is, holds something back or remains in the objective stance like a spectator—that person transforms an I-Thou encounter into an I-It one.

Buber's (1958) discussions emphasize the importance of the humanly involved nature of family nursing. However, nursing's failure to acknowledge and value the centrality of the person/nurse in relationships combined with an historical emphasis on health practitioners as detached professionals, and a current emphasis on economic interests that views families as commodities, have resulted in many nurses driving their person underground. They do not allow themselves and are not supported to engage in a humanly involved manner. For example, many nurses take up the professional veneer of objective expert as they complete 'an assessment' of a family. However, Tapp (2000) highlights the limitations of the 'expert' stance. In essence this stance of professional detachment is reflective of Freire's (1989) description of dehumanization. Freire contends that as people live or practice in an environment that does not allow their full human capacity to be expressed they become dehumanized. They lose the knowledge of themselves as people, of their power, and of the choices open to them. Freire asserts that to be human and to connect in a human way, one must be and express the person that one is. If nurses are to actualize their moral and practical commitment to families, they need to engage with people as people and work in practice environments where such engagement is possible. It is through this human-to-human process that nurses can come to understand their own meaningful human experience, access the knowledge that such understanding affords, and thereby be able to promote families' health and healing experiences (Tapp, 2000).

 ## An Example: Maureen's Story

The following story describes an experience a nurse colleague, Maureen Murphy-Dyson, had while working on a medical ward. We asked Maureen's permission to include her story because it exemplifies an I-Thou relationship. In engaging with a family, Maureen fully involved herself with the family as they lived through one of the most significant experiences of their lives. And she did so without objectifying them—without analyzing how well they were coping or trying to make them feel better.

The day I met Mr. D. was the first shift of my set. I learned on report that his death was imminent. He had a large, malignant brain tumor that was not treatable. He had declined rapidly in the last few days and was now in a confused and weakened state. He had a DNR (do not resuscitate) order. He had remained stable throughout the night, so his wife had gone home to try to get some sleep.

I did my rounds as soon as report was finished and met Mr. D. for the first time. He lay on his back with his eyes closed, in a four-bed ward. His large frame filled the hospital bed. I bent over him, said good morning, and introduced myself. He opened his eyes and a slow smile spread over his face. He was aphasic and seemed not to comprehend what I was saying, yet appeared to respond in pleasure to my talking. He clasped my hands as I spoke and searched my face intently but calmly as I chatted with him. I told him that I would be getting medications for the other patients and as soon as I finished I would help him wash up before his wife arrived. He smiled at me for a few more minutes and then he closed his eyes and dozed off.

Mr. D. slept as I gave out medications, which took about 20 minutes. When I returned to the room with towels and pajamas, I noticed that Mr. D.'s breathing was no longer audible. As I drew nearer, I could see that he was ashen and he did not respond to my voice. I drew the curtain around us. His breathing was shallow and intermittent. I felt a weak carotid pulse but I could not get a blood pressure. I leaned near him and told him I was going to be right there with him.

I stroked his hair and cheeks and he exhaled one last tremulous breath and did not draw in another.

As I waited for Mrs. D. to arrive, I removed the tubes from Mr. D. I quickly washed and shaved him, combed his hair and changed the top linen. I moved him into a treatment room and placed two chairs beside the bed.

Although I had never seen Mrs. D., I knew who she was by her demeanor. She hurried anxiously along the hall and I walked up to her and took her hand. She knew immediately that he was dead. "I'm too late . . ." Our eyes filled with tears. I gently confirmed that her husband had died a few minutes earlier. She grabbed me and held on to me. I told her how sorry I was and she asked me to come with her to see him.

Mrs. D. held my arm tightly as we entered the room. She approached her husband and looked at him. "Oh, my love," she said and she laid her face against his and wept. The side rail was down and she held him for many minutes. I stood close behind her and after a while, she turned to me and we looked at each other through teary eyes. She hugged me and I told her again what a gentle passing her husband had. She took comfort in that information because she said he was such a good man that it was only fitting that he should have such a peaceful death. Mr. and Mrs. D.'s daughter arrived and I left them alone. An hour later they emerged from his room, thanked me once again, and we said goodbye.

Seven months later, on Thanksgiving, the following letter and a small gift was delivered to the ward addressed 'To Maureen (in pink), who was on duty when G. D. passed away'.

My dear Maureen,

I have been wanting to write to you for some time. I just wanted to tell you how much it meant to me that you were with G. when he passed away. It was a consolation to me, as I didn't make it before he left us. . . . He always was early for his appointments.

When I saw the tears in your eyes, I knew that a warm and loving person had kept him company. I pray that you may never become so accustomed to death, that you will not mourn when somebody dies.

In his last years, he had become very fond of the birds that came to the feeder in our backyard, and I know that he would like you to have this little bird as a thank you from us both.

In August our second beautiful grandson was born. The new baby has many of his grandfather's facial expressions and is a bittersweet tears-and-laughter reminder that life goes on.

G. was one of a kind and will never be far from my thoughts, so that you can see how much your care meant to me.
Thank you again my dear and God bless,
Yours very sincerely
L. D.

For L. D., the woman who lost her husband, that 'moment in time' when she stood before Maureen and realized her husband had died was without doubt one of the most painful moments of her life. When Maureen first told me (Gweneth) the story and shared her letter I was struck not only by how Maureen had honoured the pain of those moments but also by the way she had been in-relation with the family. Although Mr. D. was her 'patient assignment', Maureen carried out her professional role and responsibility by deeply involving herself with both Mr. and Mrs. D. as people (not objects). At one point that meant joining with Mr. D. even though he did not seem to understand Maureen's words; at another it meant being 'with' him as he died. It also involved anticipating his family's grief and caring for them by washing and shaving Mr. D., combing his hair, and moving him into a space where his wife could have a private place to be with him. It is important to highlight how Maureen took her cue from Mrs. D.—as Mrs. D. held onto her arm, Maureen stayed with her and together they went into the room and Maureen stood quietly in the background offering unobtrusive support as Mrs. D. spent the last moments with her husband. Throughout the brief time she spent with the family, Maureen involved herself relationally by connecting human being to human being, by following the lead of both Mr. and Mrs. D., and by allowing herself to feel and express the emotion she experienced. The letter she received 7 months later shows us how Maureen's capacity and willingness to be in-relation with G. and L. D. and with her own deep emotions were not only profoundly meaningful but also resonated relationally in time and space. Even though she had only really been with them for a period of minutes, 7 months later the family still experienced this relational connection as a new grandchild was born and 'life went on'. Her brief relational connection served to support their ongoing healing.

Maureen's story exemplifies how joining relationally with people even during brief and transient moments can have significant impact on people/families; it highlights how deeply touching another does not necessarily require 'more' time but rather requires the capacity to relationally involve oneself during the time one has; and, it reminds us how important it is to be present in ways that are meaningful to the families we are with.

● Beyond Commodification of Family

Another distinguishing feature of relational practice is that while people are at the center of such practice, the contextual features of that practice are always kept in view. From Maureen's story we do not know much about the context of her practice. What made it possible for her to practice as she did with the family? Did her colleagues value her way of practicing? Did her colleagues adjust her assignment? Pick up some of her other work? Give her positive feedback for her support of the family? Were there no other patients requiring the treatment room? Because relational practice focuses not only on our relationships with particular families, but also on particular situations and our relationships to ideas and contexts, we continuously must be mindful of the ways in which our contexts of practice are shaping our thinking about families and the possibilities for practice.

The dominant view promoted by a business approach to health care is one of families as commodities (Björnsdóttir, 2001; Rankin, 2004). Rankin shows how under health care reform, managers' work is organized to focus on patients and families as units of resource utilization and expenditure. For example, during her research Rankin observed how one team leader began his shift by taking stock of the patients' charts, making the following comments on each patient in turn:

> This patient is complex, she has had a CVA (stroke) and a recent MI (heart attack), she has liver metastasis (cancer), she has a husband but there are no supports.

> This is a social admission 'Failure to Cope'. Penny (social worker) will be ticked off, but if we need a cardiac bed that will be the first one, he really should be designated ALC (alternative level of care).

Her son is in (Small Town), that's important.

This patient lives alone in (Small Town); he has a son in (Big City).

These are difficult ones. The frail elderly fractures. She has a niece who lives in (Big City).

This elderly gentleman only has a brother—that does not bode well.

Each family was evaluated as a commodity for the potential cost and cost savings to the health care system. Such a view of family leads to relationships in which nurses process families through health care as quickly as possible, limiting their relationships to the brokering of resources and the management of care by family members.

An Example: Janet's Story

A woman I know was diagnosed with advanced cancer of the bladder 1 year ago. After much deliberation, she made the decision to have a radical cystectomy. During her hospitalization, her care was less than acceptable. Many times she rang the call bell before it was answered. She was not one to ask for help often. Young nurses called her 'sweety' and 'honey' and when I visited, I would see nurses' eyes roll at the smallest request.

When the woman was ready for discharge, there was minimal instruction given to care for her stoma, and follow-up care was nonexistent. The staff were more concerned that the bed be evacuated by eleven o'clock.

Within 24 hours of returning home, the woman became confused. Her daughter was worried, as she had never been confused a day in her life. It took four visits to different physicians to have her readmitted to the hospital. All four physicians told the daughter that confusion was not uncommon for a woman her mother's age, seeming not to hear what her daughter was telling them. When one of the physicians told the woman that all the cancer cells had been removed, because of her confusion, the woman had no idea what the physician was talking about. One week later, while being treated for sepsis, the woman had a stroke, leaving her unable to speak or move the right side of her body. She had been discovered by a nurse at about 3:00 PM, was moved to a room down the hallway, and an internist was called. He came at about 7:00 PM, but did not order any tests or medications. The family was called.

A CAT scan was done 24 hours later, and results given to the family 24 hours after that. The woman was frequently incontinent, and because the staff rarely came, most of her care was left to her daughters.

The fifth day following the stroke, the physician on call came and examined the woman. He found her heart rate was 144, and she was moaning in obvious pain. After reviewing her chart he found that she had not been given ordered medications and no one had addressed the families' request for a conference.

The physician ordered morphine to make her comfortable. He spent time with the family. When shown a picture of the woman taken 3 weeks prior to the day, he could not believe it was the same woman—she appeared to have aged 15 years.

She died that night after her family left the hospital. The next morning when her daughters returned to the hospital to pick up her belongings, no one knew who she was. She had been on the same ward for 2 weeks, and not one staff member recognized her name or was aware of her death. The woman was my mother, and I one of the daughters who sat by her bed. My mother's name was Mrs. Margaret MacPherson.

This story was sent to me (Colleen) by Janet Munro, a student and an experienced nurse. Janet asked that her mother's real name be used, as her mother would have 'loved to see her name in print'. It seems especially important that her name be used, given that she died, unlike Mr. D. in Maureen's story, anonymously and alone. This story illustrates that relational practice is not only a matter of individual nurses being willing to connect relationally with those to whom they are assigned to provide care. In Mrs. MacPherson's care there was no nurse who connected, relationally or otherwise. Thus, this story highlights a whole system of failure—the family was 'bundled out the door' following surgery and left to fend on their own until her death. In the opinion of the chief coroner (Janet took her mother's case to the coroner's office), her mother's elderly appearance was the sole reason for the withholding of thrombolytic therapy following her stroke, despite the fact that she met all medical and hospital policy criteria. In her analysis of the situation, Janet wrote "Not one person acknowledged our grief; in fact, nurses seemed surprised at how upset we were. How could they know the enormous loss we were facing? They hadn't seen her playing with our children a week before, they hadn't seen the latest computer program she was developing, they didn't know about the trip she was planning. They didn't know because they didn't look past her physical appearance, making assumptions of their own. . . . There was a time when I believed that it was best not to get personally involved. How wrong I was . . . just a 2-minute interaction with anyone who asked about our mother's life, her loves, her experiences, would have made all the difference. Maybe then they could have seen the valuable life she was ending'.

Relational practice then, involves not only the capacity to engage relationally with particular families, but also the capacity to create conditions that make relational engagement between nurses and families possible.

● Relational Capacity

The most important resource each nurse brings to practice is the person he or she is. Although you might learn communication skills and techniques that can enhance your ability to be in-relation, the best way to be effective relationally is 'to be yourself'. When I (Gweneth) was doing a master's degree in counseling psychology that focused on developing advanced communication skills, I gradually became aware that although I might be gaining new behavioral skills I was losing myself. That is, it seemed to me that the strong focus on performing the communication skills correctly led me to put my own spontaneous way of being aside. Over time I became increasingly aware of how everyone in my advanced skill course began to sound the same to the point of even using the same phrases when interacting with people—phrases that had been learned from textbooks and that felt very stiff and unnatural. I began to feel more like a parrot more than a person.

That experience, combined with my experiences of teaching relational practice, has convinced me that the best way for people to develop their relational practice is

- to recognize and enhance their own spontaneous relational capacities,
- to develop the ability for intentional action.

By now it should be obvious that developing relational practice is not *only* a matter of who and how you are in-relation to particular patients and families. Rather, who you are and how you are in-relation is shaped by the colleagues you work with, by managers, by your practice environment, and by policies that govern health care delivery. Subsequently the focus of the remainder of this chapter is on helping you look within yourself to gain greater awareness of who and how you are relationally in this broad sense. Are you someone who naturally uses humour to connect with people? Are you someone who is comfortable when people express painful emotions? Are you a good listener? How do you naturally and spontaneously reach out to connect with others? For example, how do you pay attention to and honour people who might be from a different background than yours? Do you feel uncertain, intimidated, fearful? Do you tend to critically question practices that others take for granted? Do you tend to raise questions and challenges to practices that you see as unfair? Do you pay attention to your discomfort when you are directed (for example, by a policy, a more senior nurse, or a manager) to do something that does not sit well with you? As you read through this chapter, think about what you are reading within the context of those questions. And continually ask yourself: What is my natural style of communicating? What do I bring to relationships and how might I enhance what I already bring? What habits of conduct have I developed that can serve me well and what habits are constraining me?

In the next sections we discuss the capacities and skills that we believe support the ability of nurses to engage with families relationally. As you read and reflect on what we present, remember that the only 'right' way to be is yourself. The capacities and skills we offer are not offered as 'truth', rather they are offered to spark examination of your own current practice and to support the enhancement of your ability to express and live the spontaneous, compassionate person who is already living within you.

● What Are Important Relational Capacities?

Stop for a moment and try to identify someone who you would say is 'good at relationships'. It might be a nurse you have observed or someone you know or have known in your personal life. If you have difficulty thinking of someone, try to remember a time when you were with

---

TRY IT OUT 6.1.   **An Exemplary Relational Practitioner**

1. As we suggest above, *identify* someone who you would say is 'good at relationships'. Why did you identify that person? What qualities or characteristics stand out?
2. *Now identify* someone who is a nurse and is good at relationships. Think of someone with whom you have worked—perhaps a fellow student, a colleague, an instructor. What makes them good at relationships? How is this person perceived by his or her colleagues?
3. *Compare notes* with someone else. Talk to someone who has thought about this question, or talk to someone who knows the person or people you have identified. Do you both value similar attributes and qualities?

---

someone and felt understood and/or welcomed by a particular person. As you recall the person, try to identify what it was about her or him that was relational. What qualities or characteristics stand out? Try It Out 6.1 suggests that you do this and compare notes with someone else.

As we have observed nurses who we view as exemplary relational practitioners, we have noticed particular capacities they seem to bring to their relationships. These capacities include the capacity of initiative, authenticity, and responsiveness; the capacity to be mutual and 'in sync' with people; and the capacity to engage with complexity and live in ambiguity (Hartrick, 1997). We offer descriptions of these capacities in the following sections. As you consider these capacities think of them in light of your own practice—how do you live and express the capacities described? Are there other capacities you have that are not identified here? As we describe these capacities, we include examples from a study a nurse colleague, Robin McMillan (2003), conducted. Robin researched the relational experiences of community health workers who care for people/families in their homes. With the permission of her participants, she generously shared her data with us to help provide pictures of what the capacities we describe might look like in practice.

The Capacity of Initiative, Authenticity, and Responsiveness

> 66 *The first connection is to walk in the front door and take a deep breath (to get a feel of the whole). (I) Let it go into my body and cells. I can feel joy, love, anger, contentment, peace. I look around to see how they place things and what the things are. A cross, angels, collector spoons, hanging crafts, afghans on couches. I do a total assessment of what I need to know before saying 'hello' in the first minute.* 99

This quote offers an example of how people who involve themselves relationally do not just do so verbally but with all of their senses and faculties. In the quote it is possible to hear the community health worker tuning into her bodily knowing (as we described in Chapter 5) to see, hear, and come to know the family she is meeting. Overall the capacity of initiative refers to the will and exercised intent to know and join families as they are. As Thayer-Bacon (2003) contends, the first step in understanding another is to notice them—to value them enough to notice and try to understand. Thus, initiative involves a reaching out and intending toward the family—listening intently and suspending doubts or judgments long enough to make sure we have heard what the other is relating (Thayer-Bacon, 2003). This capacity involves the desire and ability to move beyond habits that block such connection and/or that hinder one's ability to see and hear what is meaningful and significant to particular people and families. It also involves the ability and willingness to recognize and challenge contextual elements that are hindering relational practice.

> 66 *If it feels right, talk. If it feels right, be quiet. If it feels right to make a little bit of a joke about something, I'll do that. If my heart starts to palpitate I go quiet because there is something wrong. There is something wrong with the conversation so I go quiet until I can sort out what's actually happening in the room, because sometimes what you think is happening is not actually happening. So take your gut instincts.* 99

Nurses who engage relationally listen carefully to families and to their own bodily knowing. They come as authentic people to be humanly present with another. Through this authentic connection, action is guided by a spontaneity and responsiveness to the experience in the moment. The quote about 'if it feels right, talk' depicts how by listening broadly and carefully it is possible to follow the lead of people/families and relationally determine one's nursing actions in the moment. When a nurse has the *initiative* to be with another in an *authentic* way, she or he is able to *respond* to the other as they are in that moment. As in the example earlier, the nurse who stayed with the family whose baby was dying came to understand that it is not a matter of finding the 'the right thing to say', but rather the focus is on being with a family, listening to the experience of the family, being informed by them, and responding by following their lead. The capacity for initiative, authenticity, and responsiveness can be experienced and/or enacted in different forms. For example, in the Box 6.1 a nurse colleague, Camille Roberts, describes how these relational capacities are central to her practice of therapeutic touch.

The Capacity to Be Mutual and 'In Sync'

> 66 *Our connection was quite odd because she didn't always understand words. She would look at you and you weren't sure if she was with you or not. So I did a pantomime like . . . we did charades. The husband would be a participant in the charades. We got her to say words playing this charades because I would be her echo. I was her voice. What I was pantomiming wasn't exactly what I was trying to say, it was more what she was telling me to do so that I could tell her husband what she wanted. It wasn't food or drink or anything like that. It was what she wanted to do in the garden or that she didn't like the blue blouse that he put on her and that's why she took a swing at him. She didn't really mean it, she just didn't like the blue blouse.* 99

BOX 6.1. **Relational Capacities and Therapeutic Touch**

The similarities I see with therapeutic touch and relational nursing practice is how one enters into relation with people and how one comes to 'know' them. For example, when one is using therapeutic touch with another, there is a knowing that extends beyond what is physically observable and measurable and what is known with the conscious mind: There is an awareness of the interconnectedness of all and an alertness to how we are part of the same open energy system. Hence, when relating to another, this underlying assumption of unity moves one to relate in a manner distinct from one based on a Cartesian objective view. Therapeutic touch begins with the centering of consciousness and it is this centered place that one works from. The impetus to help or heal is based on compassion to be with another, which to me is similar to the capacity of initiative, authenticity, and responsiveness. The concern one has for and about another speaks to a state of being that both the capacity of initiative, autheniticity, and responsiveness and the process of therapeutic touch share as a starting point. It is this openness and desire to respond that is the foundation of the exchange. The state of being of self is integral to the whole process. It is both a letting go of self and being 'in self' simultaneously, as one's consciousness becomes quiet, present, and alert to what is happening both with one's self and the other. Therapeutic touch uses the hands and the 'inner ear' to sense the energy field of the person—A 'listening' of the hands, so to speak; a willingness to be open to perceptions picked up as 'cues' in the field. This receptivity is also core to being in-relation. When receptive to another, there is an exchange, an exchange of life energy. The information gathered with one's hands, often referred to as 'cues', frequently relates to an imbalance in the field. There are several ways of picking up cues, as well as a variety of cues that present themselves in the field. For example, there can be congestion, blank areas, or overly charged, tingly areas to name but a few. Similar to field imbalances in therapeutic touch, verbal (or nonverbal) messages are often a means of relating to imbalances in life. That is, imbalance can also present itself in dialogue, as when one is relating a state of being such as pain, hurt, sadness, anger. These states are essentially times of being out of balance in one's life perceptions.

The quote here offers an example of the capacity for mutality and synchrony. This community health worker joined 'in sync' with the woman to know and respond to what was meaningful and significant to her. In spite of the difficulties in communicating, she creatively thought of a way of working in collaboration with the couple to figure out how they might address their health challenge and live in ways that were more 'right' for them. By being in-mutual-relation, it is possible to experience the commonalities of visions, goals, sentiments, or characteristics, as well as to recognize and acknowledge differences. Although mutuality supports the shared validation of persons in the relationship, being in sync allows nurses to join the rhythmic patterns of families (remember the human science theories in Chapter 3). We will be discussing the process of being in sync in more detail in Chapter 7.

The Capacity to Engage With Complexity and Live In Ambiguity

❝ *I find it easy to pick up, almost instantly where someone is and then to respond or pull back from them to get right to that real clarity of expression. I move into this efficiency place where the tasks happen in connection with what the feelings are. It's always adjusting. There is never anything that is the same, from moment to moment. If you are in the moment with someone, it's always going to be different. . . . You never know who is going to phone and talk to them and change their whole perception of what needs to be done. This is normal living. It's always a constant flow.* **"**

People who bring the capacity to engage with complexity and live in ambiguity understand that any human experience is complex and ambiguous. They are willing to trust and practice within the uncertainty of any relational moment. Their ability and willingness to engage with complexity and live in ambiguity allow them to open up to the complexities within a particular experience rather than reduce experiences to problems and seek a single, definite direction. This capacity leads them to be curious and to question the feelings, thoughts, and meanings within the situation and to seek to understand the multiple (and often conflicting) meanings of the experience for the person/family. At the same time they are able to make connections between the different elements and meanings within the experience and, with the help of the family, realize the relevance of the experience for subsequent action.

Engaging with complexity means looking beyond immediate persons/families to see how their experiences are being shaped by language, structures, organizations, cultures, policies, and so on. Although being in sync allows nurses to join the energetic and rhythmic patterns of families, engaging with complexity allows nurses to inquire about the influences shaping those patterns and to discern wider social patterns that shape experiences across many 'literal' families. Such understanding widens possibilities for intentional action beyond relationships with particular families. So, for example, a nurse on the unit where Janet's mother died might take action to counter some of the practices Janet and her family experienced, so that other families would not have similar experiences. Engaging with complexity and ambiguity also reminds us to always 'reserve judgment', that is, we may make a judgment or take an action, but we should always remember that no judgment or action is 'final'—new understandings or possibilities change our judgments and actions continuously as we inquire and follow the lead of families in rapidly changing contexts.

● Developing Skillful Relational Practice

We believe that all nurses bring these capacities to their work and have the potential to develop these capacities further. However, contextual factors have often overshadowed or hindered the expression of these capacities. Just like the nurse in the story earlier who stayed with the family while their baby died, many nurses believe they do not have the knowledge or skill necessary to 'be' in-relation during challenging situations. Moreover, the assumptions that have historically governed nursing education (Hartrick, 1997, 1999; Hartrick Doane, 2002) combined with the dominance of the disease-treatment and business approaches to health care (Varcoe et al., 2003; Varcoe & Rodney, 2002; Varcoe, Rodney, & McCormick, 2003) have led nurses to develop practices that actually constrain their own relational capacities and reduce their ability to be in responsive relation with families. For these reasons we have found that developing skillful relational practice often involves more unlearning than learning. That is, in contrast to the idea that one becomes skilled by gaining new methods and techniques (for example, communication skills) more often than not, the skillfulness of relational practice often entails removing known habits (Hartrick Doane, 2002). Varela, Thompson, and Rosch's (1993) analogy of being born 'already knowing how to play the violin and practicing with great exertion only to remove the habits that prevented one from displaying that virtuosity' (p. 251) captures how relational skillfulness is developed. Becoming a skillful relational nurse requires the ability to consciously step out of known habits (such as the disease-care assumptions described earlier in this chapter or the scarcity-driven assumptions described in Chapter 3) that are hindering you from tapping your own capacity for relational connection.

The nurse described earlier who stayed with the family during the night their baby died had to:

- step out of her habit of focusing on her own concerns and performance (that is, she had to move beyond worrying about what she was going to say, trying to find the right response),
- step out of the habit of problematizing and objectifying families (for example, move beyond thinking of these people as 'a family with a dying child' or thinking of them as 'bed blockers'),
- move beyond thinking the family situation was a problem she needed to fix or at least make better,
- move beyond her habit of thinking 'she didn't have the expertise' to be in deep relation with a family,
- resist organizational pressures to prioritize other concerns (for example, a new admission).

As she consciously stepped out of these habits, followed the lead of the family, and focused on being in-relation with them, she was able to open up to her human capacity to meaningfully relate in an authentic manner. Through her experience she not only experienced the transformative power of relationship but also gained greater confidence in her own relational capacity and a sense of trust in her ability to be with people/families in ways that are authentic, meaningful, and health promoting.

Some Things That Need to Be Unlearned or Challenged

Developing skillful relational practice involves unlearning known habits that get in the way of joining people responsively (Hartrick Doane, 2002). Following is a list of habits that may need to be unlearned.

1. *We need to unlearn the habit of looking for the master key or truth that will offer certainty in our practice.* This involves realizing that because

human life is relational, complex, and changeable there is no possible way we can know for certain which is the best way to proceed or know for certain 'what is really going on' for people. Competent, skillful practice does not rest on certainty but rather on inquiry—safe practice is grounded in a continual process of questioning how best to proceed with particular families in particular situations.

2. *We need to unlearn the habit of thinking that human experience is a problem to be solved.* Although people may identify problems in their lives, any experience involves far more than a problem. That is, there are always meanings, emotions, contextual elements, choices, and ambiguities. Therefore we need to move beyond the habit of thinking we need to 'find out what is really going on' and 'make it better' and begin trusting in families' capacities to live through difficulty. As Freire (1989) describes, 'A real humanist can be identified more by his (sic) trust in the people, which engages him in their struggle, than by a thousand actions in their favour without that trust' (p. 47). This does not mean we do not offer support for people to address problems in their lives—rather it just changes the nature of the support we offer. We move from expert 'fixers' to inquiring facilitators.

3. *We need to unlearn the habit of distancing ourselves and/or attempting to disconnect from people.* Rather than taking up a professionally distant stance and treating people as objects we are observing, or taking up our busy gait and 'doing to' people in the name of efficiency, we need to cultivate the habit of I-Thou relationships even in brief and transitory moments. This does not mean acting toward a patient as one would a friend, rather as Parse (1998) describes it means involving oneself as a compassionate stranger.

4. *We need to unlearn the habit of decontextualizing people.* The dominance of biomedicine and liberal ideology combined with a business approach to health care make it difficult at times for us to see the people/families behind the labels. 'I have 15 high risks (families) to see'; 'we had three codes going on at once'. Seeing people/families in context means seeing how their cultural, social, and economic circumstances shape their lives. Try It Out 6.2 invites you to think

---

TRY IT OUT 6.2.   A Success in Your Life

1. *Think* of a success in your life. Have you done well in school? Done well at your job? Raised a child well? Cared for a family member? Supported a friend during a difficult time? Managed a business?
2. *Reflect* on what and who made that success possible, besides yourself. For example, as a person who grew up with a violent, sexually abusive father, people have often asked me (Colleen) how I 'did it' (referring to my career or family or whatever). It is tempting to think of myself as a strong individual who survived a horrible childhood due to my 'resilience'. However, when I look around, I see all the privileges that I enjoyed—a grandmother who gave me unconditional love; a mother and siblings who suffered too, but lent strength as they could; access to education; adequate food and shelter; a few good teachers here and there.
3. *Trace* your success to the resources and people that made it possible. Did you do it alone? What can you learn about furthering your future success?

BOX 6.2. **Nursing a Hurt Community**

This year, for a change, Cathy Crowe is celebrating Thanksgiving.

Normally, October is a time of tension and anxiety for the committed street nurse. The nights are getting chilly. The homeless shelters are getting crowded. She will soon have to fight her yearly battle against hypothermia, frostbite, tuberculosis and indifference. Crowe is not expecting this winter to be any kinder than the last 15. Yet she is feeling thankful, valued and unusually optimistic.

Last weekend, she flew to Amsterdam to receive the Human Rights and Nursing Award, presented by the International Centre for Nursing Ethics to a nurse who combines professional accomplishment and social responsibility. Now, she is taking a bit of time to savour the experience and reflect on the changed political circumstances at home. Crowe left Toronto on the eve of the Ontario election. She will return, after a brief European vacation, on Saturday.

'It was a simple, quiet ceremony before 40 or 50 nurses from around the world', she said in a phone interview. 'From the first moment I arrived, I felt that people were on the same plane as I am. I didn't have to explain that fighting for a national housing program is part of nursing. I didn't have to convince anyone that homelessness is a violation of one of the most basic human rights'.

At home, she often does. People wonder why a trained nurse practitioner spends her time checking back alleys, attending inquests for street people and organizing homeless coalitions. Other health-care professionals wonder what public advocacy has to do with treating patients.

In Amsterdam, she was surrounded by nurses who had worked with refugees, orphans and victims of war. They took it for granted that part of nursing was to speak out for vulnerable groups. They honoured her efforts.

'It was heart-warming and inspiring', Crowe said. 'It will fuel my determination to keep working to end homelessness'.

She is hoping the change of government at Queen's Park will make the struggle a little easier.

Premier-designate Dalton McGuinty has promised to build 20,000 units of affordable housing, provide shelter allowances to the province's poorest 35,000 families and protect tenants from rent gouging.

Like most social activists, Crowe is encouraged, but wary.

'We have to stay 100 per cent vigilant', she said. 'It's a relief that the doors are finally open to social policy change, but we'll have to be extremely creative in the way we work with the new government'.

She fears that McGuinty is inheriting a much emptier treasury and a much more damaged social infrastructure than he realizes. She expects that it will take years—if it happens at all—to reverse former premier Mike Harris' harsh workfare rules.

For the moment, though, Crowe is relieved that she will no longer have to deal with the regime that slashed social assistance rates, cancelled public housing projects, froze the minimum wage and made being poor a source of shame.

Grateful as she is to be the recipient of this year's Human Rights and Nursing Award, it embarrasses her, as a Canadian, to stand before her peers and admit that 250,000 people in one of the world's richest countries have no place to live. It worries her that she feels more at home with nurses working in disaster zones than with her professional colleagues in Canada.

This is not the first time 51-year-old street nurse has been recognized for her work. She was awarded an honorary doctorate by the University of Victoria two years ago and given a 1998 achievement award by her alma mater, Ryerson University. She was featured in a documentary entitled *Street Nurse*, by Emmy-award-winning director Shelley Saywell.

Outwardly, Crowe is gregarious, open-hearted and bubbly. But her friends have seen the steel behind the smile.

'There have been so many difficult times, so many clashes with the authorities', said developer David Walsh, who works with Crowe on the Toronto Disaster Relief Commit-

> ┌───┐
> **BOX 6.2.** **Nursing a Hurt Community** (continued)
>
> tee. 'But she keeps speaking out. She keeps looking for new ways to raise the profile of the homeless'.
>
> Outreach worker Beric German, who describes Crowe as his 'best friend', has watched her struggle, time and again, to address the wounds that medicine cannot heal. In the mid '80s, she helped found Nurses for Social Responsibility to draw attention to the link between poverty and poor health. In the '90s, she co-founded the Toronto Disaster Relief Committee to fight for solutions to homelessness.
>
> And this fall, she is working with a new group called HOME (Housing Ontario Means Everyone) to mobilize low-income tenants to vote. 'She's always willing to stretch herself', German said.
>
> Crowe is touched by such accolades, pleased that her cause is in the public eye. But the prize she covets most, a pledge by all three levels of government to commit 1 per cent of every tax dollar to affordable housing, still eludes her.
>
> She will give thanks for life's blessings, then get back to work.
>
> *(From Carol Goar, 2003,* **Toronto Star**, *October 13.)*

about a success you have had as a way of continuing to develop your thinking about the importance of context. Seeing health and health care in context means seeing how cultural, social, political, and economic patterns shape all families, advantaging some and disadvantaging others. Read "Nursing a Hurt Community" (Box 6.2). To what extent do you think Cathy Crowe has unlearned the habit of decontextualizing people?

5. *We need to unlearn the habit of accepting systemic structures and systems as taken for granted*—as 'just the way things are'. Within the business model of health care, and the trends of health care reform, ideas are promoted that efficiency is the overriding value, that time and resources are simply 'not there' (as opposed to being used elsewhere), and that everyone (including patients) just has to learn to do with less. The public is encouraged to think that they are at fault and induced to make sacrifices (Northcott, 1994). Nurses (along with the rest of the public) are encouraged to take these ideas for granted and focus on making the best of things, rather than recognizing that these 'realities' are choices, and challenging them as such. When, for example, a hospital decides to lay off nurses at the same time as an expensive new computer system is purchased, this decision is not a 'reality', it is a *decision*. In the article "Nursing a Hurt Community", Cathy Crowe is quoted as saying that when she went to meet with nurses from the International Center for Nursing and Ethics, 'From the first moment I arrived, I felt that people were on the same plane as I am. I didn't have to explain that fighting for a national housing program is part of nursing'. We need to shift from accepting structures and systems that constrain health promotion to seeing social and political action as 'part of nursing'.

6. *We need to unlearn the habit of working in isolation.* Just as families and health are lived relationally in context, nursing work is also carried out in context. Nursing work is lived in a relational matrix

(Rodney, Brown, & Liaschenko, 2004). Whether we are aware of it or not, and whether we consciously attend to the relational matrix or not, our nursing actions are always carried out in-relation to our colleagues as well as in-relation to patients/families and the structures organizing our practice. Rather than unmindfully allowing these to influence us, we can purposefully make the most of these relations. To that end, each of the skills we outline in the following sections are intended to be taken up, not by individual nurses in relation *to* patients/families, but in concert *with* patient/families and *colleagues.*

● Cultivating the Skills of Relational Practice

As the earlier stories depict, relational practice is a humanely involved process of respectful, compassionate, and authentically interested inquiry into another (and one's own) experiences (Hartrick Doane, 2002). To deeply connect requires that nurses move beyond their habits of expertise and certainty and begin to act in ways that honour and address the complexity and ambiguity of human life. Relational connection requires that nurses turn to people/families/experiences and open themselves up to their fullness and depth. As Paterson and Zderad (1988) describe, it requires that nurses be willing to be surprised and to feel excitement, fear, uncertainty, or whatever is sparked through the inquiry process.

We believe that there are particular skills that can enhance the relational capacities you already bring. These skills include the:

- skill of letting be
- skill of listening
- skill of self-observation
- skill of questioning to look beyond the surface
- skill of intentionality
- skill of interrupting contextual constraints
- skill of reimagining.

The Skill of Letting Be

Perhaps one of the most important skills of relational practice is knowing how to 'let be' (Hartrick Doane, 2002). Situated in and constituted by powerful discourses of 'problem solving', 'alleviation', 'change', 'management', 'intervention', and 'efficiency', nurses experience tremendous anguish at the thought of being with people as they are—of letting be. The habit of striving to alleviate the problem is a difficult one to move beyond. Yet as complexity theory (described in Chapter 2) informs us, given the relational nature of life, nurses do not actually have the power or ability to effect change in any predictable or linear (cause-effect) way. Rather the power and potential for change is tapped by joining into the relational flow of health that families are living. The way one joins into this relational flow is by letting be—by not seeking to change, but to join people as they are. To develop the skill of letting be it is helpful to move beyond the dualism of either letting be or changing (Hartrick Doane, 2002). For example, many nurses interpret letting be to mean 'everything remains the same, things are not changed'. When we step out of dualistic thinking we open up to the possibility of seeing letting be as the most powerful way in which change is promoted. Letting be involves 'being open to know what is'. As we join others as they are and let be, they are invited to open up to that which they are at that moment. Inner movement occurs when life can be received as it is, without asking it to be something else (Desmarais & Hamel, 1996). Experiences open up and begin moving, and changes occur. However, as complexity theory informs us, the change that occurs is unpredictable and will depend on a number of variables. At the same time, as we let families be (and support their own process of change) we cannot only be informed by them but we are free to turn our nursing attention and action to other possibilities, such as effecting the systemic structures that constrain health and health promoting practice.

An experienced emergency room nurse, Lorna Jeffries, offers one of the simplest examples of letting be (Jeffries, 1998). Lorna described how, as she receives a patient from an ambulance, she consciously reaches out to be in-relation with the person lying on the stretcher. She has observed that by joining people in their experiences ('letting be to know what is'), people's level of anxiety and pain seems to decrease. At the same time, this presencing or letting be enables her to tune into

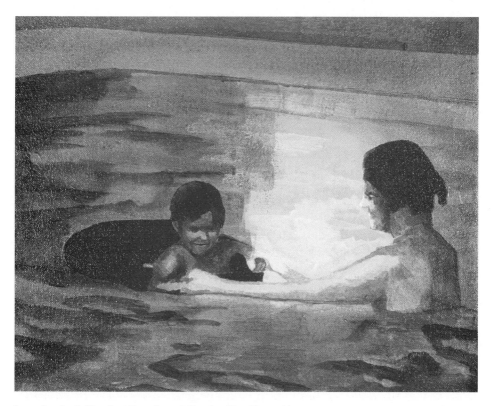

Learning by letting be. (Acrylic painting by Alex Grewal.)

what is most pressing—to learn from the person. We are not suggesting that the decrease in anxiety and pain is (from a linear cause-effect perspective) a result of Lorna's action; however, we are suggesting that given all of the other variables that contribute to the experience of coming to the emergency department in crises, her intentional relational intervention of presencing in this way and of letting be contributes to their sense of control and ease. For example, when Lorna stops (for a few seconds) in the midst of a hectic emergency department to look distressed people in the eye and relationally engage, those people have the experience of being seen, acknowledged, and valued as a person amidst the chaos—she communicates that they matter, that they are seen and that she is 'with' them. In this way, letting be is both a skill and a process. In Chapter 7 we explore the process of letting be in more depth.

The Skill of Listening

> 66 When we are listened to, it creates us, makes us unfold and expand. Ideas actually begin to grow within us and come to life. You know if a person laughs at your jokes you become funnier and funnier, and if he (sic) does not, every tiny little joke in you weakens up and dies. Well, that is the principle of it. It makes people happy and free when they are listened to. And, if you are a listener, it is the secret of having a good time in society (because everybody around you becomes lively and interesting), of comforting people, of doing them good. (Ueland, 1992, p. 104) 99

Rogers (1961) contends that listening is all the 'doing' that is necessary to promote well-being. Ueland (1992) describes listening as a magnetic force that can provide an opportunity for re-creation and discovery. Although we tend to think of listening as something we do with our ears, to truly listen requires enlistment of all of our senses. We come to know people/families not just from what they say, but from what they communicate energetically, bodily, contextually, and so forth. Therefore, listening requires opening up to hear what it is that is being communicated in multiple ways. As described in Chapter 5, our bodily sensing is a powerful way of listening and coming to know a family and situation. Listening works in concert with the skill of letting be. Unfortunately often people/nurses listen with one ear while they are busy thinking about what they want to say in response. There is a vast difference between 'listening' and 'waiting to speak'. Or we listen for the purpose of intervening to change things and/or give advice. Again, there is a vast difference between listening and waiting to act. Together using the skills of letting be and listening, nurses can offer the opportunity for people to affirm the choices they are making and/or consider options in light of their beliefs and customs and in light of their health and healing experience. The poem in Box 6.3 is a helpful reminder of how important it is to listen and let be. Try it out with the ideas in Try It Out 6.3. Building on the skill of listening, in Chapter 7 we discuss the *process of 'listening to and for'* that is central to relational family nursing practice.

BOX 6.3. **Listen and Let Be**

Listen

When I ask you to listen to me
and you start giving me advice
you have not done what I asked.

When I ask you to listen to me
and you begin to tell me why I shouldn't feel that way,
you are trampling on my feelings.

When I ask you to listen to me
and you feel you have to do something to solve my problem,
you have failed me, strange as that may seem.

Listen! All I ask, is that you listen,
not talk or do—just hear me.

Advice is cheap—10 cents will get you both Dear Abby
and Billy Graham in the same newspaper.

And I can do that for myself; I'm not helpless.
Maybe discouraged and faltering, but not helpless.

When you do something for me that I can and need to do
for myself, you contribute to my fear and weakness.

But, when you accept as a simple fact that I do feel what I feel,
no matter how irrational,
then I can quit trying to convince you
and can get about the business of understanding what's behind
this irrational feeling.

And when that's clear, the answers are obvious
and I don't need advice.
Irrational feelings make sense when we understand.

Perhaps that's why prayer works, sometimes, for some people,
because God is mute and he doesn't give advice or try to fix things.
"They" just listen and let you work it out for yourself.

So, please listen and just hear me.
And, if you want to talk, wait a minute for your turn;
and I'll listen to you.

    Anonymous

If You Are Going To Be With Me:

1. Please be patient while I decide if I can trust you.
2. Let me tell my story. The whole story, in my own way.
3. Please accept that whatever I have done, whatever I may do, is the best I have to offer and seemed right at the time.
4. I am not a person. I am this person, *unique* and special.
5. Don't judge me as right or wrong. Bad or good. I am what I am and that's all I've got.
6. Don't assume that your knowledge about me is more accurate than mine. You only know what I've told you. That's only part of me.
7. Don't ever think that you know what I should do—you don't. I may be confused but I am still the expert about me.
8. Don't place me in a position of living up to your expectations. I have enough trouble with my own.
9. Please hear my feelings. Not just my words—accept all of them. If you can't, how can I?
10. Don't save me! I can do it myself. I knew enough to ask for help, didn't I?

    Anonymous

TRY IT OUT 6.3.   **Waiting to Listen**

Next time you are in conversation—a minute from now, an hour from now, tomorrow—monitor your own listening habits. See if you can catch yourself 'waiting to speak'. See if you can force yourself to 'wait to listen'. As I was writing this, I (Colleen) took my own advice with my 20-year-old son. Instead of meeting his 'hi, Mom' with my agenda (his car loan problems), I forced myself into waiting to listen. I am not naïve enough to think this a 'magic bullet', but this time he did address and solve the problem without me even speaking!

The Skills of Self-Observation: Conscious Participation and Self-Knowing

In Chapter 5 we described the skills of conscious participation and self-knowing that are part of reflexivity. These skills are central to relational family nursing practice. As you enter into relation with a family, your ability to know and respond to them can be greatly enhanced by paying attention to who, how, and what you are doing and being. By observing oneself (for example, practicing the skills of conscious participation and self-knowing) and paying attention to the thoughts, emotions, and bodily responses one is having at any moment, the opportunity to reflexively consider those responses and more consciously and intentionally choose how to act and respond is created. Review Chapter 5 to spark your thinking and help you to further consider the skills of conscious participation and self-knowing within the process of being in-relation.

The Skill of Questioning to Look Beyond the Surface

As we described in Chapter 1, habits are powerful partly because they fit with taken-for-granted 'truths'. Throughout the preceding chapters we have offered examples that illustrate how unexamined assumptions can override relational practice. Thus a key skill of relational practice is the skill of questioning taken-for-granted knowledge and habits. This is not just a matter of questioning your own habits of thought and practice, but also questioning beyond the surface with families, colleagues, and the structures organizing your practice.

Questioning beyond the surface begins with the strategy of *seeing relations*. Looking at families and trying to imagine the context of their lives *beyond the health care encounter* is a first step. When you next encounter a family experiencing difficulty, try looking over their shoulder to imagine what might have contributed to that difficulty. For example, thinking back to Red's story in Chapter 4, what questions might have helped you bring the relation of Red's life to larger social structures into view? Looking beneath the surface at families *within the health care encounter* is a next step. As we have argued, having lived their experience, families are the best source of knowledge about themselves. Looking beneath and beyond the surface provides an opportunity to

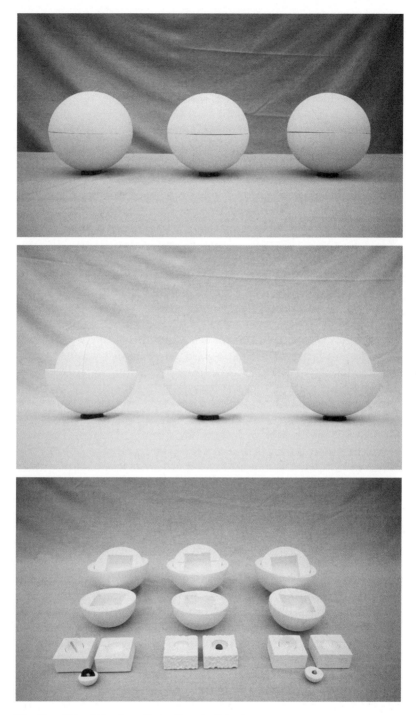

The life within. (Mixed media by Connie Sabo.)

affirm families' experience, understanding and choices. As we have shown, families also take up powerful cultural discourses and may be in the habit of seeing themselves in taken-for-granted ways (think of labels such as 'dysfunctional', 'high risk', 'disabled'). How are families seeing themselves and being seen, and how do these relations create and sustain constraining assumptions?

Noticing discrepancies is a second strategy that flows from seeing relations. Being alert to discrepancies between what you are hearing or seeing on the surface and what might lie beyond calls on your skill of self-knowing, particularly bodily knowing, as we outlined in Chapter 5. Alertness to discrepancies also calls on your contextual knowledge that in Chapter 4 we encouraged you to develop. If something does not 'ring true' or seem right, if something feels 'uncomfortable' to you, follow that lead and ask questions to figure out the discrepancy.

Noticing patterns is a third strategy that helps question beneath the surface. Pay attention to things that repeatedly signal that something taken for granted is being glossed over. For example, as a teacher, I (Colleen) have learned to raise questions as soon as someone thinks that 'education' is needed. I always question what the pattern is surrounding the request for education. For example, in a unit on which I am currently doing work, the clinical educator was asked to provide education sessions on the protocol for patients with deep vein thrombosis treatment. However, on questioning, it became clear that it was not that nurses did not know the protocol, but rather that two departments were engaged in a struggle at an administrative level regarding who should provide the service. Similarly, when someone identifies 'personality problems' or 'communication problems', I am alerted to look beneath the surface for patterns. Again, building your contextual knowledge will develop your awareness of patterns—for example, it might help you raise questions such as: What are the 'typical' ways that families with whom you work are judged or classified? What powerful cultural discourses routinely operate within your practice setting?

Finally, try routinely *posing questions* that dig beneath the surface of any situation. For example, asking 'Why do things happen the way they do?' or 'What is behind this (action, decision, policy, practice, problem)?' invariably turns up answers that are unexpected. When a man recently told me (Colleen) that he came from a dysfunctional family, I asked him how he came to think of his family as dysfunctional. Over the next 10 minutes he poured out a family history of tragedy and challenge and concluded by telling me that his family had done pretty well 'after all we have been through'. This is not to say that he changed his mind on the use of the label, but rather, that he had an opportunity to share more than the label with me. Asking what language and assumptions support any given understanding, action, decision, policy, practice, or problem also helps surface a broader understanding. Asking questions using the lenses and perspectives that we offered in Chapter 2 always turns up interesting ideas. Posing questions about gender, race, class, and history of any situation always provides new understanding.

An Example: Twos and Fours

In the emergency unit where I (Colleen) am currently doing research, policy requires nurses to categorize the acuity of patients on a scale from 1 to 5. The nurses then prioritize care, at least to some extent, in line with this scale. On the surface, this appears to be a functional sort of practice. However, my contextual understanding that economics often override nursing concerns prompts me to look beyond the surface of this practice. It quickly becomes evident that whereas the nurses talk about 'twos' and 'fours' in clinical terms ('this guy looks like he's going to pass out—I moved him up to a two'), administrators and managers talk about the scale in very different ways ('we only need one triage nurse these hours because we have mostly fours and fives'). I am also prompted to ask if rating scales are applied in ways that are congruent with forms of discrimination—for example, are elderly people routinely rated 'lower' than younger people?

The skill of looking beyond the surface is prerequisite to the skill of intentionality. When you stop waiting to speak or act, and actually listen, and when you look beyond the surface, new possibilities for intentional action become clear.

The Skill of Intentionality

❝ There are some . . . unreasonable people. People who in one sentence can disallow everything I believe in on whatever level. I can still get into that (relational) space with them because I don't take it personally. I know that in their moment, that's who they are. The accumulation of who they are is right there. And it's okay. Who am I to say it's not okay? I don't want to. I don't ever have that feeling of wanting to change anybody. If I have a desire, it's to let them feel better about their situation; who they are, what they need. And to have a clear understanding of who they are. (Community Health Worker) ❞

In essence, intentionality involves a clear and expressed congruence between espoused values and values-in-use. Intentionality encompasses:

- being aware of the values, beliefs, and theories that direct your knowing/being/doing
- exercising choice in regard to following, expanding, and/or transforming your *values, knowledge, and practices.*

As you become more intentional in your nursing work you are increasingly able to question and step out of taken-for-granted values and beliefs (such as the valuing of cure and problem resolution, valuing 'discharge' over care) and to see beyond your own concerns. Overall, the skill of intentionality enhances your ability to join families as they are, to listen and let be and to interrupt behaviors, processes, and structures that are constraining the health and healing of families. In Chapter 7 we discuss intentionality in more detail including processes that can support you in moving toward intentional action.

The Skill of Interrupting Contextual Constraints

> 66 *Even though I only have a few minutes to do an assessment when we are busy, I try to find one unique thing in every family. I try to recognize them some way, so they know I see them as people, like their kid might be good at something or have an interest, or a little piece of personality that I might pick out. But more important, I try to share things with the others [colleagues]. I say, 'hey, do you know these people have a duck farm?' 'Did you see that dad with his baby? He can look after my kids anytime!' I want everyone to see they aren't just another 'fever', or 'fracture', or 'failure to thrive'.* (Pediatric Nurse) 99

Honing the skill of looking beyond the surface and the skill of intentionality means that you can focus and intentionally act on those taken-for-granted assumptions, discourses, processes, and structures that are constraining health and health-promoting practice. The skill of interrupting (in this case it's not rude to interrupt, it's a moral obligation!) intentionally extends your skill of looking beneath the surface to sharing that skill with others. Doing so involves:

- voicing your questions
- voicing your concerns
- refusing to participate in oppressive practices
- countering with questions
- countering with alternative views.

As you look beyond the surface, share with others the questions you are raising for yourself: 'Why are we doing this?' 'How did this get decided?' 'Who is this supposed to help?' As you tune into and raise questions about discrepancies, voice your concerns: "This doesn't seem right . . ." "I'm not sure that this is the best decision . . ." When you identify practices that are not likely to be health promoting for families, refusing to participate in oppressive practices often requires that you draw on others to do so. A lone nurse can refuse to use labels such as 'bed blockers', but cannot stop 'bundling families out the door' if he or she is the only person going against the dominant practices. However, in collaboration with families and colleagues, such practices can be changed. We will say more about coalition building and emancipatory practice in Chapter 7. Countering with questions builds on the strategy of voicing your questions and concerns and involves pointing out and questioning the taken for granteds. For example, when I (Colleen) was first doing research on nursing practice in relation to violence, nurses frequently racialized the issue of violence. That is, nurses would say that they saw more violence among particular groups that they identified by race. I found it very useful to first ask nurses 'Are you thinking that violence is more a problem of [particular racial groups]?' When I directly asked about the subtle innuendoes they were making most nurses reacted with shock, saying, 'No, of course we know violence crosses every culture'. Interrupting by countering with questions sets the stage for countering with alternative views. So, for example, when I hear people labeling people who have addictions, I first ask what their thoughts are regarding what leads to addiction, and then find a way to offer an alternative view. I might say, 'Now that I know a bit about the relationship between trauma and substance use, when I see someone with an addiction I am curious about the paths that person has walked and the experiences he or she has had'. Perturbing the thoughts of others with questions and alternative views in turn sets the stage for reimagining, not as an isolated activity, but in relation with others.

The Skill of Reimagining

> 66 *One of the things I do on my way to my client is to find one really special thing about nature. Most of these people are housebound and we have to bring outdoors in. We're bringing life to them. We shouldn't be bringing anything negative or disturbing because it will leave that dirty residue with them. I always try to bring positive things to it. 'On my way to work, I saw twenty pigeons swoop down off of a tree and go down into a baseball field, where there was a beautiful seagull and the ground was frosty so it was just so beautiful'. I have to bring the outside in because what's in their house is not necessarily positive. . . . What I try to do is bring them nice things. Leave them with nice thoughts. I don't come in and say, 'Oh, God. Did you hear about the kid that got killed on the motorcycle last night?' No because that's upsetting to them. 'Gosh, I saw the most beautiful sunrise. It was a hot pink and the trees were all frosty. It's an absolutely gorgeous morning.' You don't remind them of this cold bitterness that they had in December when their family never even called them for Christmas. We remind them of tomorrow. (Community Health Worker)* 99

Reimagining involves the skill of looking beyond the surface—of looking at 'what is' while simultaneously imagining what 'might be'. Reimagining enhances nurses' abilities to create opportunities for clients to tap into their capacity and transform their health and healing experiences and to ever evolve and enhance the capacity they have to live meaningful lives. Overall, the skill of reimagining enables nurses to support families as they come to understand their current health and healing experiences, illuminate the elements that are shaping those experiences (that is, the sociocontextual) and consider how the meanings, experiences, and contextual elements might be transformed (reimagined) to support the family's capacity to live more fully (from the family's perspective).

This skill of reimagining is also closely tied to the skills of looking beyond the surface and interrupting contextual constraints. As nurses look beyond the surface and interrupt taken-for-granted contextual constraints they have the opportunity to reimagine their own relational practice and the relational contexts within which they work.

● What Guides Relational Practice?

Relational practice is highly focused and intentional; however, the goals and assumptions directing nurses are different from what guides nurses when practicing from a biomedical perspective, a perspective of liberal individualism, or a business perspective. Consistent with a socio-environmental perspective of health promotion, relational nursing practice is focused on supporting people/families as they:

- gain an understanding of their health and healing experiences in context
- clarify the meaning those experiences have for them
- realize their choice and power within their experiences
- act on their choices.

As we have highlighted, relational practice is shaped by both how you as a nurse choose to be in-relation in any given moment, by the people/families with whom you are in relation, and by the contexts within which you practice. Therefore being in responsive relation involves both personal and political skills and capacities. In each moment of your practice you make a choice about how you will involve yourself, how you will respond to the people with whom you are in-relation, and how you will ultimately promote health and healing. At the same time, as we discussed in earlier chapters, choice is a relational phenomenon. The business model currently dominating health care and the emphasis on 'efficient' disease treatment shapes your ability to exercise your choice. Therefore, we are proposing that to practice relationally you will need to be more intentional in choosing your own actions and also in joining with colleagues to effect the practice environment and create a climate in which the health-promoting quality of relationships is understood, valued, and supported.

In Box 6-3, the statements from an anonymous writer offer some food for thought with regard to how to be in-relation. In Chapter 7 we present actual processes that we have found support the living and doing of relational family nursing practice. Prior to moving onto Chapter 7, try the This Week In Practice exercise as you work in your practice area.

THIS WEEK IN PRACTICE

Who Are You Relationally?

As you go about your nursing work this week pay attention to yourself in-relation. Think of a creative way to remind yourself to pay such attention (the old string-around-the-finger trick?) and possibly make a note or two about what you notice. What habits of conduct can you identify? How do you enter into relationships? Do you find yourself distancing from people? Do you take up a professional stance? What relational capacities are strong and which ones do you find you are not expressing in your work? Are there particular situations and/or relational skills that you find more challenging than others?

CHAPTER HIGHLIGHTS

1. As you read what were you able to identify about your own style of being in-relation?

2. What are two habits that serve you well and what are two habits that constrain the way you engage in relationships?

3. What do you need to 'unlearn' in order to enhance your relational practice?

REFERENCES

Arndt, M. J. (1992). Caring as everydayness. *Journal of Holistic Nursing, 10*(4), 285–293.

Björnsdóttir, K. (2001). From the state to the family: Reconfiguring the responsibility for long-term nursing care at home. *Nursing Inquiry, 9*(1), 3–11.

Buber, M. (1958). *I and thou.* New York: Scribner.

Desmarais, G., & Hamel, C. (1996, June). *Abandon corporel. Casting new light on the experience of being human.* Paper presented at the First United States National Conference on Body Oriented Psychotherapy, Beverly, Massachusetts.

Freire, P. (1989). *Pedagogy of the oppressed.* New York: Continuum.

Gadow, S. (1985). Nurse and patient: The caring relationship. In A. H. Bishop & J. R. Scudder (Eds.), *Caring, curing coping* (pp. 31–43). Tuscaloosa, Alabama: University of Alabama Press.

Gadow, S. (1999). Relational narratives: The postmodern turn in ethics. *Scholarly Inquiry for Nursing Practice, 13*(1), 57–70.

Greenberg, E. M., McFarlane, J., & Watson, M. G. (1997). Vaginal bleeding and abuse: Assessing pregnant women in the emergency department. *MCN: American Journal of Maternal Child Nursing, 22*(4), 182–186.

Hartrick, G.A. (1997). Relational capacity: The foundation for interpersonal nursing practice. *Journal of Advanced Nursing, 26,* 523–528.

Hartrick, G. A. (1999). Transcending behaviorism in communication education. *Journal of Nursing Education, 38*(1), 17–22.

Hartrick, G. A. (2002). Beyond interpersonal communication: The significance of relationship in health promoting practice. In L. Young & V. Hayes (Eds.), *Transforming health promotion Practice. Concepts, Issues and Applications* (pp. 49–58). Philadelphia: F. A. Davis.

Hartrick Doane, G. A. (2002). Beyond behavioral skills to human-involved processes: Relational nursing practice and interpretive pedagogy. *Journal of Nursing Education, 41*(9), 400–404.

Jeffries, L. (1998). *Healing presence.* Unpublished thesis. University of Victoria, Victoria, Canada.

Jordan, J. (1997). *Women's growth in diversity. More writing from the Stone Center.* New York: Guilford.

McMillan, R. (2003). *Unveiling the invisible and uncelebrated aspects of relational practice: Enlightening conversations with experienced community health workers.* Unpublished thesis. University of Victoria, Victoria, Canada.

Moccia, P. (1988). Preface. In J. Paterson & L. Zderad (Eds.), *Humanistic Nursing* (HLN pub. No. 41-2218, 2nd ed., pp 1-iv). New York: National League for Nursing.

Montgomery, C. L. (1993). *Healing through communication. The practice of caring.* Newbury Park, CA: Sage.

Northcott, H. C. (1994). The politics of austerity and threats to Medicare. In B. S. Bolaria & R. Bolaria, *Women, medicine and health* (pp. 7–24). Saskatoon, SK: University of Saskatchewan.

Parse, R. (1998). The human becoming school of thought. A perspective for nurses and other health professionals. Thousand Oaks, CA: Sage.

Paterson, J. G., & Zderad, L. T. (1988). *Humanistic nursing* (NLN Publ. No. 41-2218, 2nd ed.). New York: National League for Nursing.

Rankin, J. (2004). Fundamentals of health management technology. Unpublished doctoral dissertation. University of Victoria, Victoria, BC.

Rodney, P., Brown, H., & Liaschenko, J. (2004). Moral agency: Relational connections and trust. In J. Storch, P. Rodney, & R. Starzomski (Eds.), *Toward a moral horizon: Nursing ethics for leadership and practice.* Toronto: Pearson.

Rogers, C. (1961). On becoming a person. Boston: Houghton Mifflin.

Tapp, D. (2000). The ethics of relational stance in family nursing: Resisting the view of "nurse as expert." *Journal of Family Nursing, 6*(1), 69–91.

Thayer-Bacon, B. (2003). *Relational epistemologies.* New York: Peter Lang.

Ueland, B. (1992, November/December). Tell me more: On the fine art of listening. *Utne Reader,* 104–110.

Van Manen, M. (1990). *Researching lived experience. Human science and an action sensitive pedagogy.* London, Ontario: Althouse Press.

Varcoe, C. (2001). Abuse obscured: An ethnographic account of emergency nursing in relation to violence against women. *Canadian Journal of Nursing Research, 32*(4), 95–115.

Varcoe, C. (2002). Inequality, violence and women's health. In B. S. Bolaria & H. Dickinson (Eds.), *Health, illness and health care in Canada* (3rd ed., pp. 211–230). Toronto: Nelson.

Varcoe, C., Doane, G., Pauly, B., Rodney, P., Storch, J. L., Mahoney, K., McPherson, G., Brown, H. & Starzomski, R. (2003). Ethical practice in nursing—Working the in-betweens. *Journal of Advanced Nursing, 45*(3), 1–10.

Varcoe, C., & Rodney, P. (2002). Constrained agency: The social structure of nurses work. In B. S. Bolaria & H. D. Dickinson (Eds.), *Health, illness and health care in Canada* (3rd ed., pp. 102–128). Toronto: Nelson.

Varcoe, C., Rodney, P., & McCormick, J. (2003). Health care relationships in context: An analysis of three ethnographies. *Qualitative Health Research, 13*(6), 957–973.

Varela, F. J., Thompson, E., & Rosch, E. (1993). *The embodied mind. Cognitive science and human experience.* Cambridge, MA: MIT Press.

Watson, J. (1988). *Nursing: Human science and human care. A theory of nursing* (NLN Publ. No. 15-2236). New York: National League for Nursing.

Wright, L. M., & Leahey, M. (1999). Maximizing time, minimizing suffering: The 15 minute (or less) family interview. *Journal of Family Nursing, 5*(3), 259–273.

Yalom, I. D. (1980). *Existential psychotherapy.* New York: Basic Books.

7 The Processes and Skills of Relational Family Nursing Practice

OVERVIEW

In this chapter we explore assessment and intervention in relational nursing practice and offer processes and strategies that can enhance nursing responsiveness to families and support the promotion of health and healing.

● Relational Inquiry as the Structure for Family Nursing Practice

> 66 *The responsibility of the nurse is not to make people well, or to prevent their getting sick, but to assist people to recognize the power that is within them. (Newman, 1994, p. xv)* 99

As we bring the different lenses and understandings of family discussed in the previous chapters together we begin to see that family, health, and 'family health' are dynamic, living experiences that are personally, contextually, and relationally constructed. This knowledge has significant implications for nursing practice. First, the broad understanding of family we have presented implies that *every moment of nursing practice involves family nursing.* Whether one is working with a literal family or with an individual who has no observable family (that is, a configuration of people) because people are constituted by their historical, cultural, and biological experience of family and situated in a world where family is the central social organizer, their health and healing experiences are shaped through and by their family experience. Therefore, all nursing practice needs to consider and attend to people's living experience of family. Second, the dynamic nature of family and health implies that family nursing practice must be fluid and ever-changing. If the experiences of family and health are varied and changeable, family nursing practice must be dynamic and creatively responsive to particular people/families in particular moments. Together these two implications highlight the importance of an approach to health care and nursing that moves beyond the service-provision model to one that is congruent with a socioenvironmental approach to health promotion.

In outlining relational nursing practice in this chapter, it is our intent to provide a roadmap that offers direction for practice without offering a prescriptive method. That is, as we suggested in earlier chapters, we offer a roadmap as opposed to designating a specific route for you to take. We believe strongly that if nursing practice is to be relationally responsive, each nurse must cultivate his or her own approach to practice in any given moment. At the same time there are particular strategies and processes that can support and enhance the capacity of individual nurses to be health-promoting, relational practitioners.

Overall relational nursing practice involves a process of inquiry. That is, when you approach family nursing practice relationally inquiry becomes the structure that underpins your nursing practice. This notion of structure is important. We want to emphasize that although in this chapter we do not offer a prescribed method or assessment tool to follow, we do offer a structure. The structure, however, is of a form that is not determined by preset nursing methods. The structure that guides relational practice is a thoughtful process of interpretive, critical, and spiritual inquiry. This process of inquiry provides a roadmap and routes to take when working with families and also suggests particular 'road signs' to look for when you are in-relation. The strength in approaching family nursing as a relational inquiry is that in doing so families and nurses can harness the power of a range of knowledges (theoretical, empirical, biomedical, technical, physiological, ethical, spiritual, and so on) as opposed to being limited by one theoretical framework and/or method. The inquiry roadmap, including the routes and processes we suggest in this chapter, sets you up to responsively engage with families by looking for particular road signs along the way. Overall nursing as a process of inquiry offers the structure for how to proceed while at the same time the fluidity to ensure that the structure and methods employed are mediated by you and the families with whom you work. As mediators of structure and method the opportunity is created for you to respond to what arises and make thoughtful decisions about how 'best to proceed' in any given moment. In this way the structure of inquiry provides concrete ways of engaging with families and also of engaging with the knowledge required for responsive, health promoting practice.

Similar to when you start out on a journey the roadmap that is offered can be useful to get a sense of direction and to help you consider possible ways of proceeding. However, just as on a trip, it is you as an individual who chooses the direction of your journey, what and how you will pack for the trip, and your mode of transportation. You determine the particular things you will note, how and where you will spend your time, in what activities you will take part, what you will ultimately experience, and so forth. For example, the roadmap of 'nursing as a process of inquiry' can be helpful by pointing out a direction when you are starting (for example, the roadmap directs you to enter into relation by inquiring into a family's health and healing experience) or at times when you are suddenly feeling a bit lost or unsure of how to proceed (for example, the inquiry roadmap gives direction for how you might go about navigating through the complexities and ambiguities of practice). However, you and the people with whom you are in-relation are the ones directing your travels. For that reason you will need to consider the processes we describe in this chapter in light of your own person and your own style of practice, in light of the people/families with whom you are working and in light of the contexts where you and families meet. We do not offer the map as a method to follow and do not expect you to practice in 'our way'. Rather it is our hope that you will enlist the processes in a way that enhances your own ability to be more responsive to the particular people/families with whom you are in-relation. Consequently, we expect that even though all nurses who read this book might be striving toward relational family nursing practice, if we were to observe you in practice, each reader would 'look' different. In common would be the values, attributes, and processes living out in practices that support families' experiences of being respected, understood and of becoming actively empowered.

● Beyond Service Provision

McKnight (1989) maintains that our current health care system is dominated by a service-provision model of health care. As a result, health care initiatives and activities (such as family nursing) most often focus on teaching people about the nature of their health problems and the value of services in addressing and/or preventing those problems. Underlying this service model of health care is the assumption that people with health 'problems' require outsiders to meet their health and healing needs (McKnight & Kretzmann, 1992).

Not only does such a model of health care contradict the principles of socioenvironmental health promotion, McKnight (1989) contends that it may also have unhealthy effects on the people it 'services'. First, an emphasis on problems highlights pathology or deficiency. Although it is possible for any person or family to be viewed from a 'half-empty' perspective, it is also possible to view them as half-full. Focusing on the problems in families' lives serves to reinforce, value, and give life to the half-empty, while simultaneously devaluing the half-full (Hartrick, 1997). A service model of health care forces nurses' attention on the pathology or problems in families. If my main job as a family nurse is to provide a service, my attention will be focused on looking for what it is that needs servicing. Although a family may have many strengths and resources, the servicing of deficiency will become the overriding emphasis of my nursing assessment and intervention. For example, scan any admission form, intake form, or initial assessment form in the health care agency where you are doing your clinical work. How do the forms set you up as

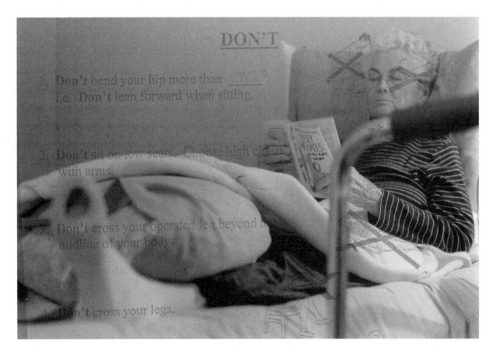

Don't. (Photograph by Gayle Allison.)

a nurse? To what do they draw your attention? How much focus is on deficiency/problems and on what service the client needs? If strengths and capacities are included in the forms, are they centrally located or are they included as add-ons? Do the forms direct you to consider the integral relationship between strengths or capacities and adversities or 'problems'?

A second possible effect of the service model of health care is that the power of the professional may push aside the expertise, technique, and capacity of people and families to address their own health and healing needs (Hartrick, 1997). A service model of health care rests on the assumption that it is nurses (and other health professionals) who possess the knowledge and expertise necessary to manage families' health and healing experiences. As a result, nursing knowledge, expertise, technique, and technology may override the knowledge and action of families. According to McKnight (1989), as the power of the professional and service systems ascends, the legitimacy, authority, and capacity of families to increase control over and improve their health (in their own lives) descends and is often forgotten.

Traditionally the nursing literature has tended to conceptually link health promotion with this servicing approach to health problems (Hartrick, 1997). This service-model, problem-oriented approach to health care is evident in the language used in many descriptions of nursing. For example, nurses speak of 'treatment and outcomes' of 'assessing, diagnosing, and intervening' to identify and address 'problems'. Often the fundamental emphasis of nursing assessment and intervention is problem focused service-provision and health promotion is seen as something an expert *nurse does* through the provision of health services to families. However, as described in Chapter 1, from a socioenvironmental perspective health promotion is not an activity of 'doing to' people but is a way of being and approaching people and nursing practice that focuses on the discovery and enhancement of people's and families' capacity (Hartrick, 1997). In contrast to a service model of care that directs attention to problems (which are often decontextualized), a socioenvironmental perspective of health promotion directs the nurse to never lose sight of what nursing assessment and intervention are fundamentally for and about—namely supporting peoples'/families' choice and capacity to live meaningful lives within their particular personal and social contexts. Therefore although nurses may well provide a service and/or may attend to the problems and adversities that exist, at the center of any assessment and intervention processes are families and their everyday lives (as opposed to centering on disease and/or treatment of problems). Once again it can be helpful to use the analogy of looking through a camera and adjusting your lens. A nurse practicing from a socioenvironmental understanding of health focuses the lens on families in context—looking for who this family and the people in the family are; what is meaningful and significant to them in their everyday lives; what capacities they have both personally and contextually; the adversities that might be constraining their power, choice, and ability to realize their aspirations (their health) and the potential actions that might be taken (by the family and nurse) to simultaneously enhance capacity and address adversity.

● Learning to Nurse Without Relying on Tools

As we described earlier, in contrast to most family nursing textbooks we are purposefully not offering a structured assessment tool or method to use when assessing and intervening with families. However, although we are not offering a predetermined structure or tool, we *are* proposing a particular way of proceeding in practice. As we described earlier, relational practice involves a skilled process of inquiry that is guided by the people/families with whom you as a nurse are in-relation. As an inquiry process relational family nursing practice involves each nurse thinking care-fully and critically about how best to come to know and respond to a particular family in a particular situation during a particular moment in time. Basically we are inviting you to take up the challenge of learning to rely on families, on your own relational capacity and skills, and on the knowledge you have (from this book as well as other education and experiences). As students learning to be family nurses it might seem a lot easier if we were to provide you with a structured assessment framework to follow or a concrete assessment tool to use. However, we believe that such a tool could well serve to limit the development of the skills necessary to support relational health-promoting practice. As we described in Chapter 1, for learning to occur it is necessary to be in a state of 'unknowing'. To offer you a predetermined tool would only serve to take you out of the complexity, uncertainty, and ambiguity that is an integral part of family nursing. Learning family nursing by relying on a tool that we created would be comparable to offering you a solid path to follow and inviting you into a stance of 'certainty'. In contrast we want you to have to be uncertain, to have to think care-fully and critically about how you might best come to know a particular family and how best to proceed in response to what arises. The reason this approach to learning is so vital is that questioning and 'uncertainty' are the media for competent, safe practice. And, whether you are a first-year nursing student or a nurse with many years of experience *we* believe that you have the capacity to navigate your way through the complex practice of family nursing if you work in-relation with people/families. Therefore, to support and guide you, rather than offer *our* method we offer some concrete processes and strategies for you to try out and try on. Ultimately it is up to you to develop the methods you will employ in your practice. To begin that development, Try It Out 7.1 invites you to develop a preamble that you might use with families to explain your approach.

The Potential Pitfalls of Assessment and Screening Tools

Before presenting the processes that we suggest can support family nursing as a relational inquiry, we believe it important to first discuss the area of assessment and screening. Professionals in the health care and nursing worlds have come to rely heavily on predetermined

TRY IT OUT 7.1.   Write a Preamble

1. *Pretend* you are a first-year nursing student and have been assigned to do a home visit with a family (maybe you are a first-year nursing student!)
2. *List* briefly some of the key ideas of relational practice (the introduction, Chapter 6, and some of the text boxes in this book provide quick reference).
3. *Develop* a brief introduction or preamble (using the key ideas you have listed) that you might use when first talking to the family to explain your stance as a nurse. What would you tell them you want to know about them? About their health? What would you say you wanted to 'do'?

assessment and screening tools or methods in their work with families. Although we are taking a different approach in this book, you will no doubt find yourself in contexts where you will either see such tools and methods being used and/or be expected to use them yourself. For that reason we want to discuss what we have experienced as potential pitfalls to avoid in the use of assessment and screening tools. Basically we want to provide an opportunity for you to critically consider how you might use such tools in your practice in ways that are relationally responsive and health promoting. To that end we offer a discussion of how assessment and screening tools are at times taken up in ways that contravene the health-promoting process. Specifically we have seen them taken up in ways that

- limit the relational connection between families and nurses,
- hinder a full and accurate understanding of families' health and healing experiences,
- make assessment an intrusive experience for families by fostering the imposition of nurses' or managerial concerns,
- decontextualize families and family nursing.

Limiting the Relational Connection

Depending on how they are taken up, structured assessment tools have the potential to come between the family and the nurse. This often occurs when nurses use the tools to provide the direction for their assessment and intervention. Guided by the structured tool nurses focus their attention on completing the outlined assessment process and/or on asking the questions outlined in each domain of the tool. Focusing in this way automatically places the nurse in the stance of detached, expert observer (remember the discussion of I-It and I-Thou relationships in Chapter 6). Guided by the tool, families become objects that are scrutinized according to the objective domains identified in the tools and then labelled, evaluated, or diagnosed according to how they 'score' on the domains. For example, in the case of 'high-risk' screening tools, people/families are often given a high-risk score that is then used to determine intervention. Not only does this stance of expert observer give rise to an I-It relationship but the interaction between the family and nurse becomes a power-over one. That is, the nurse wields the power in the relationship—it is the nurse who directs the conversation and decides what will be talked about, it is the nurse who determines what is meaningful and significant based on the questions in the assessment form, and it is ultimately the nurse who makes the final judgement about what to record when completing the form. Although when using the forms nurses may ask the family for their input and even try to be 'collaborative', the very nature of predetermined assessment tools focuses the interaction on nursing concerns. Interestingly these tools are often seen to be necessary to enable novice nurses or students who are learning about family nursing assessment to conduct a thorough assessment. Yet we have found that the only nurses who seem to be able to employ the tools in ways that are relationally consistent with socioenvironmental health promotion are very experienced nurses. This is because their experience gives them the confidence to not follow the tools so prescriptively—they are more likely to use the tool as a resource rather than a guide. In contrast newer nurses who are feeling less confident or knowledgeable tend to rely on the tools to direct the assessment. This reliance often hinders the development of their relational abilities and confidence. That is, the nurses end up developing more of a relationship with the assessment tool than with families. And at the same time, the tool allows them to not have to think as care-fully and critically about how they are being in-relation, what they need to inquire into with particular families and how they might be most responsive.

An Example: Using a CAGE

Many health care settings use an alcohol screen to identify people with problem drinking. The CAGE questionnaire is a brief questionnaire that has been researched extensively and advocated for use in a variety of clinical settings (Bastiaens, Riccardi, & Sakhrani, 2002; Chung & Colby, 2000; Fiellin & Reid, 2000; Philpot et al., 2003). It poses questions about how much the person drinks and how drinking affects the person and his or her family. However, how such a screen is used may be quite problematic. When I (Colleen) was doing research in emergency, the first time I watched a nurse administer the CAGE I was surprised. As the nurse quickly asked the questions of a man with chest pain, he responded affirmatively to all the questions. He drank more than 26 ounces of liquor per day, he felt guilty about it, he was feeling pressure about his drinking from his family, and he wanted to quit. Although the man seemed distressed during this exchange, the nurse interrupted herself while completing the screen to ask another nurse to do an ECG (electrocardiogram) for her. After completing the screen she completed the rest of her assessment and moved to the next patient without responding to what seemed to me to be a significant disclosure of concern. When the man left an hour later, I asked the nurse what had happened. She told me that his chest pain had just been muscle strain, so he was discharged. I asked, "but what about the alcohol?" to which she replied that they used to have some brochures, but at present were out of them.

What was striking about this situation was that the 'assessment' was carried out for the sake of completing the tool—the information was not really integrated into the nurse's understanding of the man's health experience and/or into how she responded to him. And this example illustrates how use of a tool can direct attention away from relational connection. The nurse asked the questions because they were on the form and she was mandated to do so, not because they were relevant to promoting his health. Even when it became clear that alcohol was of significance and concern to the man and his family, the nurse stayed in-relation with the form and failed to 'follow the lead' that the man provided. Subsequently a clear and explicit opportunity to address a significant aspect of the man's health (and life) experience was lost.

Hindering a Full and Accurate Understanding of Families' Health and Healing Experiences

As discussed in the first two chapters, any knowledge provides a limited and partial view. Subsequently, any tool is limited by the selective interests and knowledge of the people by whom it was developed. Therefore, assessment and screening tools have what Wagner (1993) terms 'blind spots'. Blind spots are things that we can't see or don't think of and therefore do not know to ask about. An example of a blind spot is the story I (Gweneth) told in Chapter 1 about not understanding how John's descriptions of living on the street were related to the children's questions about family. Because I had never experienced or known family in the way John had, I would never have thought to ask him about family as, in Ryan's words, an experience of 'unlove'. However, by listening carefully to his story (by following his lead) I gradually came to understand the connection of family to his experience of loneliness and isolation and to understand the relevance of this family experience to his overall health. By the time I heard Ryan (who we described in Chapter 5) speak, my understanding of family had widened to the point that I 'got it' immediately.

This exemplifies the limitations of predetermined assessment tools and how important it is to follow the lead of the family during assessment. By following the lead of families our assessment and intervention can be much more expansive and yet more focused at the same time. By inquiring into families' experiences we are able to expand our assessment profile and the subsequent view and understanding of a family's health and healing experience while at the same time more readily direct our attention to particular aspects that are significant to particular families. Although predetermined assessment and screening tools that are informed and developed by expert knowledge may direct our attention to aspects that are generally relevant to families, depending upon how they are used the tools (and the nurses using the tools) may be 'blinded' to other significant aspects. An example of this 'blindness' is a story told to us by a new mother.

An Example: Marilyn's Breastfeeding Worries

A nurse visited Marilyn in her home for a well-baby visit following her postnatal discharge from the hospital. To complete the well-baby visit the nurse followed the questions outlined on the agency's well-baby checklist. However, even though the checklist identified some of the aspects that were particularly significant to the family, the 'family lead' within them was not taken up and followed. For example, in following the assessment tool the nurse asked about breastfeeding but did so in a very functional way. Rather than asking about Marilyn's experience of breastfeeding and following her lead (for example, what was meaningful and significant to Marilyn was the difficulty she had when people responded negatively to her when she breastfed in public), the nurse proceeded to talk about breastfeeding according to what was itemized on the assessment tool (for example, engorged breasts, nipple care, etc.), never inquiring into and/or addressing what was meaningful and significant to Marilyn and the contextual aspects that were shaping her breastfeeding experience.

Similar to Purkis' example (in Chapter 1) of the public health nurse who did the growth and development assessment, in the above example, the nurse's reliance on the tool closed down the possibility of identifying other aspects in the family's experience. The assessment tool was taken up and used in such a way that resulted in the concerns of the nurse or the health care organization overriding the mother's concerns. Often standardized assessment tools are developed and implemented on the rationale that they will ensure a full assessment and enhance care, however, depending on how they are taken they may well lessen that possibility. For example in the case of the CAGE questionnaire it was assumed that identifying problem drinkers would allow better sedation and pain management for people with alcohol dependency. However, a colleague of ours doing research on a medical unit found that the screening results were used to predict patients who would be 'aggressive' or 'unmanageable'. Inadvertently the screening resulted in patients being labelled and stigmatized as 'alcoholics', and in some cases, in pain medication being withheld as such patients were seen as undeserving.

Making Assessment an Intrusive Experience

From a critical perspective generalized assessment and screening tools seem to be based on the assumption that as 'good patients' families should reveal any information we ask them for. Because many nurses do not stop to question this assumption, often the tools are taken up and used in ways that are experienced by families as incredibly intrusive. For example, routine screening for history of sexual abuse and/or violence for all women in labour offers a disturbing example of this assumption. Although such screening is well-intended, what often is not considered is the experiential aspect—for example, how difficult it might be for a woman who has experienced such trauma first of all to be asked about that in a routine way and second to have a stranger probing into such private areas. Based on the above assumption, nurses conduct this 'routine' screening and expect women to participate regardless of how intimate or painful that might be and regardless of how the information will be used or not used. The assumption that our health professional status gives us the right to ask families about the intimate details of their lives is highly problematic and in some ways mirrors the same invasive power-over behaviour that underlies patterns of violence and abuse. Although there is no question that we want and need to honour and attend to people's past experiences of trauma, depending on how it is done, general screening can potentially serve to hinder our ability to do so. The following example was given by a nurse who, recognizing the importance of past sexual trauma to women in labour, figured out a way that she might provide safe and responsive care, without 'screening' women and without being intrusive.

An Example: EveryWoman

Barb, a maternity nurse I (Colleen) know, was quite baffled by my interest in nursing practice with women in labour who have experienced childhood sexual abuse. I was concerned that a violence history screen that was introduced at other hospitals would be imported into Barb's unit. She asked, 'Why would we need that? I just treat every labouring woman as if she is the most sexually abused woman in the world'. She went on to explain that, for example, she tells each woman that she will always ask permission before she touches her (say, for a pelvic exam) and tells women that she does so because she knows that many women have had bad experiences as children or adults. She told me that she does not believe that she needs to have a woman 'disclose' her personal trauma history (unless she decides to) in order to provide emotionally safe care. Rather such care can be provided by engaging in a way that communicates one is willing, open, and interested in knowing anything the women would like to share that could enhance the nurse's ability to provide responsive care and by offering sensitive care without demanding disclosure. Perhaps not surprisingly, Barb finds that many women do disclose histories of child sexual abuse or adult sexual assault and that many others who do not do so explicitly, recognize and thank her for the opportunity.

Consistent with a socioenvironmental approach to health promotion, Barb leaves the control (to disclose about past sexual abuse or not and to direct nursing care) in the hands of the women themselves. Understanding that women need to make their own decisions about how much they disclose and that for some it is not something they might want to do, she has figured out a way of providing care that acknowledges and attends to their potential vulnerability without harming them further (for example, either asking about their sexual abuse history and/or treating them as though they had not had such experiences could well add to their trauma).

Decontextualizing Families and Family Nursing

Putting on a contextual lens immediately reminds us that there is no such thing as a neutral question. Often it is assumed that because the assessment tools are standardized the questions are neutral and are used and experienced in the same way by all people/families. However, phenomenology informs us that any assessment tool and/or question will have particular and different meaning for different people. A good example of this was offered by an Aboriginal health nurse who pointed out to me (Gweneth) how the standard questions that are asked in an emergency department (for example, have you had any alcohol to drink?) are often experienced by Aboriginal peoples as disrespectful, racist, and marginalizing. Because of the sociohistorical context of colonization and the social practice of racialized stereotyping (such as the linking of alcoholism with Aboriginal peoples), such questions are never experienced as neutral. Thus, the same question can be experienced very differently by different people.

At the same time, the domains of assessment and/or the screening indicators often offer a very limited, decontextual view of any family. For example, screening tools may focus nurses' attention on the deficits and/or these general indicators may be used to determine the potential of families to either do well or 'get into trouble' without consideration of the particularities of families. Failure to consider the particularities and contextual capacities of any family can result in a unidimensional view of a multidimensional experience. For example, high-risk screening tools are often used to determine whether a family should be 'followed' in the community. A family is evaluated according to high-risk indicators such as socioeconomic status, single-parent status, housing, and so forth. The potential limitations of evaluating families according to these decontextualized risk factors was highlighted by Nancy, a friend of mine (Gweneth) who felt 'outraged' when a social worker came into her hospital room following the birth of her son to 'assess' her because she was a 'single mother'. Not only did she find it surprising that her status as a single woman would be considered problematic but she found it quiet amazing that that identifier served to override recognition of all of the other capacities she had (for example, she was a mature and confident woman [nurse] who had made a decision to have a child, she had economic resources, family support, experience with children, and so forth). The inappropriateness of such decontextualized screening is highlighted even more by the fact that Nancy actually worked in the same hospital as a family support nurse! Yet as a result of the decontextualized high-risk factor of single mother, she had been 'screened' as potentially having less capacity than other women to care for her son.

Try It Out 7.2 suggests that you review an assessment or screening tool and compare it to our critique earlier. Keep this comparison in mind as you read the ideas we offer regarding health promoting relational practice.

TRY IT OUT 7.2.   **Test a Tool**

Find an assessment tool or screening tool that is used in your current area of practice, in the literature, or in a textbook.

After reading the section on Predetermined Tools, review your selected tool and ask:

- How could this tool promote or limit relational connection?
- How could this tool foster or limit learning about families' health and healing experiences?
- Could this tool be used in a nonintrusive way?
- To what extent could this tool decontextualize people and experiences or promote a contextual understanding?

● The Processes of Health-Promoting Relational Practice With Families

If health promotion is about promoting meaningful lives, then the people living those lives must be the central actors in the health-promoting process. Therefore, whether you use a standardized assessment tool or not, it is vital that you engage relationally with families—not tools. It is also important to keep in mind that family nursing is not just about what nurses do. Rather, at the center of health-promoting family nursing is what families experience and do as they collaborate with nurses to affect their own lives. Because we do not see family health promotion as limited to nursing action and believe that nursing practice must be relationally responsive to particular families in particular situations, in conceptualizing family nursing practice we have purposefully moved away from delineating a prescribed method. We have taken up Caputo's (1987) suggestion to replace method with a deeper appreciation of *methodos*, which is 'the way in which we pursue a matter' (p. 213). Rather than following a predetermined method of assessment and/or intervention, health-promoting relational practice involves joining families in collaborative relation and thought-fully inquiring into the their living experience in context and responding to what arises through that relational process. As we emphasized in Chapter 6 this 'inquiring and responding' is not equivalent to purposeless drifting. Rather, *relational practice is a skilled action of inquiry that is guided by conscious participation as opposed to structured assessment tools or linear 'problem-solving' processes.*

Because we are approaching family nursing relationally, we believe that assessment processes cannot be separated from intervention processes. As complexity theory informs us, any action (whether it be asking a question as part of an assessment process or acting in response to what the family identifies as significant) relationally impacts the family (Vicenzi, White, & Begun, 1997; Hartrick, 2001). This means that the moment one joins a family any action is potentially an intervention. For example, our experience has taught us that asking a family a seemingly simple question can have a greater effect than many strategically planned interventions. For that reason, assessment and intervention potentially are occurring in each moment of nursing practice.

Because we work with particular families in particular situations it is impossible to present a generalized prescription for action. The same action in one case may be responsive and health promoting and in another case not be—the question is how any nursing action responds to what is meaningful and significant to a particular family and how it promotes their health and healing capacity. The question 'Which action?' (that is, 'what and how do I assess and intervene?') is answered by deciding what action would be most responsive to this particular family in this particular situation. Amundson (1996) contends that when working with families such questions are ones we must:

66 *always ask, each moment, of each hour we are with our patients. How do we do therapy with this underfunded single parent, with 3*

children? With this surly young person on a path toward a career in crime? With this eloquent professional mired in a non-vital marriage? Before we even go into the room we have to think of this question. We have gone to school, to workshops, to lectures, we have read and based upon opportunity and inclination we have formed a clinical philosophy . . . (however) instead of therapeutic ambition bolstered by ideological purity we enter with the perspective of 'not knowing'. (p. 476) **99**

It is this unknowing perspective and the questioning it inspires that gives rise to ethical and competent practice.

The importance of always asking oneself what would be most responsive to a particular family at a particular moment is highlighted in the following story shared by a colleague, Helen Brown, a neonatal nursing instructor.

An Example: Sharing the Burden of Ending Tanner's Life

My husband and I were living one of those moments any parent would likely dread. Twenty-four hours following the birth of our first child, we were confronted with the decision of withdrawing life-sustaining treatment. Tanner required life support following a poorly managed birth that resulted in severe hypoxic insult to his vital organ systems. It seemed clear that the chance of Tanner's recovery from such a severe insult to his brain was unlikely. We struggled in such a short time to confront our values about the meaning of a life worth living for our child while, at the same time, worrying that the decision to withdraw life support was a selfish one. We questioned whether or not ending Tanner's life was maybe in our best interest and not his. The burden of such a decision was overwhelming. We struggled to make sense of our responsibility as his parents—should we try to minimize further suffering or believe in his slight chance for recovery? Without even knowing why, I asked the attending neonatologist what he would do if Tanner was his newborn son in the same situation. Looking back now I don't believe Andrew and I asked this question because we were hoping someone would tell us what to do. I now think we were searching to share a space with another human being as we made the toughest decision in our life together. I am sure that the space felt safe to ask this question because I knew the neonatologist to be an excellent medical practitioner and a responsive, authentic human being in his encounters with families in the NICU. The neonatologist responded by saying, 'If he was my son, I would allow him to die'.

What is interesting is that when recounting this story to a physician and some nurse colleagues, they expressed near outrage, claiming that the neonatologist clearly violated 'professional boundaries' and that 'telling us what to do' was essentially wrong. Yet in the moments of that encounter I couldn't have felt more cared for—as though I had been lifted up and carried over turbulent waters. Whatever 'boundary' the neonatologist appeared to cross was one that, in my view, required crossing as we searched to share the burden of making the decision to end our son's life. In those few moments that would change our life forever, the neonatologist entered with us into a space we feared most to tread—his willingness to do so was more important than the content of his reply. Even now, 6 years later, I remember his humanity and companionship on that dark day as much as I recall his medical proficiency. The space he made for us on that day is now an important part of the memories of being well cared for in the NICU. These memories have made it possible to both grieve and celebrate Tanner's short life.

This story arose during a conversation that Helen and I (Gweneth) had about how the 'right' way to proceed is determined in the relational moment. As I listened to Helen describe her experience I was struck by how if one took the physician's actions out of the context of the 'relational space' they would not have the same meaning. That is, by only looking at the words he spoke it may well seem that he had overstepped his authority and the golden rule of 'end of life decision making' that dictates that people need to make their own decisions. Yet consider his actions in light of Buber's I-It and I-Thou relationship (as discussed in Chapter 6). The physician could have assumed a professional, objective stance and replied that the decision was Helen and Andrew's to make—he could have turned the relational connection into an I-It one. However, as Helen described, he involved himself humanly—he entered the relational space (remember Paterson and Zderad's description of the intersubjective space in Chapter 3) and joined in I-Thou relation to be with this family in their difficulty. What is important to highlight is Helen's statement that the physician's willingness to enter the relational space and share their burden was more important than the content of his reply. In the end Helen and Andrew did make their own decision, but their ability to do so was supported by the physician's willingness to be with them as a person in that process. Again it is important to emphasize that in another situation with another family such a response might be completely inappropriate and, as the doctor and nurses who expressed outrage when hearing Helen's story purported, an overstepping of professional authority. To determine whether it was relationally responsive and health-promoting one needs to move beyond the words that were spoken and consider whether the action was in response to what was meaningful and significant to a particular family at a particular time and the way in which the practitioner's actions supported and/or constrained the family.

A Reminder!

We want to once again remind you that when we speak of 'family nursing' we are not only speaking about working with 'actual' families. Although it is possible that the processes we describe later can support assessment and intervention with literal families, they can also support health-promoting practice with, say, an individual who is going for day surgery and has no literal family. This is because given the relational underpinnings, the processes we offer are intended to help you focus on and attend to people/families in context. The processes are intended to help you tune into what is meaningful and significant to the people/families with whom you are in-relation regardless of whether those people fit the dominant family norms of Western society. In addition the processes are intended to assist you to see how the people with whom you are in-relation, their situations, and their contexts are integrally connected and shape each other. Box 7.1 offers an outline

BOX 7.1.   **Relational Nursing Practice: Assessing and Intervening Processes**

1. Entering Into Relation: Getting 'In Sync' With a Family
   - Conscious and intentional participation
   - Stopping to look, listen, and hear (smell, taste, feel)
   - Unconditional positive regard
   - Being 'in sync'
   - Walking alongside
2. Being in Collaborative Relation: Staying 'In Sync'
   - Family collaborating with nurse
   - Family and nurse working together to assess and intervene
3. Inquiring Into the Family Health and Healing Experience
   - Inquiring into what is meaningful and significant to the family
   - Keeping family at the center of view
4. Following the Lead of Families
   - Taking cues from families
   - Taking a stance of unknowing and uncertainty
   - Using theoretical knowledge to enhance sensitivity to family experience
   - Scrutinizing theoretical and expert knowledge against family experience
5. Listening to and for
   - Listening through phenomenological, critical, and spiritual lenses
   - Listening through socioenvironmental health-promotion lens
6. Self-observation
   - Participating consciously and intentionally
   - Self-knowing
7. Letting Be and Change
   - Letting be to know who this family is and what is happening for them
   - Creating the opportunity for family to come to know more about their own experience, patterns, capacities, challenges, and contextual constraints
   - Letting be as the foundation for action and change
8. Collaborative Knowledge Development
   - Drawing on family knowledge (experiential, historical, sociocultural)
   - Drawing on nursing knowledge (scientific, theoretical, biomedical, political, practical)
9. Pattern Recognition
   - Identifying underlying patterns of experience
   - Identifying family's responses
   - Identifying patterns of capacity
   - Identifying capacity-adversity patterns
10. Naming and Supporting Capacity
    - Seeing and recognizing capacity
    - Looking beyond the surface
    - Honouring the family's version of the story
    - Working with family to enhance capacity and address adversity
11. Emancipatory Action
    - Recognizing and naming inequities
    - Recognizing and naming structural conditions
    - Drawing on and sharing contextual knowledge
    - Introducing alternative discourses
    - Devoting energy to remedying structural inequalities
    - Creating coalitions

of the processes that are central to relational family nursing practice. We discuss each of these processes in the following sections. As in Chapter 6, at times we use the voices of the community health workers from Robin McMillan's (2003) research to help us exemplify some of the processes.

Entering Into Relation: Getting 'In Sync' With a Family

As described in Chapter 6, how we enter into relation can profoundly affect what we come to know and experience with families. An analogy that captures the importance of how we 'enter in' that I (Gweneth) once heard someone use was that of going on a walk in the forest (Mitha, 2000). Depending on how we enter the forest and what we are focused on, we experience the forest in very different ways. For example, if we set out to walk our two large dogs who have not had a run in a few days it is likely we will be entering the forest with a flurry of force and energy. The dogs will be noisily running through the trees and we will be walking at a clip to keep up with them. Entering in such a way we will most definitely disturb the quietness of the forest and the chirping of birds who may quickly flee on our arrival. Entering through this storm of activity we are unlikely to notice the multitude of sensations the forest has to offer us. We may fail to feel the moisture in the trees, smell the freshness of new rain or feel the peacefulness of being among the trees that are centuries old. Our activity distracts us and limits our ability to experience the forest in its fullness. On another day if we feel we would like to escape from the noise and activity of the day and set off to have a quiet walk in the forest by ourselves we are likely to experience the forest quite differently than we did previously. We may find ourselves surprised at the wildflowers we hadn't notice before, at the many shades of green that previously seemed to blend together and if we pay attention to ourselves we will likely notice how different we feel as we step into the forest and join in-relation with nature.

This forest analogy offers a way of thinking about the different ways we might enter into relation with families and how our entering shapes what we see, experience, and take away. It also highlights how 'entering in' can profoundly affect the families we are with. The analogy reminds us that a family, just as the forest, has a life and harmony all of its own and that it is important for visitors (such as nurses) to tread lightly and respectfully as they enter a family's lifespace.

Stop for a minute and think about how you enter into relation with people/families. Do you enter lightly and respectfully? Do you sometimes trample in with your busy nursing gait? Do you enter in a way that enables you to see the texture and richness of the family or do you come armed with nurse-driven assessment tools, treatments, and interventions? Think back to the nurses you discussed in Try It Out 6.1 (Chapter 6) or think of other nurses with whom you have worked. How do they appear to enter into relation with family? Try It Out 7.3 invites you to imagine entering into relation with a particular family. What would be easy for you? What would be challenging?

As discussed in Chapter 6, relationships are living processes—they are not formed, they are lived. Every moment of your practice occurs *in-relation*. The question becomes how do you practice in-relation? To be

---

TRY IT OUT 7.3.   Entering Into 'a Challenge'

1. *Pick* your favorite clinical area to think about.
2. *Identify* who the 'challenging' people/families are in that area. List the families who are commonly seen as 'difficult', 'problematic', or 'challenging'. How are they commonly labelled or identified? In emergency nursing, patients who repeatedly return to the hospital are often labeled 'frequent flyers' and seen as challenging. Patients who are angry are seen as challenging. Families who are demanding, particularly those who demand to be 'seen' ahead of others, are seen as challenging. Patients with substance abuse problems or serious mental illnesses are often seen as challenging. Elderly patients without 'literal' family to provide care are sometimes seen as problematic.
3. *Select* an example from your list of 'challenging' families.
4. *Imagine* how you would 'enter in' with such a family. What would be easy for you? What would be difficult?

---

health promoting you need to enter into relationships intentionally and consciously. Entering in in this way does not take more time, rather it just changes how you spend the time you have. It requires that you join people as they are and where they are. Rogers (1961) maintains that the primary ingredient of any relational connection is unconditional positive regard (we will say more about this in Chapter 9 when we consider the 'hard spots' in family nursing). Unconditional positive regard involves accepting people as being of unconditional worth and creating an atmosphere where judgments (for example, about good/bad/right/wrong) and expectations do not dominate. When such an atmosphere is present people are free to be open to their experiences. Therefore entering into respectful relation is fostered through unconditional positive regard and openness and by paying attention to and noticing who and what you are joining. For example, just as you would not approach a toddler in the same way as you would a 45-year-old, you also would not approach all families who are living with cancer in the same way. Similarly, you would not approach all families from a particular ethnic background in the same way. Rather, entering into relation requires that you stop, look, and listen to who, how, and what this family is being at a particular moment in time.

This 'tuning into and joining families as they are' can be termed *synchrony*. Being 'in sync' with a family involves not only paying attention to the meaning, concerns, and life situation of families but as Newman (1994) articulates in her nursing theory (see Chapter 3) it also involves being in-relation energetically. For example, walking into the home of a busy family with young children it is probably out of sync to expect to sit quietly for half an hour and discuss their situation. Rather, engaging with the children as they come and go in their interactions with their parents (rather than seeing the children as 'interrupting'); going with the flow as parenting tasks arise; engaging with the parent as he or she wipes a nose, settles a squabble or changes diapers would be more energetically in sync. Similarly, rushing into a hospital room where an elderly man is lying in bed quietly talking with his partner and his spiritual advisor (rabbi, priest, sensei, guru, minister, and so forth) and hurriedly checking an IV before rushing out of the room would be out of sync energetically. To slow one's movements would probably add only a matter of seconds to the action yet would be far less disruptive and more in sync with the family.

Relational nursing practice involves entering into families by walking along side. It involves paying close attention to both families and to ourselves so we are able to intentionally choose how we might be respectful and in synchrony with particular people/families. Through such entering in we enhance our ability to work with families in ways that are collaborative and health promoting.

Being in Collaborative Relation: Staying 'In Sync'

A central tenet of the socioenvironmental approach to health promotion is collaborative working relationships between people/families and health care professionals. In many ways 'collaboration' has become a new buzz word in health care. But what does it really mean to collaborate? As we have lived this question in our practice and worked with other nurses who are also attempting to collaborate, we have observed something interesting. Although many of us desire to be in power-with collaborative relation, our habit of being the one in charge of health care relationships and of 'health care' leads us to take charge of collaboration. If you listen carefully to nurses and other health care professionals speak and if you look at the nursing literature you will notice that discussions of collaboration are often phrased in such a way that puts the emphasis on nurses (for example, 'nurses collaborate with families' as opposed to 'families collaborating with nurses'). Although on the surface this may appear to be merely semantics we think it is quite telling about the power dynamics that continue to dominate nursing practice. Specifically it is evidence of the nursing habit to assume that health promotion is about what nurses do (that is, it communicates that health promotion is only about nursing action and ignores family action). In addition such an emphasis has remnants of the 'doing to' approach to nursing practice that Newman (1994) and Paterson and Zderad (1976) argue against. Purkis' (1997) example in Chapter 2 of the public health nurse who assessed the baby from a growth and development perspective exemplifies this 'power-over/doing-to' approach. Although the nurse talked about her practice as health promoting she was still in the expert mode of doing to. Using this example, Purkis points out that the rhetoric of health promotion has not really affected a shift in practice. Rather the expert-driven model of practice is more difficult to recognize.

In collaborative relationships the nurse is not in charge of the relating. Rather there is a mutual process where people with different forms of knowledge (such as family members and nurses) work together to inquire into and enhance the family's health and healing experience.

Inquiring Into the Family Health and Healing Experience

Although assessment is part of any nursing approach, our perspective of assessment is somewhat different from models of family nursing that delineate a particular set of questions for nurses to ask or domains for nurses to explore. Based on our understanding that family health is personally, contextually, and relationally constructed we have found assessment and intervention to be much fuller, more accurate, and less intrusive when we approach 'assessment' as a process of inquiry that is particular and specific. Rather than gathering information on a number of general domains that may not have relevance to a particular family, we begin our assessment by inquiring into what is meaningful and significant to a family. Such an inquiry is an interpretive, critical, and spiritual one and involves a process of intense exploration into the health and healing experiences of people/families. Assessment from this inquiry stance refuses theoretical closure and does not allow theoretical categorizations to dominate. That is, we do not begin with a set of questions to ask the family but rather enter in relationally to come to know the people/family in *their* health and healing experience and situation. This does not mean that we don't have or might not ask questions. Rather, as we enter-in we are sensitized by the insight our phenomenological, critical, and spiritual lens offer us as well as the knowledge and research from nursing, biomedicine, and so on. Our questions arise as our knowledge becomes useful within the context of family. Think back to the preamble you developed in Try It Out 7.1. Try this preamble with your family or friends. What does your preamble evoke? And what basis does that provide for your further inquiry?

Approaching assessment as an inquiry process illuminates the open-ended 'messiness' of human life as it is lived by including the

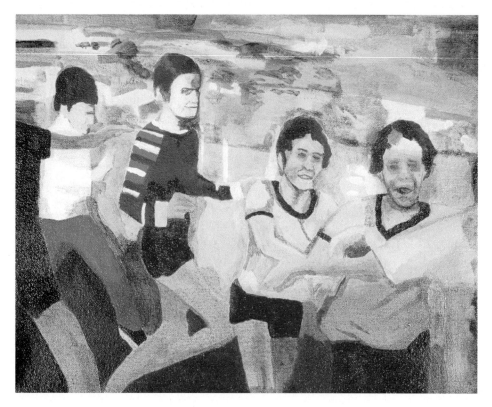

Follow the leader. (Acrylic painting by Alex Grewal.)

multiple experiences and sociocontextual factors that exist within a given family and social space. In conducting assessment as an inquiry process, nurses follow the lead of families and their health and healing experiences rather than following predetermined assessment tools or questions. A nurse approaches people/families openly, is willing to feel uncertain and unknowing. Rather than putting ones' trust in an objectively derived assessment tool the nurse puts her or his trust in people and relationships. That is, there is trust that if one engages relationally with a conscious intent to learn from the family, together family and nurse can collaboratively identify the significant patterns and develop relevant actions. We want to highlight that this process is informed by both the family's knowledge and the nurses' knowledge. Following your preamble, no actual 'questions' might be necessary to get the flow between yourself and the family started (which might be experienced by some cultural groups as much more respectful than the barrage of questions that sometimes typify Western health care encounters). However, examples of initial openings or questions include:

- "I am interested in how you have been."
- "Could you tell me a bit about what has been happening for you?"
- "What stands out as you think about things in your day-to-day life?"
- "What stands out to you as really important for me to know about your situation?"
- "What has been OK and what has been challenging?"
- "What has changed as a result of (your situation or health challenge)?"

Picking up on contextual cues (the person's appearance, the environment) is often a good starting place. Sharing your observations in a tentative manner "It seems like . . ." invites families to confirm or modify those observations. Making inclusive observations (about all family members, about the environment) invites a widening of the focus beyond a single 'patient' or family member. By approaching assessment in this way we are able to gain an understanding of people/families in relationship to their world. This contextual aspect is essential because as hermeneutic phenomenology informs us, it is only within their contexts that what people value and find significant is visible.

Following the Lead of Families

> *66 There's a kind of dance that goes on. It's as though it's cuing and the cuing prompts the next move. And then you wait, and hopefully they're usually leading, that it's coming from what they want. Not always what they need, what they want. I wait for those cues from them and then I go with that flow. (Community Health Worker) 99*

If we are to promote and support the meaningful lives of families then families need to truly be at the center of the health-promoting process. It is families who are experts in their own lives and it is they who collaborate with us. Thus, nurses must take cues from and follow the lead of families. Assessment as an inquiry process begins by following the lead of the family (for example, by inquiring into their living experience, what is of meaning and significance to them). To be able to follow the lead of families, nurses must let go of the habit of approaching people/families from a stance of knowing and certainty (for example, by immediately moving to diagnosing what is 'really going on in this family' or 'what the problem is') and take up a stance of unknowing and uncertainty. In many ways this involves what Flanagan (1996) describes as being a "confident unconfident" (p. 207). This confident unconfident is grounded in a pragmatic approach to knowledge and theory (remember Chapter 1) where knowledge is valued not because it is true but because it fosters increased responsiveness to people. Because the way we use our expert knowledge can serve to lessen our sensitivity to people, pragmatism directs us to be less confident in what we *think* we know and to approach our practice aware of the uncertainty of any truth. Because theories are valuable to the extent that they enhance the knowing and responsiveness to families *any theories guiding family assessment must be scrutinized according to how useful they are in enhancing your capacity to respond and practice in ways that promote the health and well-being of particular families in particular moments.*

An Example: Cuddling A Neonate

One of my (Gweneth) early positions in nursing was in a Neonatal Intensive Care Unit. At the time it was known that too much stimulation was harmful to babies (e.g., expert knowledge said that respiratory distress was exacerbated on touch), therefore, it was common practice to limit the amount of touching the premature babies received. This limited touching practice continued even after the babies were considered stable. The authority bequeathed to this expert 'scientific' knowledge meant that mothers and fathers were not allowed to hold their babies until they were completely off oxygen and other treatments. Although as a new nurse in the unit I attempted to plead the case for parents' right to hold their babies even briefly when the babies were out of the isolettes for tube feedings or other treatments, those who set practice policy told me that the latest knowledge informed us that allowing parents to hold their babies would not be in the babies' best interests. One of the vivid memories I carry with me from that time is holding a baby I was tube feeding as his mother (who had never held her own child) sat next to me with tears in her eyes. Her longing to hold her baby after weeks of standing by watching him struggle to live was actually palpable. All through the tube feeding I sat there feeling in my heart that this practice was wrong. The way that expert knowledge was being used did not seem consistent with responsive practice. That is, it just didn't make sense that a nurse could hold the baby without harm but his own mother could not.

Today it would be considered ludicrous for parents to not have contact with their babies—expert knowledge now tells us how vitally important that connection is to both mother's and baby's health and healing. Current research shows that skin-to-skin contact in particular improves neonate temperature control, breastfeeding success, parent-child interaction, and child development in both preterm and term neonates (Feldman, Weller, Eidelman, & Sirota, 2002; Furman & Kennell, 2000; Kennell & McGrath, 2003; Ohgi et al., 2002). This is an example of the changeability of expert knowledge—of how what we hold to be 'true' and be 'best practice' today may well be considered wrong at another time and place (Flanagan, 1996). As Rorty (1999) describes, long after you are dead, better-informed people may judge your knowledge or actions to have been a terrible mistake. Yet we treat expert knowledge as though it is a truth that offers us certainty. We assume we can rely on expert knowledge to guarantee good practice.

Having watched as expert truths have changed and evolved, we have come to believe that moving toward good practice involves shifting some of the confidence we currently place in expert knowledge to people/families. Rather than placing total confidence in expert knowledge, we need to place our confidence in people/families and more humbly recognize the uncertainty of any expert truth. This does not mean that we do not bring our expert knowledge to our work with families or act as if we don't know anything. Being uncertain is not synonymous with failing to use the knowledge we have. Rather, we are suggesting that it is important to employ knowledge with the understanding that the theories and methods of assessment/intervention at our disposal, including our own thinking, are limited. The ultimate concern guiding our practice should not be ensuring certain practice but rather ensuring we are being as sensitive and responsive to families (Hartrick, 2002c) as possible. This means that when we find ourselves in a situation where expert knowledge is somehow taking precedence over people/families, we need to critically question the knowledge that is guiding us to thought-fully consider how best to proceed. Nursing practice that is relational, competent, and ethical inquires into particular families. Because it is families who are most knowledgeable about themselves and their lives, we need to follow their lead. Nursing knowledge only becomes relevant and useable in the context of family knowledge. Therefore, families are always at the center of any clinical decision making in nursing practice.

Listening To and For

> I found nurses did listen . . . very often they heard things you didn't know you were saying. They often helped me to understand myself. (Kuhl, 2002, p. 60).
>
> Sometimes all it takes is [for nurses] to listen because by the time you have finished a conversation you know exactly what to do. (Nadia—living with an abusive partner)

In Chapter 4 you had the opportunity to begin articulating your theory of family nursing practice. As we highlighted then, the way one theorizes practice profoundly shapes how one proceeds in action. Based on your own particular theoretical perspective, as you connect with a family, you are going to be 'listening to and for' particular things. And, as your theory shifts or changes, so does what you listen for. This is why it is vital that you are as consciously aware of the theories that are guiding you as possible—so that you can intentionally choose which ones will inform your work with particular families. This also emphasizes how important it is to be continually updating your theoretical knowledge by reading current research and other theoretical knowledge. As we have continued to read and do research to inform our practice we have evolved our theoretical perspectives substantially. For example, working with Gweneth, I (Colleen) have learned to intentionally listen for capacity. Similarly, in working with Colleen, I (Gweneth) have learned to pay much closer attention to the politics of practice. As we have evolved our theories what we listen to and for when we connect with families has changed. For example, based on research we have read, we are sensitized to and intentionally listen for how families are incorporating or resisting discourses that idealize family caregiving.

Following the lead of family involves listening carefully to families and inquiring into their health and healing experiences. Although listening is certainly integral to any nursing practice, we have found that listening for particular things can enhance our ability to promote health and healing in families. The lenses described in Chapter 2 and the theories described in Chapter 3 highlight particularly important aspects to listen *for*. That is, they offer some road signs for us to look and listen to and for. It is important to emphasize that the list we offer later does not constitute a prescriptive set of questions or domains for exploration. Rather, families lead the way in relational family nursing. One does not begin with this list but dons the different theoretical lenses to expand one's ability to hear what is meaningful and significant to the family's experience. The lenses help sensitize us to what *might* be important. This sensitivity can help families and nurses recognize and articulate their health and healing experiences and the challenges they are living as they attempt to exercise their power and choice in order to live a meaningful life. It is also important to emphasize that listening to and for is not limited to verbal interaction. As Newman (1994) has described, the energetic level of communication is central to 'knowing' and pattern recognition. Listening for involves carefully attending with all of our senses and abilities. A good example of this listening with our senses is offered in my (Gweneth's) story of Don in Chapter 2 who went 'on hold' as he waited for a diagnosis. I did not 'hear' Don's diminishing spirit verbally but energetically. It was by tuning in at the energetic level (both Don's bodily communication and my own bodily sensing) that his waning spirit became evident. My awareness of his experience at the energetic level enabled me to follow his lead and inquire into his experience verbally. When one is present in this way, listening to and for may in and of itself be a powerful intervention.

Each lens overlaps with the others, each offering a particular angle on what to listen to and for. A phenomenological lens focuses our attention on living experience. As such it directs us to:

Listen for who this person/family is.
Listen for living experience. What is being communicated energetically? Bodily? Verbally? Examples of verbal observations might begin with "It looks like . . ." or "It sounds as though . . ." Questions might include:

- How have things been going?
- What has been OK?
- What has been challenging?
- What is everyday life like?

- What has changed?
- What immediately comes to mind?

Listen for what is particularly significant within peoples'/families' experience. For example, it is helpful to pay attention to what people highlight in their story, what seems to be the at the center of what they are talking about and/or what they keep going back to or repeat as they talk.

Listen for meaning. As you listen you might pay attention to the 'so what'. What does all of this mean for them? This involves listening to the details and facts of their story/description and moving to inquire into what all of those facts and details mean in their life—what is important to them/what impact are the things they are describing having on their life?

Listen for what is of particular concern—what specifically, concretely is concerning them in their everyday life. This involves listening beyond the surface (remember Chapter 6) to pick up cues. For example, sometimes what is of particular concern may not be readily obvious even to people/families. By inquiring into their experience and listening carefully, families have the opportunity to not only articulate their experience but also gain insight into their situation. For example, years ago I (Gweneth) was speaking with a man who was recovering from a myocardial infarction. In asking him how he was feeling about things, he commented that he was really going to miss french fries ('chips' to some of you!). On the surface this may seem like a fairly inconsequential thing; however, in listening beyond the surface I could hear how this was really troubling him. In following his lead and exploring that further we both came to realize that the french fries symbolized the loss of life as he knew it. As he talked we both became aware how he was feeling overwhelmed and powerless in his situation—powerless to the point that he couldn't even choose what food he wanted to eat. This example highlights how listening for significance and concern can enhance overall understanding of the health and healing experience. Questions you might consider include:

- What is it like for you?
- What is particularly important/difficult/challenging about what is happening?
- What would you really like to be able to do, change, or address?

Listening for what is not said. Using your nursing knowledge you can listen for things that they may not be saying, yet seem relevant given other things that have been said or that you have noticed. This can be helpful because sometimes families have difficulty naming all of their experience (they may not yet have found the words or may feel it isn't OK to feel the way they do) and it can be helpful to have someone else raise it and/or inquire about it. For example, Stajduhar's (2001, 2003) research on family caregivers (see Chapter 2) informs us that not all families are prepared and/or want to provide care for family members in their homes. If in listening for the families' experience this seemed relevant you might offer that knowledge and inquire into their experience (for example, by saying something such as 'Families often get the feeling from health care professionals and others that they "should" be looking after their ill members at home, yet for many families that is very difficult to do. What is your experience?')

A critical lens focuses our attention on sociocontextual structures and processes that may be shaping people/families experiences. As such it complements the phenomenological lens, directing us to:

Listen to who is speaking and for whom they are speaking. Paying attention to who is speaking 'for' or within a family gives insight into the power dynamics within a family and provides direction for nurses regarding how to proceed.

Listen for how societal norms are shaping family experience and choice. Listen for what is being taken for granted, again listening for what is not being said as well as what is being said.

Listen for the dominant narratives of family and how they are living through the stories and meanings. Discussions of the dominant views of family throughout this book are intended to alert you to the way they are played out in particular family experiences.

Listen for how sociocontextual elements are constraining and/or promoting people/families' choice and power. Listen for how economics, policies, values, norms, traditions, history, racism, ageism, and so on are shaping family experiences.

Listen for the significance of gender, age, race, ability, and so on. Discrimination based on these social categories occurs within families as well as within wider social contexts. Listen for how different values and various forms of discrimination are played out within and among families.

Listen to the ways people may be conforming to what they anticipate your expectations are, to what they might think is expected of the role of 'patient' or 'mother' or 'diabetic', and so on. How are you (and they) taking up taken-for-granted ideas and practices and reproducing and modifying them?

A spiritual lens directs our attention to the spiritual makeup of the family. A spiritual lens enables us to listen to and for the 'soul reality housed within' (Simmington, 2004) people/families' physical, interpretive, and contextual life space. It directs us to:

Listen for what it is that ultimately concerns the person/family. What concerns are at the center of their lives? What is the life force that guides them?

Listen for how people/families are moving into and through life. How are they presencing themselves within their world and what commitments are guiding their life choices and decisions? How do they relate to others, to the world around them, and perhaps to some form of the transcendent?

Listen for what it is that this person/family has 'set their hearts on'. What loyalties are at the center of their lives and what are they putting their trust, their faith, in? What leaps of faith are being taken? And, what is it they are hoping for?

Listen for how as nurses we might attend to spirit. How might we nurture the spirit-power and support people in ways that help them tap their hidden spirit-power. What is it that "in-spirits" (inspires) them and what might be depleting their spirit energy?

In concert with these perspectives, a socioenvironmental health-promoting lens focuses our attention on capacity—how people are living their power and choice in accessing resources to live meaningful lives. This lens directs our attention to also:

Listen for patterns of capacity. What inner resources do people/families have? What other resources are they drawing on? What resources do they have that they might not be seeing? What collaborative resources do you have between you? What external resources might enhance their existing capacity?

Listen for capacity-adversity patterns—What challenges have and are facing this person/family? How are sociohistorical aspects (such as those that arise with race, economics, gender) intersecting and intensifying their adverse situation? What has enabled them to live in this adversity—that is, what capacities have they accessed/enlisted as they live with the challenge of this adversity? How are they taking up certain practices within their situation?

 An Example: Following the Lead of Family to Inquire Into Their Living Experience

A number of years ago I (Gweneth) facilitated a loss and grief group for people living with Multiple Sclerosis (MS). Although all of the people in the group shared the same disease, each of them was living the disease quite differently. Not only was there variation in the physical manifestation of the disease but what the disease had meant for each of them and how it had affected their lives varied tremendously. One of the most striking features within each of their stories was how MS was truly a family experience. Although some of the people lived within a literal family and some did not, family was central to their experience of the disease. To exemplify 'listening for' I will describe the experience of one of the women I came to know through the group. Perhaps because we shared the role of mother her story of her illness experience has never left me.

As I facilitated discussions in the group I intentionally listened for who each person was and what she or he was experiencing. I learned that Sarah (a pseudonym) was married with two teenage children and had been living with MS for about 8 years. The disease had progressed quite quickly to the point that she required the use of a wheelchair and she had been left with little functional ability in her hands. Sarah was often quiet during the group discussions. Although she did not say much, it was obvious that she was reflecting deeply on what was being said by the other people in the group. One day after the group had been running for 3 or 4 weeks, the topic of family came up. As different people described their experiences Sarah quietly joined in the discussion. She began to talk about what it was like to be a mother and to live with MS, how she had at first 'fought the disease tooth and nail', refusing to let it change her life (listening for what it is that ultimately concerns her). Eventually she had given up the fight and in losing the fight she had also lost her status of mother (listening for what is meaningful and significant). I asked Sarah to tell me how her life as a mother had changed (following her lead and listening for the 'so what'; listening for what depletes her spirit-energy). She described that she had finally had to admit that she could no longer do the physical tasks that 'good mothers' did. She could no longer bake cookies, drive her children to their activities, or carry out all of the tasks she associated with mothering (listening for what is of particular concern). As I listened I began to hear what appeared to be underlying assumptions about what a good mother was (listening for how societal norms are shaping family experience and choice and listening for how certain practices are 'taken up'). Following her lead, I asked Sarah to tell me specifically what she believed constituted a good mother. As she spoke I could hear the stereotypical narrative of the all-giving superwoman mother who does it all (listening for how the dominant narratives of family are living through the stories and meanings). Her description sparked the group to have an in-depth discussion of what it was that determined a good mother—what they had experienced or not experienced as children, mothers, or spouses and what they had learned from those experiences. As part of this discussion they spontaneously began talking about the false ideal that women are expected to live up to and how no woman, regardless of whether she has MS or not, could meet that ideal (listening for sociocontextual elements that constrain power and choice; listening for the significance of gender). At one point one of the people in the group turned to Sarah and said, 'The fact that you care that deeply about not being able to do those things for your kids tells me you are a wonderful mother' (listening for spirit-power; listening for capacity in the face of adversity). In response Sarah began to cry.

A few days later Sarah phoned me to tell me how her experience in the group the previous week had opened something up inside of her that until then she had kept tightly sealed. As she reflected on the discussion and the myriad of feelings she had experienced, she had finally opened up to her deep sorrow she felt over the many losses she had experienced. She had thought that the only way to maintain control was to keep her sorrow in—her tears and the deep sense of relief she had felt in shedding them had shown her that perhaps she had the capacity to face her sorrow and live alongside her MS rather than just give up. The conversation had also sparked further reflection about how she might rethink her mothering—how she might look for new ways to 'be' a mother rather than 'do' mothering (tapping spirit-power; recognizing and naming capacity; reimagining power and choice).

The experience with Sarah and the group also served to spark a deep reflection of my own (self-observation). As a mother who at the time had three young children I reflected on how I too had taken up the societal script of the good mother. Although I had certainly attempted to carve my own path as a mother, when I looked carefully at my everyday life I began to see how the societal script was living through my own mothering actions. That awareness helped me to see how I too might draw on my capacity to choose how I lived my life as mother (clarify my ultimate concern) and how I might reimagine myself in my mothering role (reimagining power and choice). Through the experience I was reminded, once again, of how much I might learn by 'entering in' and listening to and for as I follow the lead of families.

Self-Observation

Deciding to practice relationally can be easier said than done. Trying to actually live and enact these values and principles in your everyday work with people/families can be challenging. As discussed in earlier chapters, often we have developed habits that do not necessarily give rise to such practice and these habits are not always easy to change. In addition, even if as a student you develop habits that support relational practice, you are often working in health care contexts that are disease-care focused. Consequently, you might find yourself navigating through values, structures, and policies that do not support human-centered, relationally responsive practice. Self-observation is a process that can help nurses address these habits and contexts in order to practice in ways that are relational.

Self-observation involves practicing the skill of reflexivity (described in Chapter 5) as you work with families. Remember back to the story in Chapter 6 of the nurse who spent the night with the parents whose son had been born with congenital anomalies. That story offers a good example of self-observation. The nurse initially felt very anxious about how she should proceed and even whether she could. By stopping and observing herself—by becoming aware of the anxiety that was overwhelming her, consciously enlisting existing knowledge she had about how to be in-relation with families, and reminding herself of the intent guiding her practice (that was, to bring herself to the relationship and 'be with' and respond to what the family was experiencing), she was able to step beyond her habit of feeling responsible to 'do' something and/or 'fix' the family. She was also able to see beyond her own concerns (such as how to be with the parents of a dying child) to join the family in what was meaningful to them (for example, having as much time with their son as they could). It was her process of self-observation that helped her clarify her intent, gave her direction for action, and enabled her to respond in a health-promoting way.

This process of self-observation is a central ingredient of family assessment and intervention. As you enter into relation with a family your ability to know and respond to them can be greatly enhanced by paying attention to who you are being, how and what you are thinking and doing. By observing oneself and paying attention to the thoughts, emotions, and bodily responses one is having at any moment, the opportunity to reflexively consider those responses and more consciously and intentionally choose how to act and respond is created.

Reflexive consideration of our emotional and bodily response is essential to the self-observation process, because it is often not clear to what our responses are alerting us. For example, many experienced nurses are disconcerted when I (Gweneth) invite them to try out a relational approach to family nursing. Having come to rely on predetermined assessment tools to guide their practice they describe feeling very uncomfortable proceeding in such an "unstructured" way. At times they report that even some families comment that they would 'just like the nurse to tell them what she/he wants to know'. If we took the discomfort at surface value without reflexively scrutinizing what the discomfort was alerting us to, we may only link the discomfort to the family nursing approach and assume that the approach was not suitable for certain nurses and/or for some families. However, most often when nurses *reflexively* explore their discomfort and examine what specifically and concretely feels uncomfortable (to both the nurse and family), they discover that their discomfort has been sparked by stepping out of the habits they have developed. That is, the different approach to practice has taken them outside of their comfort zone. Not only does it feel uncomfortable to be enacting their nursing role differently, but initially they find it takes much more conscious effort and is much less certain and less controlled (and therefore more anxiety producing) to enter into relation and follow the lead of the family not knowing where that lead is going to take them. Similarly families have often learned the role of 'service recipient' and may not immediately know how to respond when given the opportunity to take the lead. Therefore, initially, it feels strange. This reflexive consideration creates the opportunity for both nurses and families to understand the discomfort and make conscious and intentional choices about how best to respond to the discomfort (that is, what, if anything, they need to do differently). In this way, self-observation illuminates the meanings, concerns, and values that are shaping our experience and offers the opportunity for us to choose how to respond—to choose how to bring ourselves to our work and use the capacities we have at our disposal.

As well as offering insight into ourselves and our practices, self-observation can expand our knowledge of families and of contextual elements. Because our bodily sensations, emotions, and thoughts may be sparked in response to what is happening externally, self-observation offers a window to the world. For example, paying attention to and critically reflecting on what we are experiencing and how we are respond-ing can inform us about institutional practices and structures that might be problematic and/or in need of revision.

In Chapter 5 we described the What Can I Learn About Me game as one self-observation exercise that can promote self-knowing. In our work we have heard of nurses devising many ways to tune into and observe themselves. One example was shared by Susan Connolly, a Public Health Nursing Supervisor at the Fraser Health, Maple Ridge Health Unit in British Columbia. During a workshop I (Gweneth) conducted with the public health nurses in that region, we had talked about the importance of self-observation and the challenge of remembering to tune into ourselves in order to move beyond disease-care habits of practice and toward more health-promoting ones. To support nurses in this process following the workshop Susan, in collaboration with some colleagues, developed bookmarks that the nurses could put in their day-books to cue themselves. Each week there was a new bookmark with some new observation questions for the nurses to ask themselves. Box 7.2 offers an example of bookmark.

Another example of a self-observation strategy was described by a nurse who participated in an ethics research project our team conducted (Varcoe et al., 2003). The nurse described that she monitored her practice by asking herself each day: 'If I was a patient on this ward, would I want me for my nurse today?' Asking herself this question and realizing that sometimes the answer was 'No' helped her to more consciously decide how she wanted to be in practice and constantly reminded her to respond to the people she was caring for.

Overall the process of self-observation can be thought of as a process of 'coming clean'—of trying to honestly look at ourselves to ask what concerns are guiding us, what expectations we are bringing, and

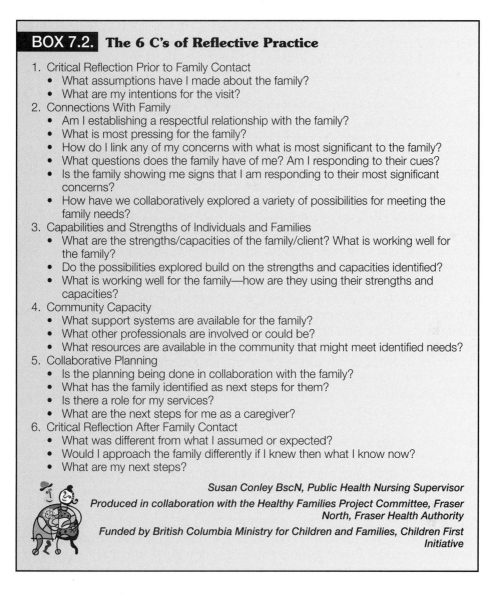

BOX 7.2. **The 6 C's of Reflective Practice**

1. Critical Reflection Prior to Family Contact
   - What assumptions have I made about the family?
   - What are my intentions for the visit?
2. Connections With Family
   - Am I establishing a respectful relationship with the family?
   - What is most pressing for the family?
   - How do I link any of my concerns with what is most significant to the family?
   - What questions does the family have of me? Am I responding to their cues?
   - Is the family showing me signs that I am responding to their most significant concerns?
   - How have we collaboratively explored a variety of possibilities for meeting the family needs?
3. Capabilities and Strengths of Individuals and Families
   - What are the strengths/capacities of the family/client? What is working well for the family?
   - Do the possibilities explored build on the strengths and capacities identified?
   - What is working well for the family—how are they using their strengths and capacities?
4. Community Capacity
   - What support systems are available for the family?
   - What other professionals are involved or could be?
   - What resources are available in the community that might meet identified needs?
5. Collaborative Planning
   - Is the planning being done in collaboration with the family?
   - What has the family identified as next steps for them?
   - Is there a role for my services?
   - What are the next steps for me as a caregiver?
6. Critical Reflection After Family Contact
   - What was different from what I assumed or expected?
   - Would I approach the family differently if I knew then what I know now?
   - What are my next steps?

Susan Conley BscN, Public Health Nursing Supervisor
Produced in collaboration with the Healthy Families Project Committee, Fraser North, Fraser Health Authority
Funded by British Columbia Ministry for Children and Families, Children First Initiative

how those are relevant and/or not relevant to the families with whom we are working.

Letting Be and Change

❝ *A lot of it is about merging. When one is aware it's easy to blend with people, to merge with them. You see what kinds of things they have, a picture on the wall . . . or a lovely family gallery they have and they start talking about their children and their grandchildren. . . . People have around them tokens of what matters to them. They've got trinkets, they've got a new bouquet of flowers, and they've got a card . . . you can tell whether they use herbal remedies or medicine . . . you see the way they do their hair. . . . I am moving into their space and I know what they are and what they feel like. When you can merge with someone that way and when they can tell that you've perceived them, then you're in their heart space. You're in that safe, really safe heart space. That's what it's all about. (Community Support Worker)* 　　　　　　　　　　　　　　　**99**

As discussed in Chapter 6 many nurses experience great angst when they find themselves in a situation where they cannot effect change. This is partly a result of nurses being educated to be change agents. We take a somewhat different approach to this notion of change. In contrast to teaching you how to intervene to create change in families, as we discussed in earlier chapters, we think one of the most important skills any nurse needs to have is the ability to 'let be' (Hartrick Doane, 2002). Rather than joining families with the intent to change them, one joins from an open, inviting stance and deep intent to come to know a family—to know who they are and what their life situation is at this moment in time. As we invite families to tell us who they are, the opportunity is created for families to open up and come to know themselves more deeply. Through such a process, experiences begin moving, and changes occur. As Newman (1994) describes, when life is received as it is, change can happen as it needs to. For that reason, letting be is perhaps the most powerful way in which change is promoted.

In Chapter 3, we described how the multidisciplinary group of practitioners in the asthma program changed their practices to be more health promoting. If you re-read that description you will see that letting be was one of the most significant shifts that occurred in their practice. For example the nurses described that at the beginning of the project they would go into a family's home armed with all kinds of information about asthma and launch into giving the information to the family. As they evolved their practice to be more health promoting they gradually found themselves letting be. They would begin the conversation by asking about the family and about their asthma experience (they would 'let be to know what is'). They would listen carefully to what was significant and meaningful to the family and then offer information when families indicated their readiness (families opened and began to move). As the practitioners became more conscious and intentional in promoting health, rather than doing asthma care, they became less and less focused on 'changing families' and more and more focused on knowing and responding to families. A central goal of that asthma program was to reduce the number of hospital admissions and by the end of the first year of the project they had managed to effect a significant decrease in admissions. Letting be is a powerful way for change to occur.

Letting be is central to relational practice for two reasons. First, it ensures that families are at the center of any action—that it is *they* who collaborate with us. As a result, letting be enables us to follow the lead of the family, to respond to what is significant and meaningful to them. The strategy of letting be moves us beyond the habitual tendency to override and control families. In essence, it helps us to get out of the way and to more effectively support families in exercising their own power and choice and effecting the changes that they wish to make in their own lives. Second, letting be takes the pressure off nurses to fix something in families and offers us a way of identifying how we might be change agents at the systemic level. As we bring our critical lens to our work with families and let be we can begin to identify social, economic, environmental, and political factors that are constraining the health of families. For example, as the nurses in the asthma program listened to families' experience of living with asthma, they learned that limited economic resources made it very difficult for some families to attend follow-up appointments. A combination of no childcare and poor accessibility to public transportation got in the way of families being able to access the support and resources the asthma program had to offer. Consequently, instead of being frustrated and trying to fix the families (e.g., lecturing them on how important it was to attend the appointments), the nurses began to identify systemic changes required to address this inequity. They began looking for ways that childcare and transportation might be subsidized to ensure families with limited financial resources would not be disadvantaged in accessing the program. Similarly, they identified a need to work closely with the emergency department to create better protocols to respond to families who came to the emergency department. This is an example of how following the lead of families can lead to collaborative knowledge that has the potential to effect systemic change.

Unfortunately because the health care system in the Western world is most often structured according to a service model of care, most nurses develop the habit of focusing on 'alleviating the problem' *in families* rather than addressing problems *beyond families* and that habit is often difficult to move beyond. Yet we have found that the more nurses try to control and change families, the less likely people/families are to respond. All people need to feel a sense of power and control in their lives and this need for control is heightened during illness or stress. For that reason, the most effective way to promote health is to join in-relation with people/families and let be to find out how best to support them in their choice and power, while simultaneously identifying how we might effect change at the systemic level.

Collaborative Knowledge Development

Collaborative knowledge development builds on letting be by bringing families' knowledge together with nursing knowledge. As nurses and families let be and begin to know the family experience, they use this knowledge to support the identification and recognition of patterns in the family's experience. This collaborative knowledge development process involves drawing on multiple forms of knowledge including nursing and other theory, biomedical knowledge, recent research findings, sociopolitical knowledge, and analysis and experiential/bodily knowledge. Central to this knowledge development process is following the lead of families. As we listen and let be these different knowledges sensitize us to hear and make meaning of what the family is telling us.

An Example: Caring for Children With Prolonged Terminal Illnesses

Rose Steele's (2002) work with families caring for children with life-threatening neurodegenerative illnesses provides an excellent example of the importance of collaborative knowledge development. She shows how 'navigating uncharted territory' the families 'struggled, often blindly, in their life journey when their child was dying' (p. 420). These families' struggles were seriously compromised by relationships with health care providers in which the families' experiences and expertise were not taken into account and by the availability of information, which families sometimes saw health care providers as withholding. There was little empirical information available on their children's illnesses, but only the occasional health care provider admitted that he or she did not have all the answers. It was these few people with whom the families had satisfying relationships, relationships characterized by collaborative knowledge development. 'Compared with most parents, those who were treated as knowledgeable partners from early on in the illness experiences described fewer feelings of anger and frustration with their primary health care providers' (p. 424).

In today's world, families bring knowledge from many domains including their experiential knowledge, their historical knowledge, their sociocultural knowledge, and so forth. Part of following the families' lead involves finding out about the knowledge they bring to any health and healing situation and how that knowledge has shaped their understanding and experience. For example, the Internet is a major source of knowledge for people today. However, the accuracy and validity of the knowledge available on the Internet is at times questionable. It is not unusual for families to form ideas about their illness situation as a result of misleading information they have gotten over the Internet. Conversely, families may not only be experts in their own experiences, some may also have more valid and reliable empirical knowledge than their health care providers. This is especially likely with long-term or chronic conditions. However, making assumptions about families' knowledge is always problematic. For example, in Steele's (2002) study many parents expended considerable effort to gain whatever knowledge was available on their children's conditions, but some did not have the resources or energy to do so. This means that part of following the family's lead involves continually asking families to 'tell me what you know about . . .' The more we follow the lead and learn from families the greater our ability is to build on their existing capacity, counter any inaccurate information that may be constraining them, tailor information and suggestions to their circumstances, and pass on the wisdom of one family to another.

Pattern Recognition

> *66 So I asked [the mom] if she could identify a pattern before [her son] comes to the hospital so she did reflect back and there is a pattern no doubt about it, and she has an action plan. But she basically leaves [taking action] until the day he's really sick and oral prednisone isn't going to help him, but [we talked about] starting the oral prednisone two days earlier and he'd never get into that state. (Nurse in an Outpatient Asthma Program)* 99

The quote here exemplifies how, as nurses enter into relation with families, follow their lead, and listen for what is of meaning and significance, both the family and nurse can begin to gain more knowledge of the health and healing situation and recognize patterns that are playing out within the family's experience and life situations. These patterns include patterns of experience, patterns of response, patterns of capacity, and patterns of adversity. The process of pattern recognition is supported through the complementary processes of letting be and collaborative knowledge development and fosters more responsive care. For example, similar to Stajduhar's (2003) research, in her research into parent's caregiving experiences Steele (2002) found that the caregiving experiences of both men and women were shaped in important ways by gender identities. Even mothers who did not want to do so stayed at home to fulfill the caretaker role. Being sensitized by this knowledge as one listens to and collaborates with the family we are able to pay attention and inquire into how such patterns might be living out in the people's/families' with whom we are working. Through such collaborative inquiry it is possible to avoid stereotyping and making erroneous assumptions that hinder relational connection.

Another aspect of pattern recognition that is central to collaborative knowledge development is identifying the sociopolitical patterns in which the family is embedded. For example, as described earlier, by following the lead of the families and listening for what was meaningful and significant in living with asthma in their everyday lives, nurses were able to hear a pattern of inequity of resources. Rather than assuming families were just not bothering to show up for appointments and becoming frustrated, by following the lead of the family the nurses learned that there were socioeconomic limitations that hindered access to the asthma program for some families. Therefore, in order to promote health in the families the nurses needed to identify and address the socioeconomic pattern of inequity that the families were living within. Try It Out 7.4 suggests that you might be able to predict and anticipate some patterns of inequity.

Through their working relationships, families and nurses can make connections between experiences and the 'so what' for action. This involves recognizing the patterns of capacity and of adversity that are simultaneously part of the family's experience. In recognizing the patterns, it is important to understand how those patterns are meaningfully experienced by the family. That is, what might be considered to be

---

TRY IT OUT 7.4.   **Anticipating Inequity**

1. *Think* about the practice area you enjoy most, work in, or would like to work in. Thinking about the people/families in that practice area, what inequities are most likely to face families in that area? There are few practice areas in which racism, ageism, poverty, and heterosexism are not issues, but additionally inequity based on geography (e.g., rural disadvantage), size (e.g., overweight), or something else might be particularly important in your area.
2. *Read* the Guidelines for Providing Good Health Care to Lesbians in Box 7.3. As you read, think about another form of oppression that families with whom you work might experience, such as racism or poverty or ageism.
3. *Reword* the 'guidelines' to provide ideas regarding how to provide 'good health care' to families experiencing the form of oppression you have been thinking about.
4. *Compare* your revisions with someone else's (a colleague or classmate).

BOX 7.3. **Guidelines for providing good health care to lesbians**

Don't make assumptions
Remember that identity does not equal behaviour
Examine your own biases—how do they affect your patient interactions?
Remember that how you ask questions may be just as important as the questions themselves.
Don't contradict your patients when they make statements about themselves; avoid arguments
Roll with resistance, giving your patient time to integrate information and develop trust in you and the process
Educate yourself about issues relevant to good health care for lesbians
If you can't support your patients' identity, refer them to someone who can
Involve your patients' significant others in decision-making and planning
Be aware of and display resources in your waiting room to let patients know you are approachable
Use inclusive language on all office forms and when talking with your patients
Ask your patients if there is something that you've missed asking about that they feel is important for you to know
Don't make assumptions

(Simkin (1998) "Not all your patients are straight"—Reprinted from, CMAJ 25-Aug-98; 159(4), pp. 370–375 by permission of the publisher. © 1998 Canadian Medical Association.)

---

adversity to one person/family may not be adversity to another. For example, one woman may cherish the caregiving role, while another might resent it, either woman might both cherish and resent it, some family members may feel it is the woman's duty, and she may or may not see it that way herself. Recognizing patterns of capacity and adversity provides significant direction for action—how to support capacity and counter adversity through emancipatory action.

Naming and Supporting Capacity

The Oxford Dictionary (1982) defines capacity as 'the power of containing, receiving, experiencing, or producing . . . (capacity includes) mental power, faculty, talent, position, character' (p. 136). These descriptors are reflective of what we have come to know about families. We have often found ourselves in awe at the strength of the human spirit and the capacity that people/families have within them. We have witnessed families experiencing life challenges such as chronic, life-threatening, or terminal illness, poverty, isolation, prejudice, and trauma. At the same time we have seen them draw on their inner power and faculties to live through those life-challenging experiences. Moreover, we have seen many people/families 'produce' positive personal and social results out of adverse circumstances and experiences.

Although often people's capacity goes unnamed or unrecognized, we have yet to meet anyone who does not have capacity and more potential capacity. Interestingly, it is perhaps during times and conditions of adversity that capacity is particularly evident. Yet it is those very times of adversity when capacity is most often overlooked or not recognized. The tendency to focus on the adversity or problem and on servicing or fixing what is lacking overrides both families' and nurses' ability to see the resourcefulness and capacity families have to effect their own life situation.

An Example: No Crib for a Bed

During a discussion I (Gweneth) had with a group of public health nurses, one nurse described her experience with a family that included a teenage mother and father and a new baby. Until the time of the birth the parents had been living on the street. On discharge the public health nurse was notified that this was a 'high-risk' family that needed careful following. The public health nurse had made a home visit and described to us what she found when she arrived. The family had just moved into a 'very run-down apartment' that had no furniture and few household items. The parents had rigged up a bed for the baby by converting an old solid-looking box into a crib. When I asked how she had found the parents and the baby, the nurse replied that the baby was in a sleeper that was old and torn but seemed to be well nourished and healthy. The parents seemed 'quite attached and interested' in the baby. What I found interesting was the varying responses of those of us listening to this nurse's story. Some of the nurses listening expressed great concern about the safety of the baby 'without a crib to sleep in'. Others talked about the teaching the parents would need if they were to be able to meet the needs of the baby. Finally, one of the more senior nurses in the group replied, 'I think their resourcefulness is remarkable'. Her comment helped turn the conversation to consideration of the capacity of these two young parents. We discussed the obvious commitment they must have to their baby and the resourcefulness they had to be able to go from living on the street to moving into an apartment. We also found ourselves marvelling at how in the course of a few weeks they had not only become parents, but had changed their entire life structure. As we began identifying the capacity we saw, the nurse who had made the home visit commented that on top of that they had seemed relaxed and happy when she was there—more so than many mothers she visits who are living in comfortable homes and who have economic resources and extended family support.

This story is a reminder of how important it is to look beyond the surface of things. On the surface these parents may not seem to measure up to parents who have more economic resources. Yet when you consider what they were willing to do and had actually done with such limited resources, it is clear that they have as much or more capacity than many families who have all of the surface fixtures that are sometimes taken for granted as necessary for a new baby. For example, a crib is often a taken-for-granted necessity for a baby and in fact, the public health nurses pointed out that ensuring there was a good crib for the baby was a routine part of their well-baby assessment. Without stopping and really thinking about it, a nurse could have easily added 'no crib' to the high-risk score. However, according to the nurse, the box was safe and secure and served the purpose well. Thus from a vantage point of capacity, the box is evidence of the parents thoughtfulness about the baby's safety and their resourcefulness in providing for the baby. This highlights how easy it is to fall into negative judgments based on preconceived taken-for-granteds and how crucial it is to consciously and intentionally question those taken-for-granteds. In addition this example highlights that if we want to find capacity in people/families we have to look for it and recognize it when we see it.

The family in this situation could be looked at through a capacity lens or through a deficiency lens. The 'story' one told of that couple could be of a family with great capacity who was living a meaningful life with their baby or it could be a story of deficiency about a family who had no resources and whose baby had to sleep in a box. What determines which story will be told is what is listened for, named, and supported. In addition, it depends on who gets to tell the story—is the family the central narrator or is the nurse? To name and support capacity in ways that are health promoting, families need to play a central role in the narrating process. Because what one family may experience as adversity may not be experienced as adversity by another, it is important that the family be the narrator of their own story. That is, relational nursing practice involves asking the family for their version of the story and then responding accordingly. This is in direct contrast to other forms of assessment where the expert nurse stands back, observes the family from her or his location, and then writes the story (for example, by completing the admission history or writing assessment notes from his or her expert view).

Collaborating with families to recognize and explicitly name capacity is perhaps one of the most empowering things that families can experience. Being situated in a health care system that is focused on problems and the servicing of those problems, combined with the powerlessness that people often experience during times of illness and adversity, sometimes families have difficulty seeing the capacity they are living. Recognizing, affirming, and/or connecting with the capacity you see living within them can potentiate people's reconnection with the power and choice they have and are living in spite of the adversity they are facing. Unfortunately, naming family strengths and capacities has sometimes been translated as yet another 'thing' to add to the assessment or intervention list—as though acknowledging family strengths is one more thing *the nurse* should do. We want to be very clear this is not what we are suggesting. Naming and supporting capacities is not one more thing to add on to an assessment or intervention! Recognizing and affirming capacity is the lens and theoretical foundation brought to every moment of practice—it is a philosophical, theoretical, and practical way of being in-relation and working with families. At the heart of this process is a collaborative, power-with, respectful, and equitable relational way of being with each other. This distinction is essential because naming family strength and capacity can be done in ways that are noncollaborative and at times even disrespectful. For example, sometimes nurses 'identify strengths of families' as part of their intervention. Depending on how that is done, identifying strengths can be comparable to an expert, benevolent nurse giving the family a pat on the back. Families have told us that they have experienced such action as very patronizing and disrespectful. Therefore, we want to emphasize that from a relational perspective, recognizing and affirming capacity may not even be something that is necessarily said/done by the nurse. Rather through their work together the opportunity is created for both families and nurses to recognize and come to know the capacities living out in the relational moment. So in the earlier example of the young family, through a conversation about 'what babies really need in their first year' the family's resourcefulness and capacity to provide this would have become readily apparent—it could have been the family, nurse, or all involved naming the capacity. At the same time the opportunity for them to collaboratively name other things that might enhance that existing capacity likely would have arisen. This process of naming capacity can be supported by bringing the different theoretical lenses to the inquiry/intervention process. For example, through a phenomenological lens it is possible to see the capacities that families are living in their everyday lives amidst the adverse situation. Similarly, a critical lens helps us identify the socioeconomic resources and limitations of people/families and how they might enhance those resources.

An Example: An Heroic Admission

Recently while I (Gweneth) was working on a research project looking at the quality of care (from an ethical perspective) on a medical oncology unit, the husband of one of the patients told me the following story and gave his permission for me to share it. Although the story has much to say about many things in health care, one of the most striking features is, for me, family capacity. I met the couple when I entered the woman's hospital room to explain the research we were doing and ask their permission to accompany their nurse throughout the day as she cared for them. The woman was lying in her bed looking very pale and quite frail. They told us that she had had a restless night that had been further disrupted when she had failed to make it to the bathroom in time. Their first request was that we bring a commode chair in so she would have easier access.

About an hour later I was standing out in the hallway and the husband approached me to say he had read the information pamphlet about the study and wanted me to know that he thought the nurses on the unit gave 'wonderful care'. 'It is the health care system and actually being able to get into the hospital to get the care the nurses have to give that is the problem', he informed me. Following his lead I inquired into their experience of 'getting into the hospital'.

He explained that his wife had been in hospital receiving chemotherapy but due to the hospital bed situation she had been discharged even though she was feeling very ill from the chemotherapy and in a lot of pain. After a few days at home and of her being 'in such pain and vomiting so badly' he tried calling the emergency department to ask if he could bring her back to be readmitted. The emergency doctor, although sympathetic, told him that the bed situation in the hospital was such that even if he brought her in there would be nothing they could do for her—that she would just end up waiting a long time to be seen and would then be discharged home. Feeling powerless, he hung up the phone and told his wife there was no help and 'we will just have to tough it out at home'. After helping his wife settle for the night he went to bed at about 1:00 AM.

The next thing he knew the phone was ringing and it was the hospital. While he slept, his wife had cut off her hospital identification band and, leaving all identification at home, had left the house in her housecoat and pyjamas and started walking to the hospital. For a well person walking at a fast clip the walk would probably have taken 45 minutes. A taxi driver stopped when he saw her and asked if she needed a ride. She accepted the ride to the hospital where on her arrival the police were called. In spite of their insistence, she refused to give her name—knowing that if she did identify herself they would just take her home. After much persistence on the part of the police and the hospital staff, she finally gave a phone number. The husband was awakened by the call asking if he was aware that his wife was at the hospital. A frantic check revealed that in fact his wife wasn't where he had left her. The nurse on the other end of the phone told him that he would have to come and get his wife. 'I said OK and hung up but it was after I hung up that I realized that if I did go down to the hospital I would just defeat her heroic effort. They would just send her home and all that she had done would have been for nothing. So I just phoned back and told them I refused to come and get her and that is how she got to be readmitted'.

In taking a phenomenological lens to this story, many capacities become evident. First, the supportive relationship between the couple that is serving as the foundation from which they are surviving this incredibly challenging situation comes into focus. The man's care and commitment toward his wife, as well as his understanding and support of her 'heroism', reveals the depth of understanding and appreciation of 'what it is like for her' to live with her cancer and through the treatment process. In taking a critical and spiritual lens to the situation, it is possible to see the capacity and hidden spirit-power the woman has drawn on to challenge the system that is seemingly refusing to provide the care she needs. Even with her existing physical limitations, she drew on her capacity and strategically thought about how she might 'march in protest' to receive the resources she felt she needed to get through this experience. What is important to highlight is how this story could be read from many different vantage points. For example, through a critical lens it is possible to challenge the discourse of the 'good patient' that does what she is told, or the discourse that says there is a 'scarcity of health care resources' and depicts the health care crisis as being due to the inevitable need to limit expenditures rather than due to corporate decisions about how to spend (Armstrong, Armstrong, Bourgeault, Mykhalovskiy, & White, 2000; McQuaig, 1998; Varcoe & Rodney, 2002). Similarly, it is possible to challenge the dominant societal narrative of family as a safe haven that 'should' look after their own and to question the values that are dominating our society and health care system and resulting in this incredibly ill woman having to leave her home in the middle of the night in a desperate attempt to receive hospital care. Finally, through a spiritual lens we are able to see the astonishing strength of spirit-power—how in spite of her diminished physical strength this woman was able tap the strength and force necessary to address her needs.

Emancipatory Action

Because the relational approach to family nursing views families in context, a major site of nursing intervention is at the systemic and structural level. As we let be and come to know what is meaningful and significant in families' health and healing experiences it is common to see structural and social inequities compromising health. Acting to reduce those inequities is often referred to as 'emancipatory' health promotion.

Drevdahl, Kneipp, Canales, and Dorcy (2001) outline a rich tradition of concern for social inequities, social justice, and emancipatory action in nursing but argue that the tendency to focus on the individual as the target of care has overshadowed emancipatory concerns. Over the past several decades, nurses have argued for emancipatory practice and claimed that nurses have a responsibility to participate in sociopolitical action (Drevdahl, 1995; Kendall, 1992; Stevens, 1989, 1992; Stevens & Hall, 1992). Not surprisingly, those arguing for emancipatory nursing practice have drawn on broad conceptions of the environment and critical social theory.

The commitment of nursing to social justice and emancipation has also been considered a moral obligation. Increasingly nursing Codes of Ethics direct nurses to attend to the social conditions of patient's lives. For example, the Canadian Nurses Association (CNA) (2002) *Code of Ethics* specifies that nurses must 'uphold principles of equity and fairness to assist persons in receiving a share of health services and resources proportionate to their needs and in promoting social justice' (p. x). Ballou (2000) conducted a historical-philosophical analysis of key professional documents and predominant published works and concluded that professional nursing practice involves a moral and professional obligation to participate in sociopolitical activities.

Despite these arguments, little has been written about what emancipatory nursing action looks like. Nurses advocating the use of critical social theory have examined the implications for research (e.g., Mill, Allen, & Morrow, 2001) or education, but few have paid attention to the implications for practice. Browne (2000, 2001) suggests that the major reason that nursing's emancipatory objectives have not advanced is that although critical theory is generally congruent with nursing's social mandate, the liberal underpinnings (remember the Chapter 1 discussion of liberal individualism) of nursing science are incompatible with critical theory.

So, what might emancipatory health-promoting practice 'look like'? If nursing is to act 'upstream', it is clear that actions must be directed not only at particular families, but also at a level beyond—at the contexts that are shaping families' experiences. Nursing practice that is knowledgeable, contextual, ethical, and emancipatory is responsive to families and the structural conditions that compromise the health and health care of families collectively. Emancipatory practice thus involves:

Recognizing and naming inequities for particular families and across families. Identifying where particular families are experiencing social inequities and drawing attention to those inequities are meaningful acts in themselves. Doing so immediately focuses energy on the inequities and assists in countering strategies that might place blame and responsibility on families for the conditions of their lives. For example, nurses in the asthma program focused on facilitating families' access rather than holding them responsible for that access.

Recognizing and naming structural conditions that compromise health and health promotion for particular families and across families. Drawing attention not only to the inequities that families experience, but also to the structural conditions that give rise to those inequities similarly focuses energy on those conditions. Such action should include drawing the patterns of inequity and structural conditions to the attention of families themselves, to colleagues, and to decision makers at various levels of policy. For example, Canam (2004) describes how a nurse working in a pediatric outpatient clinic for a particular condition drew the impact of government policies to the attention of colleagues and policy makers in order to alleviate such impact. In order to obtain government-provided treatment, the families were required to have their child receive a diagnosis. However, the waiting lists at the clinic meant that families were waiting months and years to get the diagnosis, and thus treatment for their children was delayed.

Drawing on and sharing contextual knowledge. Sharing knowledge about the contextual features of particular health problems is a powerful way to shift thinking and action. For example, imagine sharing your knowledge about the relationship between childhood asthma and socioeconomic deprivation in a pediatric clinical team meeting.

Introducing alternative discourses. In concert with sharing your contextual knowledge, alternative discourses can be introduced. For example, imagine introducing a feminist discourse into a conversation with a colleague regarding anorexia nervosa.

Devoting energy to remedying structural inequities that cross families. Remedies are not all at the level of society; not all require social action. Some remedies can be as simple as offering different hours in a diabetic clinic (remember Artur in Chapter 1?). However, some remedies require attempts to influence policy at different levels (remember the article about Cathy Crowe in Chapter 6?).

Creating coalitions. As we have argued, a lone nurse cannot 'fix' policies, organizations, and structural conditions that constrain relational practice and health promotion. Finding and working with colleagues who share your concerns strengthens action and makes meaningful outcomes more likely.

Recall the example of Barb, the labour and delivery nurse who treated all women as though they had experienced sexual abuse or trauma. In that example you can see that Barb was acting in an emancipatory way. She was operating on an understanding of gender inequity in which many women are subjected to sexual violence. She named the inequity (by telling women that she knew many will have had previous "bad experiences"), but, consistent with emancipatory action, she left the control (to disclose or not and to direct care) in the hands of the women themselves. Barb also introduced an alternative discourse (emotionally safe care) to the discourse of screening and disclosure that currently dominates nursing practice in relation to violence (Ramsey, Richardson, Carter, Davidson, & Feder, 2002; Varcoe, 2004). At the same time, Barb participated in action to block a policy from being implemented in her hospital that would require 'screening' of all labouring women for a violence history (sharing contextual knowledge and devoting energy to remedying inequity). I (Colleen) worked with Barb (together, building a coalition) on that initiative because we both believed that the introduction of such a policy would further exacerbate the very problem it was supposedly addressing. That is, forcing women to disclose traumatic experiences would be another form of gender inequity and potential harm.

Browne (2000) offers several cautions that we should heed in pursuing emancipatory nursing objectives. First, we should remain realistic, focusing on possibilities for emancipatory change rather than on expectations for actual changes. We are unlikely to change the world, but it is an objective worth pursuing. Second, we have to resist the urge to 'save' people by imposing our ideas regarding what is needed. Emancipatory actions aimed at the level of organization should continue to follow the lead of families. Finally, Browne urges that we should continually critique the ideas underlying our knowledge and practice.

● Practicing Relationally

Overall relational family nursing involves integrating the processes described earlier into everyday practice. It involves walking alongside people/families to facilitate responsive, safe, and health-promoting care. We are proposing these processes in the spirit of 'ideals'. That is, we recognize the challenge of actualizing the processes within the limitations of the 'real world' of health care. Yet similar to Paterson and Zderad (1976) we believe the processes are ideals worth striving toward. Although we may not be able to fix what is wrong in the health care world or live the ideals in each moment of practice, striving toward these ideals will support us to provide the most responsive care we can. In the next three chapters we offer examples of how these processes might be taken up within the complexity of everyday nursing practice (Chapter 8), how they might support your ability to navigate through the 'hard spots' of family nursing practice (Chapter 9), and how they are transferable to the world of nursing research (Chapter 10). Before moving on to the next chapters try out the processes we have suggested in This Week In Practice.

THIS WEEK IN PRACTICE

Practicing Relationally

Explore some of the relational processes we have presented in your clinical work with people/families this week. Regardless of where you are working and who the people are you are nursing, try to get 'in synch' with them. Similarly, try following the lead of the people— inquire into their health and healing experience and observe yourself as you do so. Does this unstructured and uncertain process feel uncomfortable? What do you notice about yourself and the response of the people/family to you? Practice 'listening to and for' through the different lenses and see how your view changes. Intentionally approach people looking for capacity and notice how that changes your response to them. Consider the relevance of emancipatory action to the situations and people you are in. What contextual elements are shaping their experience and your ability to respond? If you are not actually in a practice setting this week, identify someone with whom you have a relationship (Your grandmother? Friends? A neighbouring family?) and consciously try these ideas out when you are with them.

CHAPTER HIGHLIGHTS

1. In what ways do the processes described fit with how you currently practice or are being taught to practice?
2. How might you draw on the ideas in this chapter to enhance your work with families?
3. What do you anticipate might be the challenges for *you* in nursing as a relational inquiry process?

REFERENCES

Amundson, J. (1996). Why pragmatics is probably enough for now. *Family Process, 35*, 474–486.

Armstrong, P., Armstrong, H., Bourgeault, I., Mykhalovskiy, E., & White, J. (2000). *Heal thyself: Managing health care reform*. Aurora, ON: Garamond Press.

Ballou, K. A. (2000). A historical-philosophical analysis of the professional nurse obligation to participate in sociopolitical activities. *Policy Politics and Nursing Practice, 1*(3), 172–184.

Bastiaens, L., Riccardi, K., & Sakhrani, D. (2002). The RAFFT as a Screening Tool for Adult Substance Use Disorders. *American Journal of Drug & Alcohol Abuse, 28*(4), 681–692.

Browne, A. J. (2000). The potential contributions of critical social theory to nursing science. *Canadian Journal of Nursing Research, 32*(2), 35–55.

Browne, A. J. (2001). The influence of liberal political ideology on nursing practice. *Nursing Inquiry, 8*(2), 118–129.

Canadian Nurses Association. (2002). *Code of Ethics*. Ottawa: Canadian Nurses Association.

Canam, C., (2004). The place of advanced practice nurses in the community-based health care of children with complex health needs and their families. Unpublished doctoral dissertation. University of Victoria, Victoria, BC.

Caputo, J. (1987). *Radical hermeneutics: Repetition, deconstruction, and the hermeneutic project*. Bloomington: Indiana University Press.

Chung, T., & Colby, S. M. (2000). Screening adolescents for problem drinking: Performance of brief screens against DSM-IV alcohol. *Journal of Studies on Alcohol, 61*(4), 579–588.

Concise Oxford Dictionary. (1982). Oxford: Clarendon Press.

Drevdahl, D. (1995). Coming to voice: The power of emancipatory community interventions. *Advances in Nursing Science, 18*(2), 13–24.

Drevdahl, D., Kneipp, S. M., Canales, M. K., & Dorcy, K. S. (2001). Reinvesting in social justice: A capital idea for public health nursing. *Advances in Nursing Science, 24*(2), 19–31.

Feldman, R., Weller, A., Eidelman, A. I., & Sirota, L. (2002). Comparison of skin-to-skin (Kangaroo) and traditional care: Parenting outcomes and preterm infant development. *Pediatrics, 110*(1), 16–27.

Fiellin, D. A., & Reid, M. C. (2000). Screening for alcohol problems in primary care. *Archives of Internal Medicine, 160*(13), 1977.

Flanagan, O. (1996). *Self expressions. Mind, morals and the meaning of life.* New York: Oxford University Press.

Furman, L., & Kennell, J. (2000). Breastmilk and skin-to-skin kangaroo care for premature infants. Avoiding bonding failure. *Acta Paediatrica,* 1280–1283.

Hartrick, G. A. (1997). Beyond a service model of care: Health promotion and the enhancement of family capacity. *Journal of Family Nursing, 3*(1), 57–69.

Hartrick, G. A. (2001). Beyond interpersonal communication: The significance of relationships in health promoting practice. In L. Young & V. Hayes (Eds.), *Transforming health promotion practice: Concepts, issues and applications* (pp. 49–58). Philadelphia: F.A. Davis.

Hartrick, G. A. (2002a). Beyond behavioral skills to human-involved processes: Relational nursing practice and interpretive pedagogy. *Journal of Nursing Education, 41*(9), 400–404.

Hartrick, G. A. (2002b). Beyond polarities of knowledge: The pragmatics of faith. *Nursing Philosophy, 3*(1), 27–34.

Hartrick, G. A. (2002c). Transcending the limits of method: Cultivating creativity in nursing. *Research and Theory for Nursing Practice: An International Journal, 16*(1), 553–562.

Kendall, J. (1992). Fighting back: Promoting emancipatory nursing actions. *Advances in Nursing Science, 15*(2), 1–15.

Kennell, J. H., & McGrath, S. K. (2003). Beneficial effects of postnatal skin-to-skin contact. *Acta Paediatrica, 92*(3), 272–274.

Kuhl, D. (2002). *What dying people want. Practical wisdom for the end of life.* Toronto: Doubleday.

McKnight, J. (1989, Summer). Do no harm: Policy options that meet human needs. *Social Policy,* 5–15.

McKnight, J., & Kretzmann, J. (1992). Mapping community capacity. *New Designs for Youth Development, 10,* 9–15.

McMillan, R. (2003). Unveiling the invisible and uncelebrated aspects of relational practive: Enlightening conversations with experienced community health workers. Unpublished thesis. University of Victoria, Victoria, Canada.

McQuaig, L. (1998). *The cult of impotence: Selling the myth of powerlessness in the global economy.* Toronto, Ontario: Penguin.

Mill, J. E., Allen, M. N., & Morrow, R. A. (2001). Critical theory: Critical methodology to disciplinary foundations in nursing. *Canadian Journal of Nursing Research, 33*(2), 109–127.

Mitha, F. (2000). *Spirituality in education.* Paper presented. University of Victoria, Victoria, British Columbia.

Newman, M. A. (1994). Health as expanding consciousness (NLN Publ. No. 14-2626, 2nd ed.). New York: National League for Nursing.

Ohgi, S., Fukuda, M., Moriuchi, H., Kusumoto, T., Akiyama, T., Nugent, J. K., Brazelton, T. B., Arisawa, K., Takahashi, T., & Saitoh, H. (2002). Comparison of kangaroo care and standard care: Behavioral organization, development, and temperament in healthy, low-birth-weight infants through 1 year. *Journal of Perinatology, 22*(5), 374–380.

Paterson, J. G., & Zderad, L. T. (1976). *Humanistic nursing.* New York: Wiley.

Philpot, M., Pearson, N., Petratou, V., Dayanandan, R., Silverman, M., & Marshall, J. (2003). Screening for problem drinking in older people referred to a mental health service: a comparison of CAGE and AUDIT. *Aging & Mental Health, 7*(3), 171–176.

Purkis, M. E. (1997). The 'social determinants' of practice? A critical analysis of the discourse of health promotion. *Canadian Journal of Nursing Research, 29*(1), 47–62.

Ramsey, J., Richardson, J., Carter, Y. H., Davidson, L. L., & Feder, G. (2002). Should health professionals screen women for domestic violence? Systematic review. *British Medical Journal, 325*(7359), 314–318.

Rogers, C. (1961). *On becoming a person.* Boston: Houghton Mifflin.

Rorty, R. (1999). *Philosophy and social hope.* London: Penguin Books.

Sayers, S. (1997, June). Is the truth out there? *The Australian Higher Education Supplement,* 32.

Simkin, R. (1998). Not all your patients are straight. *Canadian Medical Association Journal, 159*(4), 370–375.

Simmington, J. (2004). Ethics for an evolving spirituality. In J. Storch, P. Rodney, & R. Starzomski (Eds.), *Toward a moral horizon* (pp. 465–484). Toronto: Pearson Education Canada.

Stajduhar, K. (2001). *The idealization of dying at home: The social context of home-based palliative caregiving.* Unpublished doctoral dissertation, University of British Columbia, Vancouver, BC.

Stajduhar, K. (2003). Examining the perspectives of family members involved in the delivery of palliative care at home. *Journal of Palliative Care, 19*(1), 27–35.

Steele, R. G. (2002). Experiences of families in which a child has a prolonged terminal illness: Modifying factors. *International Journal of Palliative Care, 8*(9), 418–434.

Stevens, P. E. (1989). A critical social reconceptualization of the environment in nursing: Implications for methodology. *Advances in Nursing Science, 11*(4), 56–68.

Stevens, P. E. (1992). Who gets care? Access to health care as an arena for nursing action. *Scholarly Inquiry in Nursing Practice, 6*(3), 185–200.

Stevens, P. E., & Hall, J. M. (1992). Applying critical theories to nursing in communities. *Public Health Nursing, 9*(1), 2–9.

Vanier, J. (1998). *Becoming human.* Toronto, ON: Anansi Press.

Varcoe, C. (2004). Violence, women and ethics. In J. Storch, P. Rodney, & R. Starzomski (Eds.), *Toward a moral horizon: Nursing ethics for leadership and practice,* Toronto: Pearson.

Varcoe, C., Doane, G., Parely, B., Rodney, P., Storch, J., Mahoney, K., Brown, H.S., & Starzomski, R. (2003). Ethical practice in nursing–working the in-betweens. *Journal of Advanced Nursing 45*(3), 1–10.

Varcoe, C., & Rodney, P. (2002). Constrained agency: The social structure of nurses work. In B. S. Bolaria & H. D. Dickinson (Eds.), *Health, illness and health care in Canada* (3rd ed., pp. 102–128). Toronto: Nelson.

Vicenzi, A., White, K., & Begun, J. (1997). Chaos in nursing: Make it work for you. *American Journal of Nursing, 97*(10), 26–32.

Wagner, J. (1993). Ignorance in educational research: Or, how can you *not* know that? *Educational Researcher, 22*(5), 15–23.

3

Family Nursing
As Inquiry

8 Family Nursing As Inquiry

OVERVIEW

In this chapter we illustrate how the theoretical lenses and skills and processes presented in the previous chapters are integrally connected and occur 'all at once' in relational family nursing practice. And, we discuss how this all at once structures family nursing practice as a process of inquiry.

f you look back through the previous chapters, you will notice that in presenting the different topics related to family nursing practice we have consistently talked about inquiry. In Chapter 1, we began by inviting inquiry into your own habits and your own knowledge of family, health, and health promotion. In Chapter 2, we suggested expanding that inquiry to develop knowledge of families by using a variety of lenses beyond the dominant lenses of biomedicine, empirical science, and economic efficiency. In Chapter 3, we advocated inquiry to develop theoretical knowledge specific to nursing. In Chapter 4, we highlighted the importance of inquiry into context. In Chapter 5, we focused on self-knowledge by exploring the skill of reflexivity as a mode of inquiry. In Chapter 6, we promoted inquiry into relationships as a way of developing knowledge about the capacities and skills of relational practice. Finally, in Chapter 7 we offered a series of processes that support inquiry and collaborative knowledge development with families. The purpose of this chapter is to bring all of the different avenues of inquiry together to illustrate how they are integrally connected and occur 'all at once'. And, how this all at once structures family nursing practice as a process of inquiry.

Given the great diversity in and between people/families and the wide range of health and healing situations families might experience, it is well beyond the scope of this or any book to provide all of the knowledge nurses might need for family nursing practice. However, we do believe it is possible to offer knowledge, skills, and processes that

- will prepare you to enter in and respond to family in ways that are competent, respectful, and health promoting
- are transferable across families and across settings.

With those goals in mind we have focused on outlining the knowledge, skills, and processes that will help you attend to particulars—to engage in particular ways with particular families in particular situations. By approaching family nursing in this 'particular' way you are well positioned regardless of who the family is or what health challenges they face. The process of 'inquiring into the particulars' helps you identify the salient aspects of a family's health and healing experience, the knowledge that is needed to address the challenges and/or adversity they face, and also the questions that need to be asked in order for you to conduct a thorough assessment and intervene in a relevant and respectful manner.

● Taking up a Stance of Inquiry

In presenting each of the different topics throughout the preceding chapters and inviting you to take a stance of inquiry to knowledge development and to nursing practice, we have attempted to portray relational practice as 'a humanely involved process of respectful, compassionate, and authentically interested inquiry' (Hartrick, 2002, p. 400). We have made a distinction between the expert stance that locates knowledge in the person/nurse and an inquiry stance where knowledge is located in the relational process of knowing. We have

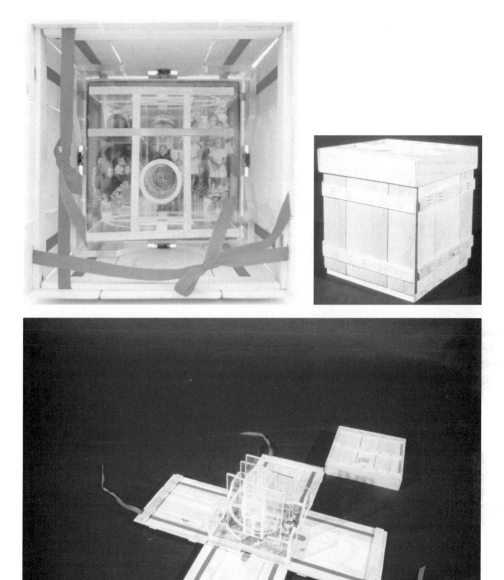

Cultural baggage. (Mixed media by Connie Sabo.)

emphasized that you are the most important resource you bring to your practice—you are the instrument of your own practice. At the same time we have invited you to move from striving to be 'an expert' who places what you already know in the foreground to becoming an inquirer who places what you *do not know* in the foreground. By taking up a stance of inquiry, you are better able to see beyond what you know already and simultaneously use your knowledge as a basis from which to evaluate existing knowledge and develop and incorporate new knowledge.

A stance of inquiry involves a dynamic process. When you enter into any nursing situation as an inquirer (rather than as an expert), you automatically take up a position of unknowing. You are ready to hold your own knowledge open to critical analysis and question. You are open to learn, develop, change, and refine your knowledge. You are open to forms of knowledge other than those you already hold and open to others' knowledge including, importantly, family knowledge. Because such a process is always open to change, you can never go wrong for long! Blunders may occur, but from a stance of inquiry, feedback is welcomed and new paths are expected! Rather than holding sole responsibility for knowledge and for being an 'expert who knows', such responsibility is shared, and importantly, shared with family. Thus, a dynamic process of knowing is congruent with, and supportive of, relational practice and collaborative knowledge development. And, in this way inquiry becomes the structure that underpins relational nursing practice. Inquiry offers the structure within which you can enact the processes that we have described in earlier chapters.

This notion of structure is important. As we described in Chapter 7, although relational practice does not occur by following a prescribed method or assessment tool, it is still structured. The structure, however, is not one of conforming to predetermined methods. The structure that guides relational practice is a thoughtful process of interpretive, critical inquiry and spiritual inquiry. As a nurse involved in such a process you become a mediator of the structure and method—you determine and shape the structure and methods of your practice rather than being driven by structures and methods determined by others. Responding to what arises, you reflexively make thought-ful decisions about how 'best to proceed' in any given moment. This nursing process of inquiry guides the way you develop the knowledge necessary to make those decisions and the way you proceed once decisions have been reached. That is, as you intervene you are simultaneously inquiring into the family's experience, your intervention and the relational responsiveness between your intervention and the family's unfolding experiences.

Within the structure of inquiry, the skills and processes we presented in Chapter 7 provide ways for engaging with families and ways for engaging with the knowledge required for responsive, health-promoting practice. In this chapter we describe possible ways to use these skills and processes to engage with families through the nursing process of inquiry. We suggest that as you enact your relational practice, you actively engage in inquiry with a wide range of knowledge. As we have suggested in earlier chapters, relational nursing practice begins with knowledge of people/families, but is informed by numerous sources and types of knowledge. We believe that in order to attend to the particularities of any family or any health and healing situation, any interaction with any family needs to be informed by multiple forms of knowledge. Each interaction must be informed by 'particular' family knowledge, empirical/theoretical knowledge, ethical knowledge, contextual knowledge, ideological knowledge, and so forth.

Our hope in this chapter is to pick up the threads from the preceding chapters, and pull them together. We began this book by asking you to consider and step outside of your taken-for-granted ways—to step out of your habits. Throughout we have tried to challenge some of the habits that we believe interfere with nurses' intentions to practice in health-promoting and responsive ways. At the same time we have been providing you with the resources to develop a new habit—that of approaching nursing as a process of inquiry.

● A Working Typology

As the literature on ways of knowing in nursing illustrates (remember the discussion of Carper's typology in Chapters 3 and 4), there are many different ways of conceptualizing types of knowledge and ways of knowing. For simplicity, we have chosen a typology of four approaches to inquiry:

- Empirical
- Contextual
- Ideological
- Ethical

These approaches are our way of bringing together multiple ways of knowing and forms of knowledge. Table 8.1 displays the processes of relational practice (as inquiry with family) in relation to different (overlapping) forms of knowledge. We have placed the processes of relational practice in the center column to indicate that they are central, but informed and complemented by the forms of inquiry we have suggested. We have chosen these approaches as we think they can enhance relational practice particularly well. We are not claiming that these are mutually exclusive or complete. Rather, these forms of inquiry overlap with each other and also with other ways of thinking about types of knowledge and ways of knowing. So, for example, White's idea of sociopolitical knowing that we discussed in Chapter 4 provides a frame for understanding empirical, contextual, ideological, and ethical knowing. We are also not claiming that the questions posed are comprehensive and complete. Questions have been posed throughout this book, and you have undoubtedly posed your own questions as you read earlier chapters. Rather, the questions are used to illustrate *some* of the ways that relational practice informs and is informed by various forms of inquiry.

Because in any moment of practice multiple forms of knowledge are operating we hope to assist you to draw more intentionally on particular forms of knowledge and to more purposefully integrate these forms of knowledge toward health-promoting relational practice. In order to do so, we suggest approaching nursing as a process of inquiry and engaging simultaneously in several forms of inquiry. Throughout the rest of the chapter we take you through such an inquiry process with the help of Helene, a woman I (Colleen) have known and worked with teaching nurses and her partner, Dana. It is our intent to illustrate how this all-at-once process of inquiry might look in practice.

| TABLE 8.1. | Bringing Knowledges Together | | | |

Empirical Inquiry	Contextual Inquiry	Processes of Relational Practice (Inquiry with family)	Ideological Inquiry	Ethical Inquiry
What am I seeing, hearing, feeling?	What circumstances have brought us together?	**Entering into relation: Getting 'in sync' with a family**	What challenges me in extending unconditional positive regard?	How do I convey unconditional positive regard?
What empirical knowledge does the family have?	What circumstances hinder collaboration?	**Being in collaborative relation: Staying 'in sync'**	What ideas hinder collaboration?	What is a good relationship?
What is of meaning and significance?	What circumstances push families from the center?	**Inquiring into the family health and healing experience**	What ideas threaten to overshadow family experience?	How are autonomy and self-determination to be fostered?
How do theory and empirical knowledge fit with family experiences?	What are the circumstances of this family?	**Following the lead of families**	What dominant ideas are shaping family understandings?	What does this family want?
Who is this family?	What circumstances shape their experience?	**Listening to and for**	What dominant ideas shape this family's experiences?	What are this family's worries?
What knowledge do I bring; what more do I need to learn?	How is my context shaping my perceptions?	**Self-observation**	What biased assumptions am I drawing on?	How am I being? How do I want to be?
What are this family's patterns of experience?	What are the patterns of capacity/adversity?	**Pattern recognition**	What taken-for-granted ideas are evident in relation?	What patterns of practice constrain/support moral agency?
What does this family want to know, be, do?	What is possible in these circumstances?	**Letting be and change**	What are the taken-for-granted directions for action?	How shall we be together?
What do families know? What do I know? How does knowledge of other families fit?	What is knowable?	**Collaborative knowledge development**	What knowledge dominates?	Given this knowledge, what are the 'best' actions?

TABLE 8.1.	Bringing Knowledges Together (continued)			
Empirical Inquiry	Contextual Inquiry	Processes of Relational Practice (Inquiry with family)	Ideological Inquiry	Ethical Inquiry
What capacities do families have?	What resources are available in the community/context?	**Naming and supporting capacity**	What ideas undermine capacity?	How can capacity be best supported?
What inequities affect this health issue and how can they be modified?	What are the structural inequities and how can they be modified?	**Emancipatory action**	What are the alternative discourses and how can practices be modified?	How can equity and justice be pursued?

An Example: Living With a Chronic Condition

Helene, a 40-year-old woman, is admitted through emergency to a medical unit of a hospital with serious dehydration, secondary to severe diarrhea, which has persisted over a period of several months. Helene has diabetes, which was diagnosed at the age of 11. She has been in renal failure for a number of years, but at present has a fully functioning transplanted kidney. After being on hemodialysis for several years, she had her first kidney transplant. This first transplant failed quite quickly. However, 3 years ago, Helene received a second renal transplant that continues to work effectively. At present, Helene is being admitted with the diagnosis of diarrhea and dehydration, NYD (not yet diagnosed). In addition to the listed problems, Helene has had significant coronary artery disease, for which she had six bypass grafts in coronary artery bypass graft surgery about 6 years earlier.

On admission to the medical unit, Helene is pale, thin, and tired-looking. In fact, she looks exhausted and distressed. She is quite weak and struggles to get on a bed pan, which she requests as she is moved from the emergency stretcher to her bed on the unit. On admission to the unit, Helene's vital signs are as follows:

Temperature 37.7
Heart Rate 128 bpm
BP 95/40
Helene's blood work is as follows:

FK506	13.3	[normal]
Sodium	148	[135-148 mmol/L]
Potassium	3.7	[3.6-5.0 mmol/L]
Chloride	129	[100-112mmol/L]
Bicarb	7	[22-31 mmol/L]
WBC	9.5	[4.0-11.0 G/L]
HGB	160	[120-155 G/L]
MCV	93	[82-100 Fl]
RBC	5.2	[3.9-5.3 T/L]
HCT	0.48	[0.37-0.47]

Platelets	191	[125-400 G/L]
Neutrophils	6.9	[2.3-7.7 G/L]
Lymphocytes	1.5	[0.8-3.1 G/L]
Monocytes	1.1	[0.2-0.8 G/L]
Creatinine	183	[40-120 umol/L]
Urea	4.4	[2.5-8.0 mmol/l]
Magnesium	0.18	[0.70-1.05 mmol/L]
Glucose	3.6	[3.5-6.0 mmol/L]

Helene's monthly blood work for the 4 months prior to admission showed:

HGB	155, 163, 167, 165
WBC	6.0, 7.2, 6.1, 6.1
Platelets	179, 199, 204, 213
Creatinine	86, 79, 75, 76
Potassium	4.7, 4.4, 4.7, 4.4

On admission, Helene was on the following medications:
Mycophenolate 1 G BID
FK 506 (Tacrolimus) 3 mg BID
Prednisone 5 mg OD
Zocor 40 mg OD
Aspirin 325 mg OD
Insulin 23 units (N); R 2-5 units; and regular prn through the day

---

As you review Helene's story, approach the story as a process of nursing inquiry and look for the particulars.

- What do *you* take particular notice of?
- What information in the story did *you* give precedence to?
- What is missing from this story?
- What is the emphasis of the partial knowledge that this story conveys?
- What does the story tell you about Helene as a particular person, at this particular time?
- As a 'family' nurse practicing from a relational perspective what do you find yourself wanting to know more about?

Stop for a minute and think about how this presentation of information is reasonably typical of the kind of information nurses receive about patients and families every day. In line with dominant forms of knowledge and ways of knowing, nurses are presented with an abundance of biomedical and empirical knowledge, knowledge generated by other disciplines. It is, of course, the task of nurses not only to use this knowledge, but also to generate nursing knowledge on which to base their practice. And, in order to practice relationally with families, nurses must acquire other knowledge in the process of collaborative knowledge development. But what knowledge do you need and how do you go about developing this collaborative knowledge? Let's begin this nursing process of inquiry by considering inquiry with family. Helene is admitted to the unit accompanied by her partner. How might Family Nursing As Inquiry with Helene and her partner begin? What questions might you as an inquiring nurse ask in order to come to know Helene and her partner? What other knowledge(s) might you need that you don't already have?

Inquiry With Family

In relational nursing practice, inquiry *with* family is not about asking families a series of preset questions. Rather, questions that support inquiry with family follow the lead of family. Following the lead of family, the questions are not questions to ask *of* families, but questions to ask *with* families. For example, as I (Gweneth) read the story and think about how I might begin my inquiry given my desire to enter into relation with Helene and her partner in a meaningful way, I find myself wanting to follow the lead of their decision to be admitted to hospital. I am curious about Helene and her partner's experience. What has led to Helene's admission on this particular day—what was it that she/they were experiencing (what was/is of particular meaning and significance to them), and what are they hoping for in this admission? It is important to emphasize that taking the stance of inquiry does not involve simply asking questions so they can be answered. Rather, as I think about which questions to ask with the family I am 'looking over their shoulder' to see what might be relevant in the context. For example, given the information earlier, I know that Helene has lived with several chronic health challenges for a number of years and probably has a lot of experience managing her health situation—thus my curiosity about why they chose admission today, what was happening for her/them? In posing the questions I am also aware that any answers will likely be partial and provisional and subject to change. That is, the 'story' that is told today may well change and/or be modified tomorrow as the family's situation changes.

Inquiry Questions That Might Be Asked

Inquiry in relational practice involves inquiry into self, other, and context all at once. Although they are occurring all at once, it is useful to think about questions that you might address as you foreground yourself, others, and the context.

To begin, what questions might you ask of yourself as you inquire with family? Consult the center column Table 8.1, and notice that the questions in the following list are ones that have been posed in earlier chapters. As you enter into relation, get in sync with family, and take up the processes of relational practice, you might ask yourself:

- *How* am I . . . with this particular family? Am I taking an I-It or an I-Thou stance? How am I experiencing this family (bodily/self-knowing)? How am I seeing this family (as a problem, a challenge, an opportunity)?
- *What* am I . . . with this particular family? What role am I taking—expert, supporter, inquirer, listener, gatekeeper, facilitator?
- *Why* am I . . . taking these stances and roles with this family? What biases, habits, assumptions, ideologies are shaping my practice?
- *Where* am I . . . going with this family? What is my intention? What are the likely impacts of any course of action? How is this family experiencing me?

TRY IT OUT 8.1. **Asking Questions**

1. *Select* a colleague or classmate—preferably someone who works in or is interested in a different practice setting than yourself.
2. *Review* the general inquiry questions we have posed.
3. *Take turns* stating the questions in your own words, each thinking about your own context of practice. What are the similarities? What are the differences? What do you learn?

If you have Helene in mind as you read these questions, what would be *your* likely stance toward her? How might *you* feel? What would you expect of yourself? What would you be most worried about? What would you likely do first?

Questions about the self in relation to other leads logically to begin asking questions about other, that is, about family. In your study and practice you will encounter assessment guides and screening tools that specify exactly what questions to ask families. In taking a stance of inquiry, even if you draw on these tools, we think that it is important that you

- put your conversations into your own language (remembering that you are your most valuable resource and that your 'best' approach draws on your own way of being),
- take your lead from families,
- tailor your inquiry to the context.

Families you encounter during a brief interaction in an immunization clinic versus those you encounter during the first of many, long interactions in a palliative care setting will have very different concerns. Try It Out 8.1 invites you to think about some of these differences. Some questions that focus on family and seem logical throughout the processes of relational practice include asking:

- *Who* is this particular family and how could I get to know them in their situation?
- *How* is this family receiving me/being with me? How do they expect me to be? How do they understand their experience?
- *What* is of particular meaning and significance to this family? What is important to them? What are they hoping for? What are they 'setting their hearts on'? What capacities does this family have? What do they know, and how do they know it? What do they expect of me?
- *Why* is this family experiencing what they are experiencing?
- *Where* has this family been and where are they going?

Inquiry With Helene and Dana

Helene summarized her expectations of nurses in two words: competence and empathy. Having been diabetic since age 11, and having had so many hospitalizations, interactions with health care providers, and experiences within the health care system, Helene is very knowledgeable about both her own health and particular health issues, and about how health care works. Although she does not expect health care providers to know as much as she does about diabetes, or her experience of diabetes, she does expect them to know the limits of their knowledge and to know enough to provide a basis for their decisions. As importantly, Helene would like empathy. By this she means a sense that health care providers might strive to imagine what it might be like to be in her shoes (or at this point in time, her hospital slippers).

On admission, Helene said there were three things of meaning and significance to her:

1. She wanted to get the diarrhea and dehydration under control
2. She wanted to know what the cause was.
3. She wanted to maintain control of her insulin regulation.

As noted, Helene is very knowledgeable about herself, her health, and health care. Helene has worked very hard to maintain a delicate balance of insulin control, and at this moment in time, her severe diarrhea and dehydration and inability to eat or absorb much food has drastically reduced her insulin needs. What she wants is for nurses and other health care providers to take her knowledge of her blood sugar regulation into account and to leave her to continue to regulate her own insulin. Dana, Helene's partner, shares Helene's worries, but she is also worried about being able to support Helene. Dana needs to work, but she also wants to be with Helene as much as possible. Helene's parents live thousands of miles away, and their relationship to Helene is not always experienced by Helene as supportive, leaving Dana's support even more crucial.

In addition to her own knowledge and experience base, she and her partner, Dana, have been together for more than 10 years, and Dana has been at Helene's side through hemodialysis, two transplants, an MI, two strokes, and much more. They would name the strength of their relationship as an amazing capacity, and they would name their chosen 'family' of their network of friends as another important capacity. Together, Helene and Dana have been through Helene's many acute illnesses, but they have also lived with the knowledge that Helene's life will always be dominated by health concerns and hospitalizations. For example, although her transplanted kidney is functioning well, the reality is that at some point the kidney will fail, and Helene will be faced with a return to dialysis with or without the possibility of another transplant. They live life as well as they can, within the ever-present limitations of Helene's health.

Questions about the family's experience, how it came to be, where they have been, and where they are going lead logically to bringing the context into the foreground. Questions that might be asked about the context include:

- *How* has this (family/self/relation) come to be?
- *Why* has this come to be?
- *Where* will this context push this family? Where will this context push me in relation to this family?
- *What* adversity arises? What is collaborative knowledge development in this situation? What are the targets for action?

In relation to Helene and Dana, posing the questions of how and why this immediate situation came to be surfaces Helene's complex history of multiple health challenges. Helene's dehydration and diarrhea cannot be understood without understanding this history. Further, understanding how she has handled the problem to date cannot be understood without understanding this history. Helene remained at home, trying to keep herself hydrated despite chronic severe diarrhea over the past several months for a complex set of reasons. Helene tries to minimize her hospitalizations, partly because she would (understandably) prefer to be at home, partly because, due to her immunosuppressive transplant drugs, she does not like to risk exposure to iatrogenic infection, partly because she knows she will have to fight to retain control of her insulin management as well as other decisions if she is hospitalized, and partly because she receives excellent physiological monitoring through her regular monthly visits to the renal clinic where she sees her nephrologist and has blood work done. Further, in the past 2 weeks she visited the emergency department twice regarding the diarrhea and was sent home with little more than prescriptions for Imodium.

When asked what influence the context has on her immediate experience and her likely relationship with nurses, she instantly expresses concern that on a general medical floor, the staff are usually unfamiliar with chronic renal disease and transplant functioning and medications. She worries that lack of knowledge might lead health care providers to make mistakes—for example, by prescribing or administering drugs that are incompatible with her immunosupressants. She also finds it a challenge to be cared for by health care providers who do not know her personally, in contrast to her long-term relationships with renal unit staff.

● Collaborative Knowledge Development

Understanding this source of adversity and knowing (at least partially) what is of immediate significance and concern to Helene and Dana highlights the importance of collaborative knowledge development in her situation. How might you help Helene gain confidence in your competence and knowledge? At the same time, how might you admit the limits of your knowledge? How can you convey empathy? What do you need to know to help her get the diarrhea and dehydration under control (for example, what has she already tried, what can she drink, how bad is it at present, what makes it better, what makes it worse? What possibilities do you know of that she has not yet tried?). How can you contribute to identifying the cause of the diarrhea? What can you do to facilitate her control over her insulin regulation? How might you foster Helene receiving the support she needs/wants (for example, from Dana, their friends, yourself, other staff)? As you can see, targets for action likely include:

- increasing your own knowledge where gaps exist (for example, perhaps you do not know much about immunosuppressives),
- choosing actions to reduce diarrhea and foster hydration from among those that have either previously worked or not been tried (forget the Imodium, it didn't help),

---

BOX 8.1. **Three Overarching Questions**

Who is this particular family at this particular time and in this particular situation?
What more do I need to learn and know to attend to those particularities?
What actions would be most responsive to this particular person/family?

- ensuring that the insulin orders enable Helene to decide and administer her own dose of insulin,
- resisting other influences that impede Helene's control over decisions that affect her.

Other targets for action can be identified depending on the context. If there are, for example, policies in place that prevent Helene from deciding and administering her own dose of insulin, such policy becomes a target for action that emerges from this collaborative process.

In nursing as inquiry the three overarching questions (see Box 8.1) are always Who is this particular family at this particular time and in this particular situation? What more do I need to learn and know to attend to those particularities? and What actions would be most responsive to this particular person/family? In thinking about what you now know about Helene, what else might be important for you to know? What further inquiry will you undertake with Helene and Dana? What more can you learn from them? What further knowledge of the context do you require? What empirical knowledge is required to collaboratively develop knowledge and action with this family?

Empirical Inquiry

Empirical inquiry to support relational practice is not only disease, illness, and problem focused. Examine the column under empirical inquiry in Table 8.1, and compare that column to the processes of relational practice. A relational approach demands a wider empirical inquiry in at least three important ways:

1. A wider range of empirical data is required.
2. Empirical data must be interpreted in light of other forms of knowledge.
3. Collaborative knowledge development and the use of other forms of knowledge direct further empirical inquiry.

First, a wider range of empirical observations are needed to get and remain 'in sync' with family. That is, while 'standard' empirical data are often offered or collected, relational practice directs your attention to more *particular* features of a situation. So, for example, what observations can you make about Helene in relation to her environment (is she wary, relaxed, relieved, embarrassed, and so on), in relation to Dana, in relation to you? Dana is likely to question you about Helene's lab work results and medications, for example, so how might you interpret such questions? (As a challenge to your expertise? As overstepping Helene's autonomy? As an opportunity for collaboration and learning on your part?) What will be important about your response? In turn, what does the empirical data suggest about what is of meaning and significance to Helene and Dana? For example, you might think that Dana's insistence on knowing Helene's kidney function tests suggests that she is worrying that Helene's transplant is failing. Your knowledge that although being dehydrated is not good for kidney function it will not necessarily provoke transplant failure will allow you to respond to the concerns in a knowledgeable and meaningful way. What does the empirical data suggest for further collaborative knowledge development?

Second, empirical inquiry in relational practice suggests using empirical data in concert with other forms of inquiry. Empirical knowledge can be evaluated in light of other knowledge. So, in Helene's situation, you already have some understanding of her experience that provides a basis for understanding her empirical data. To take a very simple example, how do you interpret her blood pressure? First, if asked, Helene would tell you that her blood pressure tends to be in the range of 130/85, so you know that this current BP is exceptionally low for her. A cursory inspection of her lab work tells you that her low blood pressure is at least in partly due to dehydration. In particular, her elevated sodium, chloride, and hemoglobin suggest significant dehydration. Do you think that her hypotension is being masked to some extent by her concern and level of stress? Such analysis would leave you even more alert to the consequences of hypotension and provoke further inquiry. For example, does she become dizzy and faint when getting up?

Third, further empirical inquiry is guided by the collaborative knowledge development process. Continuing with Helene's example, the process of collaborative knowledge development leads to understanding that knowledge regarding diarrhea in the context of diabetes and immunosuppression is critical to providing responsive care to Helene. Indeed, in addition to investigating various infections as causative, her physicians immediately began to investigate the possibility that diabetic neuropathy was the explanation for her diarrhea. What other empirical information might enhance understanding and pattern recognition in relation to Helene and Dana? Study of the experience of living with chronic conditions such as diabetes or renal failure might be very helpful in sensitizing you to what might be the challenges they face, and the capacities that might be supported. For example, a group of researchers led by Paterson and Thorne (Paterson, 2001; Paterson, Russell, & Thorne, 2001; Thorne et al., 2002) have extensively researched the experiences of diverse people living with chronic conditions, illustrating both the complexities of chronic illness and the ways in which health care providers are often disempowering, despite good intentions. Similarly, a study of the process of renal transplant, particularly the challenging dynamics of families' experiences of being asked to consider organ donation (for example, Langley & Shaw, 2002; Molzahn, Starzomski, & McCormick, 2003), might provide some basis for 'pattern recognition' in understanding Helene's experience.

Finally, empirical inquiry in turn suggests further inquiry of other forms. Try It Out 8.2 invites you to expand your empirical knowledge together with other forms of knowledge. Again, the question that an

---

TRY IT OUT 8.2.   **Expanding Knowing Through Empirical Inquiry**

1. *Consider* the empirical information you have about Helene including her vital signs, her blood results, and the list of medications.
2. *Think* about this knowledge in relation to your own current knowledge as a nurse.
   - What inquiries would you need to undertake to relationally respond to Helene and Dana?
   - What knowledge would you need to develop further to both interpret this information and understand it in a relationally relevant way? For example, would you need to look up the medications to learn more about them? Once you looked up the medications, how might this expanded empirical knowledge inform your response to Helene? How might you enlist it to inform your nursing actions? How would you connect it to other existing knowledge you have and that Helene and Dana might have? How would knowing more about the medications enhance your ability to 'follow the lead' of Helene and Dana? For example, might you ask 'I understand that many people on prednisone long term find that their appearance changes—did that happen to you?'

---

inquiring nurse needs to ask continually is 'What more do I need to learn and know to act most responsively?' For example, knowledge about families' experiences of transplantation could in turn provide background for further inquiry with family. How did the decisions about transplantation get made in their family? Is there any relationship between this experience and the fact that Helene does not experience her parents as supportive? Such knowledge might also suggest further contextual inquiry. For example, how does a successful transplantation affect economic status through policies such as disability pension eligibility? It is important to emphasize, however, that in relational practice you do not merely ask any questions that might come to mind as a result of *your* knowledge and/or concerns. Rather, the *particular* questions that are asked are determined by 'following the lead of the family' and 'listening to and for' what seems to be of particular significance and meaning as you collaborate (e.g., with the family and other health practitioners) to develop knowledge and act in a relationally responsive manner.

Contextual Inquiry

In Chapter 3 we outlined contextual nursing practice and suggested building contextual knowledge of families, of family health, of nurses in context, of the health care context. In that chapter, we focused on development of general contextual knowledge. We also emphasized in Chapter 4 the importance of your own social context to the processes of self-observation. Now we suggest bringing that general contextual knowledge and self-knowledge together with other forms of knowledge in approaching particular families in particular situations from a stance of inquiry.

Although it seems logical that the context would be central in contextual inquiry, as with all inquiry in relational practice, contextual inquiry is directed toward the self, other, and context all at once. Therefore, it is useful to pose questions that reflect and explicitly take the relational nature of family nursing into account. As you enter in with family, it is useful to begin by asking: 'What circumstances have brought us together?' As you consider how to stay in sync with family you might ask 'What circumstances hinder collaboration?' Each of these questions directs attention, not just to the circumstances external to yourself and the family and your relationship, but also to how you and the family are together within that context. If you imagine yourself as Helene's nurse, how would the circumstances differ if you were a student new to the medical unit or if you were a nurse with 10 years of experience on that unit? What would be different if you had an elderly mother who had been refused a kidney transplant because of age-related eligibility criteria? What would be different if you were a home care nurse meeting Dana and Helene in their home rather than in a hospital setting?

Paying Attention to the Sociopolitical Context

Inquiring into the family experience and following their lead invites paying particular attention to the sociopolitical context of health care as it affects particular families' lives and experiences and the sociopolitical context of particular families' lives and experiences. Beginning questions might be 'What circumstances push families from the center?' What are the circumstances of this family? In Helene's situation, the very circumstances of being a person with a chronic condition (several actually) on an acute medical unit might push her concerns to the side. Other acute priorities on the unit at a particular time might overshadow Helene's and Dana's concerns. Again, we want to emphasize that you can 'be relational' and be in a hurry. Nurses can communicate their busy-ness with disconnection, or with connection.

In listening to families, contextual inquiry leads you to listen for the circumstances that are shaping the families' experience. In Helene's situation, most salient to her circumstances at the time was the fact that Dana (an accountant) had a contract that required long hours of work, making visiting difficult.

Paying Attention to How Context Is Shaping Capacity

Integral to all contextual inquiry (indeed all inquiry) is self-knowledge. In particular the question of how the context is shaping your perceptions is important. If you were to encounter Helene in emergency prior to her admission to the medical unit, how do you think your focus would be shaped differently than if you encountered her after admission? If the medical unit was overrun by a virulent infection, would you see Helene somewhat differently (for example, thinking both of the fact that she is immunosuppressed and what such infection might mean for your workload with other patients).

Identifying patterns turns attention to the 'spirit' and life force that shapes Helene and Dana's health and healing. What is it that ultimately concerns them? How do they enter into life with each other, with family and friends, and with other forms of power? What are the patterns of capacity/adversity within their current life context? Such inquiry might turn attention to the obvious strength and power Helene and Dana must have within them to have lived through the many health challenges they have faced. Similarly, it might highlight the wealth of knowledge they bring having lived with both diabetes and renal failure for so long. For example, Helene has developed capacity in terms of knowing herself well enough to 'know' what symptoms she needs to attend to and how to attend effectively. Dana has developed capacity in knowing how best to support Helene, and together they know how to keep their relationship and their relationships with their network of friends intact through repeated 'life and death' experiences. Recognition of this family capacity turns attention to how contextual factors are enhancing and/or constraining such capacity. For example, how well does an acute care hospital setting facilitate nurses drawing on patients' knowledge of their own health when they have been living with chronic conditions? How does it support and/or hinder the expression of their spirit-power? Similarly, you might pay attention to the adversities that seem to have particular significance and meaning. What is it that seems to be the most difficult part of their health experience? How might you collaboratively tap other contextual resources and capacities to enhance their already existing capacity? From the story it is evident that Helene and Dana have a supportive and loving relationship and that as a couple they also have the support of friends and community. As we mentioned in Chapter 7 often it is during times of adversity (such as illness) that capacity is most evident. As a nurse caring for this family you might pay attention to how they draw on these and other capacities to live in and through the health challenges. This 'paying attention to capacity' will enhance your ability to support and foster it.

Compare this pattern recognition (knowing) we have just suggested with what typically passes for knowledge about family. For example, how would the knowing generated by the above inquiry compare with the knowledge that Dana and Helene are Jewish (or Muslim or atheist or Buddhist or Christian and so on) or that Helene practices a certain form of breathing meditation?

Inquiring into Helene and Dana's experience through a capacity lens asks questions of possibility. It asks what is possible in these circumstances. Practice is limited in very real ways by the circumstances of both families' lives and of practice. For example, it was not possible for the public health nurse in Chapter 7 to provide a crib for the baby whose young parents were using a box, but it was possible for her to understand the box as resourcefulness and share that understanding with the family and with other nurses. In Helene's case, it is not possible for the nurse to identify the cause of her diarrhea, but it is possible for the nurse to be responsive to Helene's concern about the cause and to be responsive to her concern about maintaining control over her care. By focusing our inquiry on what is possible, we promote a half-full approach to practice.

Contextual inquiry for collaborative knowledge development turns attention to questions such as 'What is knowable?' In Helene's case the actual cause of her diarrhea is not 'knowable' at this time, creating tension and uncertainty. Collaboratively deciding how that uncertainty can be lived and what resources can be drawn on provide a basis for action. In Helene's case, her long relationship with the renal health care team is a critical resource to her, even though this crisis may not be physiologically related to her renal function—she knows and trusts this team and relies on their involvement to ensure that any intervention to

> **TRY IT OUT 8.3.** **Expanding Knowing Through Contextual Inquiry**
>
> 1. *Imagine* that you are assigned Helene as a patient. Entering into relation with Helene and Dana, understanding that they are concerned about her being a patient on a general medical ward is important contextual knowledge. What does this knowledge lead you to want to inquire into? For example, what questions are you raising about yourself? What are you curious about with regard to policies and protocols that might shape how much control Helene has over her treatment while on the ward? Given that Helene has identified competence and empathy as the two expectations she has of nurses, how might you proceed?
> 2. *Discuss* your views with some colleagues or classmates and inquire into their views.

deal with her current health problems will not threaten her transplant or compound her preexisting chronic health issues. A key concern of Helene's is that her nephrologists be informed and involved in decisions regarding medical treatment. The structural inequities that Helene drew to attention included that the medical unit had fewer staff per patient, that there were fewer ways in which families were accommodated (less space, no family friendly policies), and that the staff were not as highly educated compared to those on the renal unit (where all nurses and physicians had additional specialty education). Given Helene's expressed concerns about competence, combined with these contextual features, demonstrating competence and building trust would be key features of a meaningful and 'good' relationship with Helene. Try It Out 8.3 invites you to explore your ideas about the context.

Ideological Inquiry

Because we simultaneously are affected by and affect our contexts, considering context leads you to consider how people are taking up and living out the practices and features of their context. Allen and Hardin (2001) demonstrate how 'social organization is not produced by external structures operating upon or causing people to adopt certain behaviours. Rather social structure is an *effect* of taking up practices and reproducing and modifying them' (emphasis in original, p. 163). Throughout this book we have pointed out how taken-for-granted ideas can shape thinking and practices, and we have encouraged the uncovering and challenging of such ideas. We now illustrate how this ideological inquiry is an explicit part of your approach to family nursing practice. Ideological inquiry is particularly important in advancing knowledge toward social change (Rodney, 1998). Rodney contends that 'ideological inquiry can provide us with the theoretical and empirical tools necessary to challenge what is taken for granted in health care delivery and social policy' (p. 5).

In a relational approach, ideological inquiry is directed toward self/other/context, considering how certain practices are being taken up, reproduced, and modified. Ideological inquiry can be guided broadly by four questions:

1. What ideologies am I living and how am I taking them up?
2. What ideologies is the family living?

3. What ideologies dominate this context?
4. How are we living these ideologies together in relation?

Again, Table 8-1 offers some more specific questions in relation to the
processes of relational practice.

Analysis of your own ideologies relevant to family nursing practice
began at least as soon as you started reading this book. Examining your
ideas about family, health, and health promotion automatically required
you to consider the ways in which you take up, enact, and modify dominant ideologies. Similarly, your own spiritual and/or religious beliefs are
a form of ideology. Considering what ideologies you might be living draws
on the process of self-observation to consider what assumptions and
biases you are living in your practice.

The Ideology of Compliance

When you consider what ideologies you might be living in relation to
Helene, your particular understandings, for example, about people who
have diabetes, come into play. A popular ideology in use with people
with diabetes (and renal and cardiac disease for that matter) is the ideology of compliance. Nurses have used the idea of compliance in various
ways (Murphy & Canales, 2001). Murphy and Canales analyzed the
nursing literature and characterized nursing authors' use of the idea of
compliance as either 'evaluative', 'rationalization', or 'acceptance'. That
is, nurses writing about compliance accepted the idea, rationalized its
use, or evaluated and tried to modify its use. Although they used various
definitions, and often did not define the term compliance, nurse authors
usually used the term to mean the extent to which patients/families
followed the wishes, orders, or advice of health care providers. In other
words a nurse governed by the ideology of compliance assumes that
'good patients' should follow the treatment protocols and regimes
provided by expert health care providers.

'Evaluative' literature has been critical of use of the term compliance
because of its inherent assumption of patients/families yielding to more
powerful health care providers, and because through its use nurses are
complicit with disempowering patients/families and keeping them in line
with the biomedical model. 'Rationalizing' literature offered some critique
of the term, but used the term despite the issues of paternalism,
coercion, and acquiescence. Murphy and Canales thought this contradiction was ironic because the authors who rationalized use of the term
wrote as though their critiques somehow distanced them from the associated assumptions and issues. Finally, Murphy and Canales found that
most authors simply accepted the term without apparent awareness of
the long history of controversy raised in both medicine and nursing. We
agree with the 'evaluative' authors, and with Murphy and Canales, that
the use of the term compliance perpetuates current systems of
domination. For example, in my (Gweneth's) research with people living
with diabetes, participants described how often health care providers'
efforts to get them to comply with diabetic regimes seemed to take precedence over all other aspects of care (Hartrick, 1998). Moreover, they
reported that when their blood sugars were 'out of whack' the nurses

---

TRY IT OUT 8.4.   **Example Ideologies**

1. *Think* of a practice setting of your choice. In what way is the *idea* of 'compliance' used? The *word* compliance is not used to the same extent in all settings, but the *idea* may be found to be operating in most health care settings. In mental health, compliance with medication is a common theme. In maternity nursing, the term might not be used but the idea of compliance might be operating in relation to women's breastfeeding practices. In public health, the idea might be most visible in relation to parents' immunization practices, and so on.
2. *Describe* a situation in which the idea could be seen to be operating in this practice setting. Describe the situation in a story, and tell the story to someone (or write about it if you prefer).
3. *Examine* the power dynamics in the story. How is power operating, and how does the ideology of compliance figure in those dynamics?
4. *Compare* the story as told with how it might be told if the processes of relational practice were used. What is similar? What is different? What happens to the ideology of compliance?

---

would often assume they had not been following their regime and would respond negatively toward them. They found it particularly frustrating that even when as 'good diabetic patients' they had been 'complying', the nurses would 'not believe' them. What was particularly frustrating about this was that it was during these times of uncontrolled blood sugars that they as 'patients' needed the most support and help from nurses—yet because the nurses placed such emphasis on compliance and assumed uncontrolled blood sugars were a result of noncompliance, the nurses would become distant, less responsive, and at times even finger-wagging toward them. Try It Out 8.4 invites you to consider how the idea of compliance is used in practice and to consider its use in relation to the processes of relational practice. Can the idea of compliance be used in health-promoting practice where the idea is that families are supported in taking control of their own health and healing?

Working Around Ideology to Meet Families With Unconditional Positive Regard

An important question to consider when examining the ideologies you are living is the extent to which they shape your ability to meet families with unconditional positive regard. For example, if you think of a family as noncompliant, are you as able to extend unconditional positive regard as if you think of that family as acting responsibly in terms of their own health? Similarly, if patients are making choices that are in opposition to your own particular religious beliefs how does that shape your ability to be with them in ways that honour *their* ultimate 'spiritual' concerns? This is a critical sort of difference (we will say much more about difference in the next chapter) and is just as important whether you are from the same or different religions than the families with whom you work.

Considering what ideologies families are living requires getting in sync with families and actively listening for how dominant ideas are shaping families' understandings and experiences, including their health care experiences and experiences of you. For example, in the story of Sarah who was living with multiple sclerosis (see Chapter 7), it was possible to hear the dominant ideology of the superwoman mom shaping her experience. In Helene's case, dominant ideas about medical units (as nonspecialized with less technology and less-educated staff in comparison with other types of units) may shape Helene and Dana's perceptions of the unit and its nurses. It is important to keep in mind that the goal is not to achieve some 'right' way of thinking. We all live multiple contradictory taken-for-granted ideas. We can, for example, critique the ideologies of a youth-oriented society at the same time as working to look youthful. I (Colleen) feel pleasure at compliments that I don't look my age, while at the same time I am perturbed that aging women are not seen as attractive and recognize that such compliments arise from that youth-oriented preoccupation. Rather than aim for a right way of thinking, the goal is to have a greater critical awareness so that we may more consciously and intentionally choose and act within and around the ideologies.

Such a critical awareness requires that we inquire into the ideologies that are available and operating in the wider sociopolitical context. For example, Simmington (2004) contends that Western society's practice of religion and models of helping often focus more on maintaining the particular system of religion or helping practice than addressing the needs of the human soul. The strength of the ideological structures may lead us to lose sight of the human being and of human wholeness. Similarly, returning to the idea of compliance, different practice settings will take this idea up differently, and to greater or lesser extents. When I (Colleen) was practicing in coronary care units, the idea was pervasive. Patient and family teaching was geared toward optimizing compliance with lifestyle changes prescribed by health care providers. However, there was a recognition that such changes were still within the control of the family. When I began working with nurses in particular nephrology units I was taken aback at not only how pervasive the idea of compliance was, but also how patients and families were 'punished' for noncompliance. For example, both nurses and patients told me that patients who came in to hemodialysis 'overloaded' (with too much fluid, sometimes from drinking too much or eating the wrong things) were punished in various ways—being made to wait, being verbally chastised, or by having the fluid removed rapidly in ways that caused discomfort. Compliance was a dominating ideology in those nephrology settings and was so normalized that it was difficult for the nurses to see the harmful impact of that ideology, never mind to think differently.

Ideological inquiry identifies directions for action. Critical analysis of how taken-for-granted ideas are shaping thinking and experience for both yourself and families opens up possibilities for understanding things differently and for helping others to understand things differently. Remember Sarah in Chapter 7 who was living with multiple sclerosis (MS) and the way the support group helped her open up to new possibilities for understanding mothering? Ideological inquiry identifies patterns in the ways practices are taken up, and the possibility of naming and supporting the capacity of redefining situations and experiences. In

Helen Brown's experience of a physician telling her what he would do if Tanner were his son (Chapter 7), Helen refused the taken-for-granted idea that physicians should not give their opinion in end-of-life decisions. In so doing she interpreted his words as highly supportive. It is important to emphasize that the goal of ideological inquiry is not 'consciousness raising' with families. In relational practice the goal of ideological inquiry with families is *not* to help families see things right. Rather, in congruence with the idea of letting be and change, as Banks-Wallace says, drawing on Collins' (1990) notion of womanist thought, the goal is 'to affirm and re-articulate a consciousness that already exists' (Banks-Wallace, 2000, p. 36). When Helene was on hemodialysis, she did not need me (Colleen) to point out the ideology of compliance, but found it affirming that I too could see the dynamics operating. Indeed Helene helped me see how even in my critiques I was still using the idea, giving it 'currency'.

Taken-for-granted ideologies often reflect values in operation (Rodney, 1998). Thus, ideological inquiry is inextricably linked to ethical inquiry, the final form of inquiry to which we now turn.

Ethical Inquiry

Ethical inquiry is ultimately an inquiry about the questions 'What is good?' and 'How shall I do good?' In nursing, this translates into 'What is good practice?' and 'How shall I do good in my nursing practice?' A relational approach offers processes to assist in deciding how to do good. Again, examine Table 8.1 and compare the column on ethical inquiry with the column about processes of relational practice.

Principle-based biomedical ethics—meaning principles such as autonomy, beneficence, malificence, and so on—that have been used widely to understand ethics in medicine (Evans, 2000; Wolf, 1994) have also dominated nursing ethics (Storch, Rodney, & Starzomski, 2004). However, nurses and others are progressively developing ethical theory particular to nurses and nursing issues. There are several important interrelated trends in ethical theory that are particularly helpful to relational practice. First, 'relational' ethics has supported the development of the idea that nurses are moral agents who enact ethical decisions within a relational matrix (Bergum, 2004; Donchin, 2001; MacDonald, 2002; Mackenzie & Stoljar, 2000; Rodney, Brown, & Liaschenko, 2004). That is, various authors have challenged the idea that moral agents are independent decision makers and have shown how nurses make ethical decisions *in-relation* with others. Second, contextual ethics (which is related to relational ethics) has supported understanding that moral choices are made *in context* (Hartrick Doane, 2002; Hoffmaster, 2001; Rodney, Pauly, & Burgess, 2004; Winkler, 1993; Wolf, 1994). That is, just as a family can only be understood in context, the ethical issues that arise and the decisions that are made can only be understood in context. Third, contextual ethics informed by feminist and postcolonial ideas has emphasized that race, sex and gender, class, history, colonialism, and other features of the sociopolitical context must be taken into account in understanding and making moral choices in nursing and health care

(Brown, Rodney, Pauly, Varcoe, & Smye, 2004; Shaha, 1998; Sherwin, 1992, 1998). For example, in my research in emergency, I (Colleen) saw nurses deciding what care patients deserved in concert with their colleagues as well as in relation to unit 'norms' (Varcoe, 2002; Varcoe, Rodney, & McCormick, 2003). In congruence with emergency unit culture, nurses labelled patients who repeatedly returned to emergency as 'frequent flyers' (see Malone, 1996) and judged those patients to some extent according to the opinions of their colleagues and in accordance with organizational pressure to get patients out of the unit quickly. Further, assumptions based on class and race were evident in those judgments. Understanding that these practices are not merely a consequence of either interpersonal relationships or the context acting on individuals (Allen & Hardin, 2001) means that nurses can make choices that contribute to shaping health care culture.

A fourth trend in ethical theory has been the linking of ethics and spirituality. As Niebuhr (1972) and Hague (1995) have described, morality is a spiritual endeavour and similarly spirituality is a moral endeavour. Simmington (2004) contends that an ethical environment is one in which 'the total well-being of our patients, including their spiritual well-being, is honoured and advocated' (p. 466). Simmington asserts that healing and wholeness are spiritual concepts and that movement in the direction of healing and wholeness is movement in the direction of evolving spirituality. Subsequently, to practice ethically nurses must question whether the social, cultural, and religious trends that inform ethical decision making are supporting people's spiritual life and/or are they interfering with spiritual expression? 'To act ethically . . . is to do all we can to remove barriers that interfere with the ability of individuals, groups and the collective to live their lives fully . . . while our own spiritual journey, and those of the people we walk beside, may not be without pain, it is up to us to ensure that it is also not without joy' (Simmington, 2004, p. 480).

Ethics As a Way of Relating in the World

As the relational and contextual nature of nursing has gained recognition, it has become increasingly evident that the rational models of ethical decision making that have traditionally dominated nursing are inadequate to support nurses in their everyday practice. As a result, different suggestions for addressing this inadequacy have been made. These suggestions have included grounding ethical practice in nursing theory (Yeo, 1989), developing a philosophy of ethics that evolves from nursing practice (Bishop & Scudder, 1990), articulating a nursing ethic based on care (Watson, 1988; Fry, 1989; Gadow, 1990), understanding human experience within relationships as the foundation for ethics (Bergum, 1994; Pauly, 2001), and developing a feminist ethics (Liaschenko, 1993; Sherwin, 1998). What each of these approaches to ethical nursing practice has in common is the emphasis on the everydayness of morality (e.g., that every minute of nursing practice involves ethics) and an understanding of ethics as a deeply personal process that is lived in the complexity and ambiguity of everyday nursing work.

During the past 4 years we have been part of a team of researchers in the School of Nursing at the University of Victoria that has undertaken research in ethics, experience we have drawn on throughout this book. Having found existing ethical theory and ethics education in nursing inadequate to offer nurses the knowledge and skills they require to navigate their way through the complex, ambiguous, and shifting terrain of everyday nursing practice, we undertook projects with the potential to inform ethical nursing theory, assist us to reconceptualize nursing ethics, and inform our rethinking of ethics education in nursing (see http://web.uvic.ca/nursingethics). Through our work as a team we have come to believe that at the center of ethical practice is a particular way of relating in the world. This way of relating is grounded in an ethic of social justice (meaning a conscious concern for the welfare of all human beings that moves beyond individuals to families, groups, communities, and societies) and the understanding that people, knowledge, decisions, and actions are relationally and contextually derived. This means, for example, that what constitutes ethical practice in one context or with one family may not be ethical in another. As we have described earlier, to practice relationally (and thereby practice ethically) requires that the particularities of people/families, situations, and contexts be taken into consideration. And, just as inquiry is the structure that guides relational practice, so inquiry is the structure that guides ethical practice in nursing.

We believe that the relational inquiry process of nursing that we have described throughout this book provides a theoretical and practical foundation for ethical practice in nursing—for 'doing good' in practice. Relational practice focuses on relations both among and between people and between people and their environments or contexts. Relational nursing practice is based on the idea that nurses enact their practice (and their moral agency) in relation to others and to contexts—that nurses are not autonomous in their decisions but make decisions in relation to others and to what is going on around them. Thus, these trends mean that ethical inquiry can support relational nursing practice in helping to answer the questions 'What is good practice?' and 'How shall I do good in my practice?'

We hope this book has stimulated your thinking about what good nursing practice is. We do not believe that good technique is sufficient for good nursing practice, nor is practice based on biomedical knowledge alone sufficient, no matter how comprehensive that knowledge is. Good nursing practice is not simply the 'correct' or best actions of individual nurses. Rather, good nursing practice requires relationally responsive practice, multiple knowledges, and collective action. Try It Out 8.5 invites you to develop your vision of good nursing practice with family.

Again, as Table 8.1 suggests, bringing ethical inquiry together with the processes of relational practice requires attention toward the self/other/context. Asking yourself 'How do I convey unconditional positive regard?' requires paying attention to your own values and how they are living in your practice. Similarly, answering the question 'What is a good relationship?' in your nursing practice requires examining your values. Is a good relationship to you one in which you offer unconditional

> **TRY IT OUT 8.5.** **Your Vision of 'Good' Practice with Family**
>
> 1. *Think* of a story from your practice, from class, from personal experience, or from the literature that represents something important to you about 'good' practice with family. Create a written summary of the story (a paragraph or two).
> 2. *Analyze* the story in terms of facts, values, and emotions. Create a written summary of your analysis (another paragraph or two).
> 3. *Create a vision* statement for yourself (yourselves, if you want to do this with someone else) that reflects what you have learned from the story and that will provide you with direction for your future practice. This product could take a variety of forms—for example, a picture, a poem, a story, a piece of representational art, or a short essay.

positive regard? Is it a matter of taking control or acting as expert or following the lead of families? Directing the question 'What is a good relationship?' toward 'other' suggests understanding what families want from a health care relationship. Directing the question toward the context means analyzing both what is seen as a good relationship in that particular context and what is a good context for relational practice. For example, what is considered a good relationship with a dying person within the culture of a palliative care unit might be quite different than within the culture of a prison. Quite different practices may be 'normalized' and taken for granted within these contexts. Such questions surface the ways in which families and contexts influence 'good relationships' so that rather than operating in an unconscious way, nurses can more deliberately and intentionally make choices about how they take up ideas and practices.

Given that autonomy and self-determination are fundamental to any code of ethical practice, the question 'How are autonomy and self determination to be fostered?' is routine. However, a relational understanding of autonomy means that any person's or family's autonomy and choice can only be understood in context. This means, for example, that understanding a person's wish to die requires understanding that wish in context and in relation to what it is that ultimately concerns that person and family—to their spiritual life centers. Does the person not wish to be a burden to his or her family members? Or does that person wish to die only because of physical pain that is not being (and potentially could be) relieved?

Understanding moral choices in context suggests turning back to other forms of inquiry. How are autonomy and self-determination being lived in relation to the dominant ideologies that you are exploring (the ideology of compliance serves as a good example here, too) and/or in relation to the empirical inquiry you are undertaking? So, following the lead of families and asking 'What does this family want?' and 'What are this families worries?' requires taking other forms of inquiry into account. For example, what does this family want within what is known and what is considered possible?

Ethical inquiry provides significant direction for action. The questions 'How am I being?' and 'How do I want to be?' reflect both analysis of your own values and of the relational context. These questions also suggest the possibility of being more intentional in your practice based on an analysis of your values in relation to the values of the families with whom you work and the values operating within the context of practice. These questions lead directly to the question 'How shall we be together?' Given this knowledge and analysis, you can determine the 'best' actions you can take and how you might best support capacity, equity, and justice.

● Conclusion

In presenting Helene and Dana's story we have attempted to show possibilities—to illuminate family nursing as a process of inquiring into particulars. From this example it becomes evident that multiple knowledges inform any nursing moment and that there are also multiple routes that one might take to come to know families and respond in ways that are relevant and health promoting. Approaching nursing as a process of inquiry frees you up to 'follow the lead of the family' and to simultaneously open up to multiple ways of knowing. In the next chapter we consider how relational family nursing practice can support 'connecting across difference' and facilitate navigation through the 'hard spots' of family nursing.

THIS WEEK IN PRACTICE

Try Your Own Example

Throughout this chapter we have been using Helene and Dana's experience to consider Family Nursing As Inquiry. This week in practice, try a different example and try out the relational inquiry process.

1. *Choose* a person or family with whom you are working.
2. *Consider* how you might structure your nursing practice to be in line with a process of inquiry.
3. *Try out* the different modes of inquiry including empirical, contextual, ideological, and ethical inquiry. As you try out the different modes of inquiry 'all at once', consider how these different modes of inquiry are informed by the theoretical perspectives presented in Chapters 2, 3, and 4. How, for example, do the nursing theories in Chapter 4 inform your empirical inquiry—how might it shape what it is you inquire into? For example, consider Newman's notion of patterns of energy—how would that shape what you look for empirically and how you interpret and enlist the empirical knowledge available? Similarly, how might postcolonial theory or feminist theory inform empirical inquiry? How does a poststructural lens help you see ideological practices? As you 'play' with the ideas and processes remember that there is no 'right' answer. After you have experienced some of the ideas and processes have a conversation with a classmate or colleague who has also tried them out. What did you each experience? What similarities did you find? What differences?

CHAPTER HIGHLIGHTS

1. How does this stance of relational inquiry compare with the nursing stance implied or advocated in your other studies in nursing?
2. How does this approach fit with what you would want and expect from caregivers in relation to health and illness in your own family?
3. What do you anticipate would be the challenges and advantages of purposefully taking up relational inquiry as your approach in practice?

REFERENCES

Allen, D., & Hardin, P. K. (2001). Discourse analysis and the epidemiology of meaning. *Nursing Philosophy, 2*(2), 163–176.

Banks-Wallace, J. (2000). Womanist ways of knowing: Theoretical considerations for research with African American women. *Advances in Nursing Science, 22*(3), 33–47.

Belenky, M. F., Clinchy, B. M., Goldberger, N. R., & Tarule, J. M. (1986). *Women's ways of knowing: The development of self, voice and mind.* New York: Basic Books.

Benner, P. (1984). *From novice to expert: Excellence and power in clinical nursing practice.* Menlo Park, CA: Addison-Wesley.

Benner, P., Tanner, C. A., & Chesla, C. A. (1996). The social embeddedness of knowledge. In P. Benner, C. A. Tanner, & C. A. Chesla (Eds.), *Expertise in nursing practice* (pp. 193–231). New York: Springer.

Bergum, V. (1994). Knowledge for ethical care. *Nursing Ethics: an International Journal for Health Care Professionals 1,* 72–79.

Bergum, V. (2004). Relational ethics and nursing. In J. Storch, P. Rodney, & R. Starzomski (Eds.), *Toward a moral horizon: Nursing ethics for leadership and practice.* Toronto: Pearson.

Bishop A. H., & Scudder J. R. (1990). *The Practical, Moral and Personal Sense of Nursing: a Phenomenological Philosophy of Practics.* Albany: State University of New York Press.

Brown, H., Rodney, P., Pauly, B., Varcoe, C., & Smye, V. (2004). Working the landscape: Nursing ethics. In J. Storch, P. Rodney, & R. Starzomski (Eds.), *Toward a moral horizon: Nursing ethics for leadership and practice* (pp. 154–177). Toronto: Pearson.

Carper, B. A. (1978). Fundamental patterns of knowing in nursing. *Advances in Nursing Science, 1*(1), 13–23.

Chinn, P. L., & Jacobs-Kramer, M. (1988). Perspectives on knowing: A model of nursing knowledge. *Scholarly Inquiry for Nursing Practice: An International Journal, 2*(2), 129–139.

Collins, P. H. (1990). Black feminist thought: Knowledge, consciousness, and the politics of empowerment. 2nd ed. New York: Routledge.

Donchin, A. (2001). Understanding autonomy relationally: Toward a reconfiguration of bioethical principles. *Journal of Medical Philosophy, 26*(4), 365–386.

Evans, J. H. (2000). A sociological account of the growth of principlism. *Hastings Center Report, 30*(95), 31–38.

Fry S. (1989). Toward a theory of nursing ethics. *Advances in Nursing Science 11,* 9–22.

Gadow S. (1990) Existential advocacy. In Pence T. & Cancral J. (Eds). *Ethics in Nursing: An Anthology* (pp. 41–51). New York; National League for Nursing.

Grant, A. (2001). Knowing me knowing you: Towards a new relational politics in 21st century mental health nursing. *Journal of Psychiatric & Mental Health Nursing, 8*(3), 269–276.

Hague, W. J., (1995). *Evolving spirituality.* Edmonton Department of Educational & Psychology. University of Alberta.

Hartrick, G. (1998). The meaning of diabetes: Significance for holistic nursing practice. *Journal of Holistic Nursing, 16*(4), 420–434.

Hartrick, G. (2002). Beyond behavioural skills to human-involved processes: Relational nursing practice and interpretive pedagogy. *Journal of Nursing Education, 41*(9), 400–404.

Hartrick Doane, G. (2002). Am I still ethical? The socially mediated process of nurses' moral identity. *Nursing Ethics, 9*(6), 623–635.

Hoffmaster, B. (2001). *Bioethics in social context.* Philadelphia: Temple University Press.

Langley, V. L., & Shaw, M. (2002, February). A day in the life: The donor and her family. *Urologic Nursing, 22*(1), 13–24.

Liaschenko J. (1993). Can Justice coexist with the supremacy of personal values in nursing practice? *Western Journal of Nursing Research 21,* 35–50.

Liaschenko, J. (1997). Knowing the patient? In S. E. Thorne & V. E. Hayes (Eds.), *Nursing praxis: Knowledge and action* (pp. 23–53). Thousand Oaks, CA: Sage.

Liaschenko, J., & Fisher, A. (1999). Theorizing the knowledge that nurses use in the conduct of their work. *Scholarly Inquiry for Nursing Practice: An International Journal, 13*(1), 29–41.

MacDonald, C. (2002). Nurse autonomy as relational. *Nursing Ethics, 9*(2), 194–201.

Mackenzie, C., & Stoljar, N. (2000). *Relational autonomy: Feminist perspectives on autonomy, agency and the social self.* New York: Oxford University Press.

Malone, R. E. (1996). Almost 'like family': Emergency nurses and 'frequent flyers'. *Journal of Emergency Nursing, 22*(3), 176–183.

Molzahn, A. E., Starzomski, R., & McCormick, J. (2003). The supply of organs for transplantation: Issues and challenges. *Nephrology Nursing Journal, 30*(1), 17–27.

Murphy, N., & Canales, M. K. (2001). A critical analysis of compliance. *Nursing Inquiry, 8*(3), 173–181.

Niebuhr, R. (1972). *Experiential religion.* New York; Harper Row.

Paterson, B. (2001). Myth of empowerment in chronic illness. *Journal of Advanced Nursing, 34*(5), 574–582.

Paterson, B., Russell, C., & Thorne, S. (2001). Critical analysis of everyday self-care decision making in chronic illness. *Journal of Advanced Nursing, 35*(3), 335–342.

Pauly B. (2001). *Weaving & Tapestry of Nursing Ethics: Philosophical Grounding and Future Directions.* Unpublished manuscript. University of Victoria, Victoria.

Polanyi, M. (1962). *Personal knowledge.* Chicago: University of Chicago.

Rodney, P. (1998). Towards ideological inquiry. *Canadian Association for Nursing Research/Association Canadienne pour la Recherche Infirmière, 9*(1), 5–6.

Rodney, P., Brown, H., & Liaschenko, J. (2004). Moral agency: Relational connections and trust. In J. Storch, P. Rodney & R. Starzomski (Eds.), *Toward a moral horizon: Nursing ethics for leadership and practice* (pp. 154–177). Toronto: Pearson.

Rodney, P., Pauly, B., & Burgess, M. (2004). Our theoretical landscape: Diverse approaches to health care ethics. In J. Storch, P. Rodney, & R. Starzomski (Eds.), *Toward a moral horizon: Nursing ethics for leadership and practice* (pp. 154–177). Toronto: Pearson.

Schaefer, K. M. (2002). Reflections on caring Narratives: Enhancing patterns of knowing. *Nursing Education Perspectives, 23*(6), 286–294.

Schultz, P. R., & Meleis, A. I. (1988). Nursing epistemology: Traditions, insights, questions. *IMAGE: Journal of Nursing Scholarship, 20*(4), 217–221.

Shaha, M. (1998). Racism and its implications in ethical-moral reasoning in nursing practice: A tentative approach to a largely unexplored topic. *Nursing Ethics, 5*(2), 139–146.

Sherwin, S. (1992). Feminist and medical ethics: Two different approaches to contextual ethics. In H. Bequaret Holmes & L. Purdy (Eds.), *Feminist perspectives in medical ethics* (pp. 17–31). Indianspolis: Indiana University.

Sherwin, S. (1998). A relational approach to autonomy in health care. In *the politics of women's health: Exploring agency and autonomy* (pp. 19–47). Philadelphia: Temple University Press.

Simmington, J. (2004). Ethics for an evolving spirituality. In J. Storch, P. Rodney, & R. Starzomski (Eds.), *Toward a moral horizon. Nursing ethics for leadership and practice* (pp. 465–484). Toronto: Pearson Prentice Hall.

Smith, M. C. (1992). Is all knowing personal knowing? *Nursing Science Quarterly, 5*(1), 2–3.

Storch, J., Rodney, P., & Starzomski, R. (Eds.). (2004). *Toward a moral horizon: Nursing ethics for leadership and practice.* Toronto: Pearson.

Sweeney, N. M. (1994). A concept analysis of personal knowledge: Applicaton to nursing education. *Journal of Advanced Nursing, 20*, 917–924.

Thorne, S., Paterson, B., Acorn, S., Canam, C., Joachim, G., & Jillings, C. (2002). Chronic illness experience: Insights from a metastudy. *Qualitative Health Research, 12*(4), 437–453.

Varcoe, C. (2002). Inequality, violence and women's health. In B. S. Bolaria & H. Dickinson (Eds.), *Health, illness and health care in Canada* (3rd ed., pp. 211–230). Toronto: Nelson.

Varcoe, C., Rodney, P., & McCormick, J. (2003). Health care relationships in context: An analysis of three ethnographies. *Qualitative Health Research, 13*(6), 957–973.

Wainwright, P. (2000). Towards an aesthetics of nursing. *Journal of Advanced Nursing, 32*(3), 750–756.

Watson J. (1988). *Nursing: Human Science and Human Care.* New York: National League for Nursing.

White, J. (1995). Patterns of knowing: Review, critique, and update. *Advances in Nursing Science, 17*(4), 73–86.

Winkler, E. (1993). From Kantianism to contextualism: The rise and fall of the paradigm theory in bioethics. In E. Winkler & F. A. Coombs (Eds.), *Applied ethics: A reader* (pp. 343–365). Cambridge, MA: Blackwell.

Wolf, S. (1994). Shifting paradigms in bioethics and health law: The rise of new pragmatism. *American Journal of Law and Medicine, 20*(4), 395–415.

Yeo, M. (1989). Integration of nursing theory and nursing ethics. *Advances in Nursing Science, 11*, 33–42.

9

The Hard Spots in Family Nursing: Relational Practice as Connecting Across Differences

OVERVIEW

In this chapter we invite you to engage with the complexities and urgencies of difference in everyday family nursing practice and to consider 'difference' within the context of your own practice. We invite you into the difficulties and challenges that are part of connecting across difference, so that you might imagine your own possibilities for action.

● Difference: The Center of Hard Spots

At this point our intent is to explore how the inquiry process of relational practice might be taken up within the 'hard spots' of family nursing. By hard spots we mean those times and situations where nurses experience difficulty, find it challenging to be in-relation with particular people and/or feel a sense of powerless or frustration at the actions of others. Specifically we want to explore the hard spots that arise as we are required to connect across difference. As hermeneutic phenomenology informs us, we are all situated and constituted 'differently'. Therefore, any interaction we have as a nurse is ripe with difference. These differences involve differences in values that occur not just between and among individuals, or between health care providers, but between groups set apart by position, power, and experience—that is, between groups with different opportunities to impose their values.

First, we consider difference as a relational concept and relational practice as a way of connecting across difference. We invite you to consider the complex interplay of challenges to relational practice and how these might be thought of as differences to be connected across. Turning to consider particular forms of difference, we begin with the most obvious and familiar, and perhaps the most challenging difference— that of 'cultural difference'. One of the predominant ways that difference is thought and talked about in Western countries and nursing is in regard to 'culture'. In these discussions of cultural difference culture is often confused with ethnicity or race. In this chapter, we move beyond this limiting view of culture and beyond a 'recipe approach' to nursing practice in which nurses learn about 'others' and how to deal with 'them'. Rather, we take a relational approach to consider culture and other forms of difference that are often encountered in family nursing practice. In so doing we draw your attention to the similar patterns between cultural difference and other forms of difference. Throughout the chapter we invite you to explore how relational practice as inquiry might enhance your ability to be health promoting with diverse families, particularly those who experience stigma and marginalization due to poverty, mental illness, physical (dis)abilities, racism, heterosexism, and so forth. It is not our intent to offer a solution that you can use in every situation. Rather, our intent is to create an opportunity for you explore how you might form your judgments and determine your actions consciously and intentionally in particular situations. Our overriding goal is to bring the murky terrain of 'connecting across difference' to the forefront of everyday relational family nursing practice.

● Locating the Hard Spots of Difference Relationally

Stop for a moment and consider the way we talk about problems and families within the nursing and health care world. Labels that come readily to mind include 'at-risk families', 'dysfunctional families', 'childbearing families', 'underserved families', 'grieving families', 'marginalized families', 'families living with chronic illnesses', 'poor families', and 'families living in poverty'. Consider the power of these categories or labels. The way in which we think and talk about families, and think and talk about problems in relation to families shapes our approach to families. The way we 'locate' problems through our language and the ideas we use further shape our approach. A common practice of languaging, both in our everyday conversations in the health care world as well as in the professional literature, is to locate the problems and hard spots *in* families. That is, the problems or deficits are thought of as arising from families themselves and/or the health challenges that they face. Examples include 'This family is not complying with treatment', 'This diabetic patient isn't eating like he should', and so forth. These problems and hard spots can be thought about in this way, or, they can be thought about as arising from the context of families' lives or the context of health care practice, from our own values and practices as health care providers, or from all of the above simultaneously. Certainly there are real problems that families face, and families do present challenges to nurses. And sometimes, as some of our earlier examples have shown, our assumptions and practices as nurses present challenges to families! However, locating problems *in* families can promote blaming families for their health problems and obscure the challenges that families face. Similarly, locating 'the problem' with nurses blames nurses for whatever the hard spots are and suggests that practice with families is entirely within nurses' control. Locating problems only within the context of practice can overlook the capacity of families and nurses and absolve both of responsibility for action and change.

Overall locating problems in one or the other of these ways leads to the conflation of responsibility and blame. For example, health care providers may blame a person with diabetes or heart disease or kidney disease for dietary decisions. And, often in this blaming process contextual factors such as economic hardship, a controlling family member, or a variety of other factors that constrain the person's choices may be overlooked. As responsibility and blame become intermingled nurses' response-ability within the hard spots of nursing is hindered.

Therefore, in turning to consider the hard spots and challenges within family nursing, we have conceptualized them in a relational way—that is, we see hard spots as arising when particular families and particular nurses in particular contexts experience differences between them. By conceptualizing difference relationally we are able to look at differences and problems from multiple vantage points simultaneously. Difference implies more than one perspective and thus draws attention to the place *in between* different perspectives. Using the relational approach we have proposed in earlier chapters, we see dealing with these hard spots as requiring relational connection. That is, dealing with the hard spots requires 'connecting across difference'. Viewing and approaching difference relationally promotes responsibility rather than blame; understanding rather than defensiveness; connection rather than guilt or anger; and responsiveness rather than a sense of powerlessness and frustration.

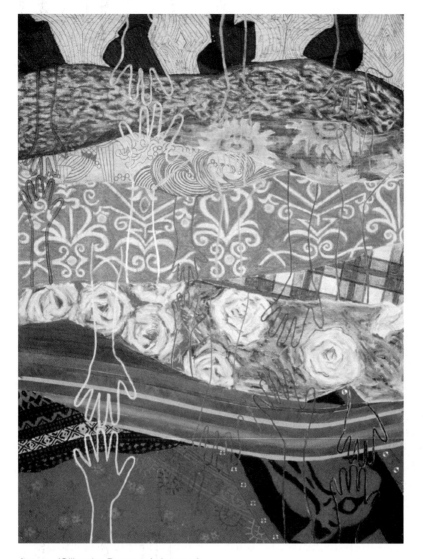

Agape. (Oilbar by Danaca Ackerson.)

● Relational Practice As Connecting Across Difference

Using a relational approach to think about difference suggests 'looking for the join' (Bhabha, 1994). That is, if family nursing is enacted in-relation, then the meeting space (the join) in between differences where ambiguity and ambivalence reside is the focus of practice. 'Differences', whether they are differences in values, beliefs, privileges, practices, concerns, or experiences, both challenge and offer us the greatest opportunities to learn about ourselves, learn about others, and learn about contexts. In this way differences offer a prime site for knowledge development and growth. 'Joins' or places where differences come together (think of plumbing, or duct work, or grafting one plant to another) can be places of weakness or places of strength greater than that of the original material.

An Example: What's the Point?

The power of locating difference relationally was highlighted during an experience I (Gweneth) had with a group of nurses with whom I was working who wanted to develop their health-promoting practice with families. One of the nurses described the frustration she felt working with people who were living with Chronic Obstructive Pulmonary Disease (COPD). She stated that after 20 years of work she had reached the point of wondering 'what the point was'. She described how no matter what 'she did' people did not seem to respond. Not only did they not show up for their appointments at the out-patient clinic where she worked, but they also continued on with behaviours (such as smoking) that were obviously detrimental to their health. Following her lead I inquired into her frustration and what it was for *her* that was particularly frustrating. She responded by describing a woman with whom she was currently working, what she had done to try and promote health, and how the woman had not responded. She was frustrated that all of her time and hard work had been 'for nothing'. To explore this 'difference' between the nurse and the woman, I suggested that we play it out relationally through a reenactment. She could take up the woman's part (to help her experience the difference from another vantage point) and one of the other nurses could take up her part as the frustrated nurse. The intent was to not only provide an opportunity for her to experience the difference from the patient's location but also to simultaneously explore the difference relationally. As the simulation went on, as 'the patient/nurse' she became more and more resistant to the nurse with whom she was in-relation. And, it was obvious to all of us watching that there was no 'connecting across difference' occurring. After about 5 minutes 'the patient/nurse' suddenly stopped and exclaimed to the nurse who was talking with her, 'This is horrible, it's not that I don't want to comply I just find it so hard to even think about doing what you are asking of me—it is so overwhelming to think of making the changes you are telling me I need to make. You have no idea how it will change my life and I am not sure I want my life to change in that way'. The patient/nurse then turned to the rest of us with a look of total amazement on her face exclaiming, 'It is so clear to me now why people have not responded—what I am telling them is what is important to me as a nurse, not necessarily what is important to them!" Experiencing this relational disconnect from another vantage point (and from a vantage point where she as a patient had less power), the nurse had been able to see that it was the relational disconnect that was at the center of her difficulty. She had been locating the problem in 'the noncompliant patient' and at times even in herself (e.g., 'Why can't I get these patients to change') rather than in the relational space 'between' them. She had been blaming the patient and taking responsibility for failing to affect the changes she envisioned. Once she shifted her attention to the relational space between them she was able to see a way that she might relationally connect across the difference. For example, she could see that the join that was between them was their shared desire for the woman with COPD to live a full and meaning-ful life. And she could see that rather than joining with the woman and collaboratively working toward that goal, as a nurse she had been working from her own personal assumptions about what a full and meaningful life might be (e.g., get well physically). Her nursing assumptions about how best to create a full life with COPD (e.g., give up smoking and fully comply with the COPD program) had dominated the relationship and prevented her from joining relationally with the woman to 'follow her lead' and find out what was of particular meaning and significance to her. As she gained insight into how she might join and work relationally with people living with COPD, the differences suddenly seemed workable.

Looking for the Join

In this example, the power of focusing on the join, the space in between differences becomes evident. Focusing on the join created the opportunity for significant differences to be acknowledged and attended to, allowed the nurse to move away from an adversarial relationship with the woman (a contest of wills, working 'against'), clarified responsibility, and offered a way of working 'with' the woman to promote health. In Chapter 6 we argued that relations are *transactional.* That is, each element (for example, each person, idea, experience, context) is affected and in some way altered through the relational transaction. Approaching difference by looking for the join offers the opportunity to connect across differences and experience the power of the relational transaction to promote health and healing. Although we are different from the people with whom we are trying to relate, when we think of the boundaries between us as lines that *join* us—rather than lines that separate us (Wilbur 1985)—and enter into a relational space, it is possible to find a space or common ground from which to work together. Thinking of the contexts in which we work as both affected *by* us and affecting us orients us to working on the joins that connect us to those contexts rather than taking their influences for granted. At the same time such relational connection offers opportunities for personal learning and growth. In contrast, locating the problem in people/families, in ourselves, or in the context often serves to create a wider gulf. Moreover, labelling people according to the differences (e.g., as a noncompliant COPD patient and being blind to everything else that is meaningful and significant in their life world) serves to reduce, devalue, and at times degrade them by 'lessening' all that they are.

● Challenges to Relational Practice Are the Challenges of Crossing Difference

When we think about the hard spots in family nursing from a relational perspective we are compelled to think about situations in which our ability to be in-relation is challenged. And, conceptualizing difference relationally, the hard spots can be seen as differences to be connected across. So, in any challenging situation, it is important to identify the differences that are operating and to remember that differences do not just arise from a single source (self, other, or context), but rather from multiple simultaneous sources.

Relational practice requires that you connect across difference by joining people as they are and where they are. Unfortunately this may be easier said than done. Rogers (1961) maintains that the primary ingredient of any relational connection is unconditional positive regard. As we have said in earlier chapters, unconditional positive regard involves accepting people as being of unconditional worth and creating an atmosphere where judgments and expectations do not dominate. Entering into respectful relation is fostered through unconditional positive regard and openness and by paying attention to and noticing who and what you are joining. When such an atmosphere is present people are free to be open to their experiences.

Before proceeding on with your reading, stop for a moment and try to come up with three differences where you might have the greatest challenge in approaching people with unconditional positive regard. What differences might challenge *your* ability to enter into relation with people as they are and respond with unconditional positive regard?

Families That Challenge Your Ability to Be In-Relation

Situations that nurses commonly find challenging include families whose members harm themselves—for example, through smoking, substance use, or suicide—or families whose members harm each other—for example, through smoking, substance use, violence, abuse, or neglect. Recently, I (Colleen) was working with a student who was caring for a patient that 'pushed all my buttons' (meaning raised all my personal sensitivities). The patient was a man who was in prison for the murder of his girlfriend. With my interest in and concern about violence against women, I found it very difficult to support the student who was also struggling over how to provide care to this man. Despite the fact that he was under guard on the medical unit, I was concerned for the student's physical safety and, when she began to speak empathically about him, I found myself concerned for her emotional safety. I immediately assumed the man was manipulative, and had to seriously confront myself regarding the extent to which I was so biased against him that I could not entertain any positive ideas about him. I had to sort out that although my values of nonviolence and gender equality were challenged, I was blaming this one person for all male violence and failing to consider how he might have come to be a violent person. Basically I had to name my discrimination. After actively reflecting on my biases I concluded that viewing this man through anger, hostility, or negative judgment and letting this view shape my suggestions to the student about how to approach his care would contradict other values I hold (such as unconditional positive regard) and would not be health promoting for anyone. I was not entirely successful in adjusting my attitude, but I tried to encourage the student to convey positive regard for him as a person without condoning violence. Ironically, in the face of the student's acceptance of him, the man became quite upset and confided remorse that the student was convinced was genuine. Although the challenge in this situation could appear to have arisen from the man himself, I contributed to the challenge of difference (and extended it to the student). Anticipating your own biases and hot spots allows you to think ahead to how you want to be with particular families, rather than simply reacting based on habit. As you read through the rest of this chapter try and imagine situations that you might find most challenging and try to think through how you would ideally prefer to act.

Colleagues That Challenge Your Ability to Be In-Relation

Whereas some challenges appear to originate from particular patients or families, other challenges appear to originate from colleagues. As we have argued, practice is enacted *in-relation*. Thus, our colleagues shape our practice and how closely we practice according to our values. As the influence of our colleagues on our practice varies with power relations, students are particularly challenged by differences. The following story was told to us by a fourth-year nursing student during an ethics research project.

An Example: Bouncing Back and Forth

I listened to a child's . . . chest, who was in for pneumonia and he was due to be discharged that day or the next day. And I had listened to his chest in my assessment and he was clear in my opinion. . . . And he had been ordered Ventolin. And I didn't think he needed it. . . . So I discussed it with the medical student who had ordered it. . . . 'Oh give it to him anyway' was the response.

And, so, I went to the RN, and I said, 'This is the issue and I don't think he should get it'. And she said, 'Well, go and talk to the medical student again'.

So I went again to the medical student, and I said, 'I don't feel comfortable giving this Ventolin, I don't feel he needs it'. Because I think that kind of medication, unless it's needed does some major flip-flops with the heart rate and all sorts of things. It's pretty traumatic to have this mask thrust in your face . . .

And again, the medical student said, 'I think he needs it, give it to him'. So I went back to the RN and I said, 'You have to give it to him, I'm not giving it to him'.

And I felt very confident that my opinion was correct. And, so I felt frustrated in the end, because as it turned out, I was in the room with him and the parents when the RN gave him the Ventolin and she just walked out. She put the mask on with him screaming and fighting and carrying on and I was the one who was distracting him in the end while he had to sit there for 15 minutes.

Notice how the student is drawing on empirical knowledge (Ventolin '*does some major flip-flops with the heart rate*') and combining ethical knowledge about autonomy with experiential knowledge about children ('it's pretty traumatic to have this mask thrust in your face'). But clearly in this situation, knowledge is not enough. The power dynamics are such that the student is unable to practice in a way that she knows to be health promoting. Despite her efforts, the child not only received the unnecessary medication (and was thus needlessly exposed to its side effects), but the student ended up participating. The student took a stand and refused to give the medication, but rather than supporting her, the RN simply gave the medication herself and thereby dismissed the student's concerns.

Differences with colleagues are a continuous feature of practice. In this situation there are differences in values, and differences in power. And as the example illustrates, you will not always be entirely successful in living your values. However, naming the differences in any given situation (difference in power and values, for example), being clear about your values (which this student was), naming the relational hard spots, and building alliances are helpful in working the hard spots. There are more than individual differences at play in this example—so identifying additional differences (in this case, did the unit culture foster adherence to medical orders regardless of appropriateness? Was 'getting the meds out' valued over safe administration of medications?) provides a better basis for action. Similarly, using the language of ethics (for example, saying that it is unethical to give a harmful medication unnecessarily) might have given the RN in the story more pause. The student may have been able to draw on others as allies (her instructor, other nurses), after, if not during the incident. As you enter any work place, your ability to practice across difference can be enhanced by anticipating where the challenges may lie between you and the culture of the workplace and the individuals with whom you work, and also by anticipating where useful allegiances may be forged.

Contexts of Nursing Practice That Challenge Your Ability to Be In-Relation

As the earlier examples suggest, challenges that appear to originate with families and health care providers are also influenced by the contexts within which practice occurs. For example, Simmington (2004) describes how the health care context typically leads nurses to view the people they care for as physical beings who happen to have a soul as opposed to spiritual beings having a physical experience. Thus, when people are struggling with spiritual questions the health care context leads many nurses not to see or understand the significance of their spiritual concerns (e.g., their god values) and how they are shaping people's choices and actions.

In a current research project we are involved in on two quite different nursing units (medical oncology and emergency), there are remarkable similarities with regard to the impact of contextual constraints on nursing practice. For example, in both, the geography fragments and disrupts nursing work and makes it difficult to match nursing skills to the care patients and families require. As is the case in emergency units in Britain, Australia, the United States, and the rest of Canada (see, for example, *Australian Nursing Journal*, 2002; Dunn, 2003; Lipley, 2002; Spooner, 2002) the emergency has long waiting times due primarily to fiscal reduction of hospital capacity that prevents admitted patients being transferred from the emergency. This leaves patients awaiting hospital admission in stretchers where acute emergency patients are supposed to be; acutely ill patients in the hallway being cared for by ambulance attendants; pediatric emergency patients being cared for by float pediatric nurses with no emergency training; and patients with chest pain sitting in the waiting room. In the medical oncology unit, palliative care patients are intermixed with a range of people with other conditions including those receiving chemotherapy treatments, people with acute medical conditions, and people with dementia requiring long-term care. Given the range of patient care needs and the differing workloads those needs entail, rather than being assigned to a particular room, the nurses are assigned to care for people who are dispersed around the unit. It is not uncommon for a nurse to have patients at either end of the ward. On both wards, the geography and overwhelming workloads makes consistent connection with patients (e.g., even timely response to call bells) amazingly challenging.

Despite these challenges, the nurses on these two units have high-lighted two ingredients essential to dealing with contexts that challenge relational practice—team relationships and political action. In both these units, the sense of team and collegiality is what makes the situation tol-erable for the nurses. And, their relationships (the join between colleagues) make possible the actions they are taking to improve the quality of their work environment (working on the join between the nurses and their practice contexts). An assessment of the context of any practice setting in which you work will help you to anticipate possible challenges to your ability to practice ethically, and possible resources and capacities on which you can draw.

Context of Families' Lives That Challenge Your Ability to Be In-Relation

In addition to the context of practice, the context of families' lives shapes your ability to promote health and be responsive. Policies and resources to which families have access can profoundly shape their possibilities, and in turn, your possibilities. As we have shown throughout this book, social determinants of health, particularly poverty, shape health in profound ways. For example, recently, while trying to get off drugs, Sheryl, a woman I (Colleen) knew, died of an overdose of heroin, partly because of a series of problematic policies (Paterson, 2003). Sheryl desperately wanted to get off drugs and was on a pilot program using morphine as a gradual way to decrease addiction. When funding for this program ended abruptly, she applied for a methadone program. On a waiting list for weeks, she tried to 'get clean' herself. She had lost partial custody of her two young daughters and thus her social assistance income had been cut to the point that she could no longer afford an apartment, factors that undoubtedly made her struggle more difficult. Finally she was offered a detox bed, but in order to qualify for the methadone program, she needed a 'hot' urine sample (with evidence of drug use in her urine). The day before admission to detox, as a way to get her urine 'hot', Sheryl did heroin after several weeks of being 'clean' (and therefore with a reduced tolerance). Sheryl—actress, mother, daughter, singer, friend—died.

Again, taking stock of the context of the lives of the families with whom you work allows you to anticipate the differences you will have to cross and challenges you will face, and helps identify areas for action in advance. The policies that contributed to Sheryl's death are obviously based on different understandings of addiction than a health-promotion perspective would support. This story is told with the permission of her parents in hopes that some good might come of her needless death. We wonder how the nurses in the detox center feel telling people with addictions about the policy (one said it is equivalent to telling an alcoholic to go drink a case of beer before he or she can get treatment). And, we wonder how the expertise of nurses and families might be used in policy decisions.

The Complex Interplay of Challenges

Differences, and challenges to relational practice, will arise from the complex interplay of people and contexts. Regardless of how you begin to define any given challenge, in most situations closer scrutiny identifies multiple differences, differences that arise not just from families, colleagues, contexts, or your own limitations, but rather from self and others (families and colleagues) in-relation and in context. In preparing to work across difference and meet the challenges to relational nursing practice it can be helpful to:

- anticipate your own biases and hot spots (enhancing self-observation). Imagine situations and differences that you might find most challenging and try to think through how you would ideally prefer to act,
- anticipate where the challenges may lie between you and the culture of the workplace and the individuals with whom you work (enhancing pattern recognition).
- identify where useful allegiances may be forged (enhancing emancipatory action),
- anticipate possible challenges to your ability to practice posed by policies and resource availability (enhancing emancipatory action),
- identify the possible resources and capacities on which you can draw (enhancing naming and supporting capacity).

In thinking of how you might go about consciously and intentionally engaging in the processes listed here, it is important to remember that relational practice is not about 'getting it right'. Rather, it is about involving yourself relationally to inquire into and question self/other/context and imagine possibilities for action. Freire (1994), whose work has been foundational to the field of critical thinking and critically informed practice, describes that from a critical perspective 'correct thinking' is to be curious, to create and re-create. In this way, correct thinking and practice involves tapping into and using your creative, imaginative potential to revise, adapt, expand, and alter both yourself and the contexts that shape families and nursing practice (Hartrick Doane, 2002). It involves courageously holding yourself open to be in the flux of relational difference and inquire into how you might proceed to most responsively connect across difference. As you read the example Barbara in May, try out the activities we identify earlier. For example, as you read try to anticipate your own biases and hot spots that might arise if you were the nurse in the situation that follows. Try to anticipate what challenges might arise

BOX 9.1. **Referral to HBPP Program**

Date of Referral: May 2, 2005   Referring physician: Dr. Joy Samson
Patient's name: Barbara Shultz   Consultants:
DOB: July 22, 1980   Dr. James Roy (OB/Gyn)
Para II Gravida 0   Dr. Alissa Singh (Psychiatry)
EDC: Dec. 18, 2004
Pre-pregnant weight: 49 kg   Current weight: 49.5 kg
Complications: twins, schizophrenia

Reason for referral: This 25-year-old Gravida-II, Para-0 with schizophrenia shows evidence of inappropriate behavior and possible hallucinations. Psychotic symptoms were controlled with medication prior to this pregnancy, but currently has poor compliance with medication regimen. Lives with mother who supports noncompliance. In addition, this patient has anemia and poor nutrition. Referred to HBPP for close monitoring of mental and physical health. Considering involuntary admission for monitoring.

Medications: Olanzapine 12.5 mg/day PO
Haldol 2 mg/day PO
Multivitamin with iron PO OD

Lab value	Normal Value
Hgb 110 G/L	120–155 G/L
Iron 63	63–165
K^+ 3.6 mmol/L	3.5–5.0
Na 140	139–146

between you and the different people in the situation, including other health professionals, what allegiances might you want to foster, what policies or lack of resources might challenge you, and what capacities you might draw on. This situation was reported to us by one of our students.

An Example: Barbara in May

It is 2:00 PM on a beautiful Monday in May as Chris arrives at the home of Barbara Shultz. Barbara is a 25-year-old woman who has been referred to the Healthiest Babies Possible Program (HBPP) by her physician. Box 9.1 presents the referral slip that Chris received. This program is designed to reach out to women who are pregnant and who may be isolated or in need of support. As a nurse in the program, Chris does home visits—counseling women, providing food and vitamin supplements if needed, and making referrals to other health care professionals. This is Chris's second visit to Barbara; the initial visit was on Wednesday the previous week. Barbara lives with her mother in a two-bedroom townhouse in a suburban area populated mainly by young families.

Approaching the townhouse door, Chris notices Barbara sitting in the living room, staring out the window. Barbara's mother, Adele, opens the door and invites Chris in. Chris enters the living room where Barbara sits in an easy chair. Barbara is thin and pale and there is a small bulge under her nightgown—evidence of the fact that she is 20 weeks' pregnant and expecting twins. Barbara was diagnosed with schizophrenia in her late teens. Adele gestures toward Barbara and, with a very concerned look on her face, says, 'You have to talk to her. She's been like that most of the time—very far away'. She brings a chair for Chris to sit near Barbara, and heads into the kitchen.

Barbara was referred to the HBPP program by her family physician 2 weeks earlier. After her first visit with Barbara, Chris called the referring physician who added more detail about her concerns regarding Barbara. First, on the advice of her family, Barbara had stopped taking her medications. Prior to her pregnancy and through the first weeks, she took Olanzapine 12.5 mg/day PO and Haldol 2 mg/day PO. The physician had discussed the importance of continuing to take the medications, but was unsure whether or not Barbara would or could do so, especially as her mother, with whom she lives, was worried about the effect of the medications on the fetuses. In addition, Barbara had missed her last two appointments with her psychiatrist. The physician and psychiatrist are considering involuntary admission of Barbara to the hospital.

Following her first visit to Barbara the previous week, Chris had felt very uneasy. Chris had difficulty communicating with Barbara, and although Barbara claimed she was now taking her medications, Chris was not sure whether to believe her. During that visit, Barbara had been unwilling or unable to talk about her pregnancy. She seemed alternately uninterested in and agitated by Chris's efforts to converse with her. As Chris had left that day, Adele followed outside and provided more information—that Barbara is married, but hasn't seen her husband in 3 months. Her husband has a job up north. Adele informed Chris that her daughter has been sleeping a lot and at strange hours. She is eating a reasonable amount, but mostly junk foods.

Before leaving, Chris had asked Adele about the family's financial resources. Adele said that Barbara has not been working for the past several years, and Adele herself works as a clerk in a nearby produce store. Because Barbara is married and her husband is working, she is not eligible for social assistance. Barbara's husband had sent money to her every 2 weeks at first, but no checks have arrived in the last month.

Today, Chris begins by asking Barbara how she is feeling. Barbara stares out the window. 'Were you able to eat some lunch today?' Chris asks, hoping to get at least a little information, and perhaps to find a way to get Barbara to talk. Adele has been standing in the door. 'She hasn't eaten anything today—except some cookies, chips, and pop. I told her that she has to eat better food for the sake of the babies. I don't think she actually cares what happens to them'. Barbara does not respond.

'Did you see Dr. Samson yesterday?' Chris inquires.

'I couldn't get her to leave the house', replies Adele. 'When I try to get her to go in the car, she gets very agitated, and thinks I am trying to get her to go to school—besides, they want to lock her up. They wouldn't lock her up if we lived up the hill (referring to a wealthy area nearby)'.

This example offers an illustration of the incredible complexity of everyday nursing practice and offers an opportunity to see how connecting across difference begins with an attitude and way of being and a willingness to take risks. Moreover, it requires a willingness to be in difficult places/situations and in conflict. The differences evident in Chris' visit with Barbara and Adele and the situation as a whole creates considerable discomfort, and as our usual habit as nurses is to reduce discomfort, Chris may be tempted to escape (give them some pamphlets and multivitamins and leave!), or ignore differences and smooth things over ('I'm sure Barbara will be fine now that she is back on her medications'), or to respond with some quick and easy answers (a phone call to the physician to get the involuntary hospitalization in process?). Hanging in there with the discomfort and ambiguity takes courage and patience.

So let's consider this situation more closely. What differences are evident as you read? Look at the referral slip reproduced in Box 9-1—what perspectives dominate? And how might the processes of relational practice help you work across these differences? Some obvious tensions Chris must take into account are between the mother (Adele) and daughter (Barbara) and between the physician and family. Tensions between the physician and family point to differences based on wealth, position, and ability. Adele thinks that their relative poverty disadvantages her family in relation to the physicians, and Barbara's mental illness limits her autonomy. Some less obvious tensions with which Chris must contend are the difference in value of women and fetuses. The program for which Chris works is entitled The Healthiest Babies Possible, not, for example, The Healthiest Mothers Possible, or The Healthiest Mothers and Babies Possible, or The Healthiest Families Possible. The program's title suggests a valuing of babies (over other family members/aspects of family). This might not be the intention, but the language of the title points to a possible tension that might be relevant as Chris sorts through how to be with this family. For example, if the focus of the program is babies' health, we are curious about how a nurse is supposed to proceed if, as in this case, the nursing concern for 'best babies' is in tension with the choices the mother is making. That is, it seems that Barbara's mental health has come under increased scrutiny (by her mother, the physicians, by Chris) because of the value of the fetuses she carries, more than out of concern for Barbara herself. How might this particular nursing concern constrain Chris' ability to connect across difference with Barbara?

As we have outlined in previous chapters, rather than directing Chris to 'fix' the problem, relational practice directs the nurse to get in sync and focus on inquiring into the *family* health experience, looking intentionally for patterns of adversity and capacity. From a relational perspective, it is impossible to address the goal of best babies without 'joining' the entire family situation. In dealing with difference in this process, rather than making a choice—to side with Barbara's mother, or with Barbara, or with the fetuses, or with the physicians—a relational approach directs Chris to enter in from a stance of inquiry, to look for the join both within the family and between the family and the health care workers. That is, how as a family is their individual well-being intricately tied together and how might Chris proceed relationally to foster the join between them and thus their well-being? From the information in the example earlier, what tensions and ambiguity can you already identify? What values and desires might everyone in the situation hold in common and be able to join around? Try It Out 9.1 invites you to try your imagination out with this situation. Think about this situation as we turn to considering specific ways in which difference is often thought about in practice.

> **TRY IT OUT 9.1.** **What Can You Imagine?**
>
> With two classmates or colleagues, role-play the parts of Adele, Barbara, and Chris outlined in the example. Role-playing can be as simple as having a conversation about the situation with each person beginning by saying "If I were (name of the person they chose), I would say . . ." Or, you could actually act out the parts. Work with the person taking the role of Chris to allow her/him to follow the processes of relational practice—that is, using a stance of inquiry follow the processes outlined in the previous chapter. Take note of 'differences' as you go. If you have a fourth classmate or colleague avail-able, have that person watch and give feedback. As you engage in the role-playing, think about how taken-for-granted ideas about mental illness might be shaping how you are thinking about Barbara and about the well-being of the fetus? For example, in research in which I (Colleen) was involved, we found that mothers with mental illnesses were viewed as a danger to their children by service providers, in the media, and in the way policies were developed and implemented (Greaves et al., 2002).

● Culture As Difference: From Sensitivity to Safety

Difference most commonly is talked about in nursing and health care (and in the world more generally) as *cultural difference*. However, talking about cultural difference is a tricky business because:

- What is meant by difference is culturally bound.
- Even though people often assume they share a common understanding, what is meant by culture and how it is understood is contentious and variable.
- Related to these two problems, culture is conflated (combined and confused with) with ethnicity and race.

This confusion allows dominant perspectives free rein and supports strategies of 'cultural sensitivity', which locate the challenges of cultural difference with those who are from nondominant groups. Thus, in order to deal with cultural difference relationally, we argue that difference must be taken seriously and that culture must be understood relationally, distinguishing culture, ethnicity, and race.

Taking Difference Seriously

From the perspective of liberal individualism (remember Chapter 1), difference is conceptualized as something to be celebrated, digested, and/or transcended. In contrast, Moosa-Mitha (2004) contends that from an antiracist perspective, difference cannot be digested or assimilated but must be seen as something very tangible that needs to be taken up and attended to seriously. We share the views of antiracist scholars who highlight that to attend to difference it cannot be covered over and/or transcended. Rather, to take difference up seriously, practitioners need to actively and reflexively scrutinize themselves in light of the differences living out in particular practice situations—they need to critically consider what the differences are and how the differences might be attended to within the health promoting process.

Part of taking difference seriously is recognizing that differences can run very deep. In other words, differences can be very profound and significant; therefore, connecting across differences is not a trivial matter. There are differences among people with regard to very fundamental issues, such as how one sees and understands the world. Throughout this book, we have been offering you different views of reality, contrasting, for example, a Cartesian view with a pragmatic view (remember Chapter 1). Similarly, families will have different views of reality. For example, Little Bear (2000), drawing particularly on the Aboriginal people of North America Plains, describes that in North American Aboriginal philosophy 'existence consists of energy. All things are animate, imbued with spirit, and in constant motion. In this realm of energy and spirit, interrelationships between all entities are of paramount importance, and space is a more important referent than time' (p. 67). He explains how such ideas lead to a holistic and cyclical view of the world in which the centrality of repetitive patterns puts the emphasis on processes (rather than products) and on 'happenings' rather than objects. Time is also dynamic, but goes nowhere, time 'just is'. He further explains that Aboriginal languages do not make use of dichotomies—there is no animate/inanimate, so that everything is more or less animate, and thus, 'if all are like me, then all are my relations' (p. 68). If you think back to the description of the Cartesian view of the world that dominates health care and consider it in light of this example of the North American Aboriginal view, it becomes obvious that there are significant differences between the two views. This is just one example of the different perspectives that people may hold and the significance of those differences to how people may view themselves, others, and the world. And it illustrates that to be health and healing promoting, nurses must attend to difference. That is, differences cannot be overlooked, discounted, erased, or trivialized—they must be taken seriously.

Understanding Culture Relationally

Critical consideration of difference is particularly crucial in terms of culture because what is meant by culture and how culture is understood is quite varied. Culture is often seen simply as shared values, beliefs, and practices, or is equated with ethnicity or nationality. Culture is frequently thought of without taking power into consideration and seen as a thing that belongs to particular groups of people. We critically consider each of these ideas and then offer alternative ways of thinking about culture.

Culture As Shared Beliefs

Culture is often seen very narrowly as a collection of shared beliefs. Razack (1998) says that the view of culture that has the widest currency is one in which 'culture is taken to mean values, beliefs, knowledge and customs that exist outside of patriarchy, racism, imperialism and colonialism' an understanding that 'reduces all facets of social life to issues of culture' (p. 58). If culture is seen in this way then difference is seen as being outside of patriarchy racism, imperialism and colonialism. Stephenson (1999) argues that in health care such narrow definitions trivialize culture, focusing attention only on traditions that differ from the dominant norm and turning attention away from the webs of social and political influences that also comprise cultures. To illustrate, Stephenson uses the example of a 5-year-old girl who died of chicken pox in the United States. Her parents were undocumented immigrants from Mexico who did not speak English, did not have money, and did not know where to go for help, and thus did not seek care until too late to prevent her death. However, a reporter asked what it was about Mexican *culture* that led them to delay treatment. This example echoes the experience that I (Colleen) have had doing research on violence against women. Many people ask me, 'What is it about their [referring to any number of groups] culture that leads the women to stay with abusive men?' With a narrow understanding of culture, broader contextual issues are overlooked, and at the same time, problems that arise from those broader contexts are associated with the culture of individuals. Although the chances of entering or leaving an abusive relationship are influenced by economic independence for *all* women, this influence is only seen as 'cultural' in racialized groups.

Culture As Ethnicity or Nationality

As suggested in the earlier examples, culture is often described in ethnic or nationalist terms and confused with ethnicity or nationality. Often, in doing so, culture is seen only as relevant to people who differ from the dominant group. Thus in Canada, where we are quite proud of our 'multiculturalism', Indian culture, Chinese culture, Thai culture, Vietnamese culture, and so on are made visible (and often associated with 'lesser than') while the dominant Euro-Canadian culture goes unremarked as the norm. Razack (1998) points out that culture talk is a double edged sword in that it 'packages difference as inferiority . . . yet is important for contextualizing oppressed groups' claims for justice, improving their access to services and for requiring dominant groups to examine the invisible cultural advantages they enjoy' (p. 58). For example, sometimes culture is significant and needs to be named in order to illuminate discriminatory practices that are related to culture, but at other times, culture is not the most useful way to understand people's experience and meaning. In fact, there are times when 'naming' culture obscures the adversity people are experiencing. For example, in Stephenson's story of the little girl who died of chicken pox, attributing her death to 'Mexican culture' overlooks the families' poverty, language barriers, and unfamiliarity with services and immigration status; blames the parents; and is discriminatory as a consequence! Therefore, we want to highlight the importance of not normalizing and/or essentializing (turning a particular difference into the essence of a person or group) difference and culture. Given the phenomenological understanding of people as situated and constituted, no two people who share an ethnic background can be lumped together and seen as having the same culture. For example, a colleague who is originally from Pakistan described how she is seen differently depending where she is. In Canada she is seen as being from

Pakistani culture in that she originates from Pakistan, speaks English with a certain accent, at times dresses in clothing from Pakistan, and so forth. Yet when she returns to Pakistan she is seen as a white Westerner because people there see her as having Western ways and a Western accent. What this points to is the fluid nature of culture and of cultural identity and the limitations of categories and generalizations.

Culture and Power

The third reason why we need to be critically aware of how we are naming culture is that culture often is considered without paying attention to power. That is, culture, particularly when seen as a collection of shared beliefs, is seen to exist independent of social and economic circumstances. Swendson and Windsor (1996) claim that culture has been used both to explain and deal with 'others' in Western capitalist societies. Therefore, structural issues, such as poverty, unemployment, access to care, and so on are thought about as cultural issues, and as choices about a way of life, rather than as unwanted life circumstances.

 ## To Illustrate

Have you ever heard about certain groups who don't make eye contact? Or for whom avoidance of eye contact is a 'cultural norm'? Eye contact, Razack (1998) points out, is 'a perennial favorite as a marker of the perils associated with cross-cultural encounters' (p. 57). However, Razack shows how seeing eye contact as cultural overlooks the affects of power, racism, and colonialism, and the fact that eye contact is being judged within a context of white supremacy, usually by members of dominant groups. To what extent is avoidance of eye contact (with white people) by racialized groups a safety strategy? To what extent is it an aversion to what racialized people might see in the eyes of white people? She also shows how a focus on cultural behaviours (she is talking in particular about the criminal justice system), such as avoidance of eye contact (which is often considered as indicative of guilt by those with the power to judge), draws attention away from systemic oppression. Thus, in her example, discriminatory justice system practices (such as disproportionately high arrest and incarceration rates of Aboriginal people and people of color) are explained as cultural misunderstandings rather than as a consequence of institutionalized racism.

Culture and Groups

Finally, culture is often seen as being *located in groups or people*, rather than as being *lived between* groups and people. Locating culture in groups means seeing it as a thing that people have. Allen (1999) argues that culture is not an object; 'there is no such "thing" as culture' (p. 227). Instead, culture is created, culture is lived, and culture is always in process. In the words of Stephenson (1999), 'culture is a process that happens between people'; culture is a relational process. Thus, to engage relationally in family nursing practice is also to engage culturally.

Understanding 'other' cultures is usually a haphazard affair. As we go about living, surrounded with all sorts of stereotypes and sensationalized and eroticized images of others, there is little direction regarding how to achieve understanding that crosses the differences of culture. Allen (1999) argues that culture is *always* 'perspectival', meaning that culture is always viewed from a particular perspective—no one can stand outside of their own values, beliefs, attitudes (all of which can be thought of as 'cultural') to view difference. Thus, as with engaging across any difference, in 'connecting across culture' it is important to begin with interrogating our own perspectives. Try It Out 9.2 invites you to depict your various cultures. After completing the activity, think about your cultures as relational. Do you share the same culture with your parents as you do

---

TRY IT OUT 9.2.   **What Are Your Cultures?**

1. *List* some of the 'cultures' to which you belong. In the figure, I (Colleen) listed a few of the cultures I can think of that are important in shaping my perspective. I left out 'Western culture' as it seemed too obvious, and 'paragliding' culture because it seemed less relevant to this purpose, and 'martial arts' culture because I have left it somewhat behind. I also left out 'native' or Aboriginal culture because, although my father was Aboriginal, I am not part of any Aboriginal culture.
2. *Depict* your cultures in a Venn diagram (see the Figure) or in some other way.
3. *Shade* those cultures according to the extent to which those cultures are dominant relative to the larger culture in which you live.

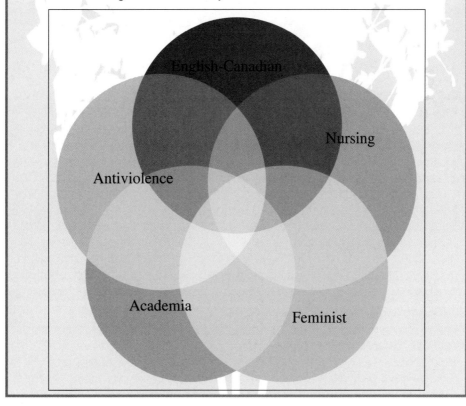

with your friends or with any children you know? Do you enact your culture differently depending on whom you are with?—for example, nursing and non-nursing friends? Can you begin to see your culture as a relational process?

Multiculturalism and Cultural Sensitivity

In the past two decades or so, Western nursing has begun to grapple with the idea of cultural difference. Nurses have developed a number of useful ideas and have taken several approaches. In recognition of diversity and the need to cross differences, nurses have taken up the ideas of multiculturalism and advocated being 'sensitive' to cultural difference. In Canada, as in many other former colonies with diverse populations, including the United Kingdom (Culley, 1996) and Australia (Swendson & Windsor, 1996), multiculturalism has become policy, and this policy has been widely disseminated in state organizations, including health care settings.

Multiculturalism is based on understanding culture as shared beliefs, as a thing that belongs to groups of individuals, groups that are often identified by ethnicity, nationality, or religion. In nursing the ideas of multiculturalism are used to focus on bringing culture into nursing care. Thus, nurses are encouraged to learn about different cultures (note the implied norm and the implication that culture is a group thing) and be more 'sensitive'. In health care and nursing, multiculturalism is an approach that deals with problems of difference as being mismatches between minority and dominant cultures. Dealing with difference is seen as a matter of being more sensitive to others and of reducing the prejudices of individuals.

An Example: The Multicultural Corner

A year or so ago, I (Colleen) picked up a health care organization newsletter that had a feature entitled 'Multicultural Corner' that is 'designed to help health service providers become more aware of the cultural sensitivities of patients, clients and residents'. In this edition of the newsletter, Indo-Canadians were featured. This one-page feature listed the 'Countries of Origin' as 'Pakistan, India, Sri Lanka, Bangaladesh, Nepal, Fiji, East Africa, United Kingdom and Hong Kong'; 'Religion and Religious practices' as 'Sikhism, Hinduism, and Islam' with information about practices such as hair cutting and prayer beads, and a list of languages ('English, Hindi, Punjabi, Guharate and Urdu. Most speak English.'). The page also had information under the categories of 'Family Support', 'Hospitalization', 'Diet', 'Death', and 'Child Care'. The Family Support section read:

- Extended families are common.
- Family spokesperson is usually the most established male (i.e., language skills, financially established, seniority in family).
- Role of women—caregivers, nurturers, generally submissive but respected.
- Elderly—have authority and are accorded respect, help with childcare, arrange marriages, provide advice.

The Hospitalization section contained items such as:

- 'lots of support from family and friends',
- 'expectation that friends will visit to show concern and caring (if it's a problem, talk to the family spokesperson)',
- 'cleanliness is important',
- 'embarrassment and resistance to have male health care professional look after patient'.

The section on Diet makes points such as 'vegetarianism is common' and 'feasting may be observed'.

The intention of this multicultural corner publication was to help nurses and others to provide more sensitive care. However, it is very likely that the intent was undermined because of the approach taken. First, the document lumped an incredibly diverse group of people into one category. This kind of categorization begs the question of who is doing the categorizing. To what extent can this information possibly apply to potentially millions of diverse families? Second, it offered a very stereotypical and overly general view. To what extent could most of the hospitalization statements, for example, be applied to most people? For example, think back to hermeneutic phenomenology and the ideas of situated and constituted that highlight how as individuals we are constituted by the multitude of experiences and locations we live. This means that an Indo-Canadian person who came to Canada as an adult will be constituted differently than someone who came as an infant and/or someone who was born and grew up in Canada. Although they may share particular sociocultural experiences and even traditions, there will also be significant differences between them—thus their cultures will be different. Can such standardized information lead to being more 'sensitive'? And, how might the information lead to unwarranted assumptions about individual people/families? Finally, whose interests are most served here? For example, one of the worst possibilities is that the document could be used to provide a short cut for nursing practice. Based on having this information nurses can think they 'know' what is important to 'those people' and not have to inquire into the particularities of the people/families for whom they are caring. In the document, friends visiting 'to show concern and caring' is identified as a potential problem, pointing to tensions that commonly arise in this particular health care organization (health care providers often complain that people they identify as Indo-Canadians have 'too many visitors') and suggesting that the interests of providers should supersede interests of families.

Although multiculturalism has drawn attention to diversity, it uses narrow understandings of culture and thus overlooks social inequities and structural determinants of health. And it reduces all practices to culture and overlooks other influences, such as gender roles or economics, which might be similar across cultures. With a narrow definition of culture (as shared beliefs or practices) the historical impact of colonization, immigration, and racism is also overlooked. When trying to bring culture into care as an 'add-on', it is easy to confuse culture with ethnicity (think of the Multicultural Corner newsletter example). When the problem is defined as mismatches between minority and dominant cultures, political and economic forces are overlooked. For example, in the Multicultural Corner, immigration policies that disadvantage women and contribute to confining them to caregiving roles do not figure in the description of the role of women; similarly the many Indo-Canadian women who are leaders, professionals, and so on are discounted. Also, when the problem is defined as mismatches between minority and dominant cultures, the different culture becomes the problem (for example, too many friends visiting) and the solutions become bringing others into line ('talk to the family spokesperson'). Finally, focusing on 'prejudiced individuals', another hallmark of multiculturalism and cultural sensitivity, overlooks how racism is deeply embedded in language, structures, and institutions. A nurse shooing Indo-Canadian visitors out the door is not just an individual practicing in a discriminatory manner; he or she is acting in concert with ideas sanctioned by the organization.

The Limitations of Cultural Sensitivity

Cultural sensitivity is one of the central practices of multiculturalism. Cultural sensitivity, or being more sensitive to others' values and beliefs, is the dominant way that dealing with racial difference (under the banner of cultural difference) has been conceptualized in health care and service delivery and is an idea that has been widely taken up in nursing. Based on the narrow understandings of culture that underlie multiculturalism and the confusion of culture, ethnicity, and race, however, cultural sensitivity is highly inadequate in that it overlooks and obscures issues of racial supremacy and inequality and the way that cultural relations are embedded in and shaped by sociopolitical and economic contexts (Culley, 1996; Swendson & Windsor, 1996).

Cultural sensitivity implies that those operating from the dominant norm and who wield the power ought to be sensitive to difference. This sensitivity requires no social action. Sensitivity to cultural difference, when culture is seen as values and beliefs, means sensitivity to values and beliefs, but not sensitivity to context and the structural determinants of health. Perhaps our overriding concern with the idea of cultural sensitivity is how it gives rise to a recipe-book approach to culture such as in the multicultural corner publication above. Nurses are encouraged to learn about others' values, beliefs, and practices (Chinese do this, African Americans do that, Jews think this, Muslims think that) as recipes to guide practice with others. Naturally, this places the dominant white Eurocentric norm at the center and leaves the culturally sensitive practitioner open to generalizations and stereotypes based on race, class, religion, and so on. Working from the ideas of multiculturalism and sensitivity, it is perhaps not surprising that, as Gray and Thomas (2002) have concluded, nurses have taken up a very limited view of culture, and focused on difference, particularly racial/ethnic or religious differences, without bridging those differences. Clearly, such an

approach is not congruent with relational nursing practice or with emancipatory action.

Crossing Cultural Difference in Nursing: Beyond Cultural Sensitivity to Cultural Safety

Recently nursing scholars have introduced the idea of 'cultural safety'
as a tool for emancipatory practice in diverse contexts. Cultural safety
begins with an understanding of culture as embedded in historical,
economic, and social contexts. The idea of safety is predicated on an
understanding of 'unsafety' as anything that diminishes, demeans, or
disempowers the cultural identity and well-being of an individual or
group (Wood & Schwass, 1993). Promoting safety requires actions that
recognize, respect, and nurture the unique cultural identity of people/
families, and safely meet their needs, expectations, and rights.

Nursing educators initially introduced the idea of cultural safety in
Aeotara/New Zealand to facilitate health care interactions between the
indigenous Maori people and Pakuha (the nonindigenous, predominantly
white immigrants) (Papps & Ramsden, 1996; Wood & Schwass, 1993).
The idea has since been explored as a way of promoting ethical practice
within ethnically diverse populations (Anderson et al., 2003; Browne &
Fiske, 2001; Polaschek, 1998; Reimer Kirkham et al., 2002; Smye &
Browne, 2002). Box 9.2 outlines the central ideas of the evolving concept
of cultural safety.

Cultural safety involves the 'recognition of the social, economic and
political position of certain groups within society . . . and is concerned
with fostering an understanding of the relationship between minority status and health status. The intent is to change nurses' attitudes from
those which continue to support current dominant practices and
systems of health care to those which are more supportive of the health
of minority groups' (Smye & Browne, 2002, pp. 46–47). The concept of
cultural safety not only turns attention to the attitudes and practices of
individuals, but also directs attention to examining how dominant
organizational, institutional, and structural contexts shape health and
social relations and practices, and prompts the unmasking of the ways

---

BOX 9.2. Cultural Safety: Central Ideas

- The social, economic, and political position of groups within society are understood
  to influence health and health care.
- Minority status (based on race, ethnicity, sexual orientation, class, gender, age, and
  so on) influences health status.
- Nurses have an obligation to support the health of minority and nondominant
  groups.
- Care should be respectful and preserving of human dignity.
- 'Cultural' and power differences between nurses and clients should not jeopardize
  the care clients receive.
- Stereotyping and discrimination must be challenged.
- Structural inequities should be challenged and remedied.

policies and practices may perpetuate neocolonial approaches to health care (Smye & Browne, 2002).

Culturally Safe Relational Practice

The ideas of cultural safety are congruent with and parallel to the ideas of relational practice. Rather than directing nurses to learn about other cultures (where we can never know enough) and fearing cultural faux pas, cultural safety helps us focus on understanding the complex dynamics of contexts within which culture is embedded. Taking difference seriously is facilitated by following the lead of family because families will let us know what is of meaning, significance, and importance to them, whether we define these things as different (from ourselves or an implied norm) and whether we label these things as cultural or not. We believe that culturally safe practice requires intentional connection across difference within relational inquiry.

● Connecting Across Difference: Attitude to Action

In approaching difference you can:

* attempt to ignore or overlook difference,
* use difference with (examined or unexamined) value judgments to see families and people who are different from yourself as 'those people',
* engage difference with intentional value judgments to see families and people as different from yourself, but of value as human beings, that is, as worthy of your unconditional positive regard.

The latter is congruent with a relational approach, and is what Canales (2000) proposes in her discussion of 'inclusionary othering' as a way of connecting across difference. Canales defines othering as the way we engage with 'others' (those perceived as different from self) and further defines exclusionary othering as a process that uses power within relationships for domination and subordination. She conceptualizes inclusionary othering as a process that attempts to use power within relationships for transformation and coalition building, in other words, as a way of connecting across difference. Canales suggests engaging with others perceived as different from oneself in an actively inclusionary manner. Like other postcolonial and feminist authors such as Collins (for example, 1990, 1993) and Lugones and Spelman (1983), Canales advises nurses to work to know the other's world, to reconceptualize meanings and understandings, and to connect with others as allies and in friendship. Browne and her colleagues (2002) suggest that in order to connect across difference, nurses:

* begin with working toward the development of a critical consciousness of one's own power, knowledge, and privilege,
* explicitly name discrimination, with attention to the language we use to refer to others,

- actively reflect on generalizations and biases that may inform action,
- actively attend to patient's and families' claims of discrimination.

We believe that these strategies will allow nurses to enact the processes of relational practice (Chapter 7) in a meaningful manner across differences.

Developing Critical Consciousness of One's Power, Knowledge, and Privilege

Seeking to cross differences, 'looking for the join', means acknowledging differences beginning from one's own location. Acknowledging differences in turn means abandoning neutrality. Taking a neutral stance is problematic because such a stance overlooks or obscures differences that can be the basis for connection. Rather than acting on assumptions of neutrality, such as the assumption that the 'playing field is level' (meaning that everyone has the same opportunities) or the 'we're all the same' assumption, differences in values, beliefs, experiences, and practices have to be taken into account if the differences are to be crossed.

In order to talk about 'difference,' comparisons have to be made. And making comparisons is never a neutral act but rather is a political act; making a comparison involves defining one thing in terms of another. 'They haven't learned Canadian values yet', 'They don't understand parenting in the same way we do'. Comparisons are most powerful and potentially problematic when the comparison is implicit—that is to say, when the comparison is with some implied but unnamed 'norm'. For example, in relation to people with COPD, one nurse said 'they don't seem to know what's good for them', implying that 'we', the health care providers, know better. The comparison with the dominant group isn't obvious, but in a powerful way certain groups are being defined in a way that makes them 'other than'.

Comparisons are also most problematic when you think that you are being neutral ('I treat all my patients the same'; 'every family gets the same care here'; 'I don't see colour, I just see people'). Here, neutrality is dangerous because it makes blind spots and implicit norms more difficult to see. Thinking you are neutral obscures differences, privileges, and disadvantages and their impact, and overlooks both the struggles people have in living with disadvantage and the advantage privilege affords. For example, if you try to deal with racism by not seeing colour or seeing yourself as beyond racism, you paradoxically blind yourself to discrimination based on skin colour and to the way racism is institutionalized (embedded in the structures of society). Thinking that you are neutral leaves you open to stereotyping and overgeneralizing, both of which dramatize difference and separation (Canales, 2000). When comparisons are made using stereotypes ('women are emotional', 'welfare families are lazy and dependent') those stereotypical representations often define the identity of those being compared in favour of dominant groups ('women are more emotional *than men*'; 'welfare families are lazier *than those with employment*'). Rather than approaching difference from a position of neutrality, examining the basis (perspective) from which you are making comparisons (the skill of self-knowing and process of self-observation) means that you can approach difference and comparisons with greater critical awareness. It is important to emphasize that we are not suggesting that you stop making comparisons. Rather, we are advocating for you to pay attention to the comparisons you are making and the basis you are using for those comparisons, that is, your own power, knowledge and privilege.

In earlier chapters you were invited to think about your own social locations and positions. Here we turn your attention to your specific sources of power, knowledge, and privilege. People writing about difference maintain that an examination of the practitioner's motives is the first step in connecting across difference (see, for example, Collins, 1993; Lugones, 1987; Lugones & Spelman, 1983; Nye, 2000). Approaching difference from an unexamined position of privilege in order to benefit (should we say 'rescue' or 'save'?) others, simply reinforces power and privilege differences and does nothing to bridge those differences. Lugones argues that friendship (caring about other human beings) is the only valid reason to seek to cross worlds separated by privileges such as race or class. To this Nye (2000) adds the reason of awe, 'awe at the mystery and complexity of human existence' (p. 108).

In 1988, Peggy McIntosh wrote a paper entitled 'White Privilege: Unpacking the Invisible Knapsack'. In it she describes how she realized that although as a white person she had been taught about racism as something that puts others at disadvantage, she had never been taught to think of white privilege as something that put her at advantage. She described white privilege as 'an invisible package of unearned assets which I can count on cashing each day, but about which I am meant to be oblivious' (p. 1). McIntosh proceeded to begin to identify the ways in which she enjoyed her unearned privilege and the ways she was encouraged to be oblivious to the 'special provisions, maps, passports, codebooks, visas, clothes, tools and blank checks' that she could pull from her invisible, weightless knapsack (p. 1). She included things such as, 'I can turn on the television or open to the front page of the paper and see people of my race widely represented' and 'If my day, week, or year is going badly, I need not ask of each negative episode or situation whether it has racial overtones'. Try It Out 9.3 invites you to look in your

---

TRY IT OUT 9.3.   **What's in Your Backpack?**

The first step in connecting across difference is to practice with an awareness of your own privilege. At a minimum as a nurse you have the privileges of education, of speaking the first language of your country with fluency, and of special access to health care through your knowledge. In relation to the families with whom you work you also likely have a relative position of power. What else is in your knapsack?

Make a list of the privileges you carry in your knapsack. What automatic benefits do you have by virtue of your able-bodied-ness, intellectual abilities, language skill, education, accent, skin color, gender, size, income. It is much easier to see our own disadvantages than our advantages, so resist for the moment the desire to list all the disadvantages you may have endured.

knapsack and identify your privileges. Not all of you will have had the advantages of 'white privilege', not all will have had enough to eat all your lives, or spoken the dominant language of your country as your first language. Although we do not think that there are parallels between advantages based on race with those based on gender, sex, class, and so on, these forms of advantage intersect as do forms of marginalization, and so all are important to identify.

Nurses are often in a position of power relative to families and individuals they see as patients. Nurses usually have more knowledge about the health care system and sometimes have great influence over the access that families have to health care. Nurses have advantages of education, employment, and language skills, which may position them as relatively powerful in relation to families. Nurses also are often in a position of power relative to families and individuals because they see them at times of crisis or vulnerability.

However, nurses are not always relatively more powerful than the families with whom they work. Nurses are diverse in terms of their experiences, social locations, knowledge, employment positions, and so on. In fact, one of the hard spots is when patients and families are abusive, manipulative, or disrespectful toward nurses. Relationally, nurses' relative positions of power due to their knowledge, skills, and employment intersect with other forms of privilege and oppression, such as gender, class, and race.

An Example: A Challenging Clinical Placement

Kara entered the four-bed room. The hostility was palpable. 'You!' shouted the elderly man sitting by his wife's bed. 'My wife needs help and where have you been? She's supposed to have a private room'. Kara ignored him as she took a new IV bag to another patient's bed. 'You! My wife needs some water. Get her some water'. Kara shuddered, thankful that her instructor, trailing behind her, could not understand the rude demands.

Kara was a student who I (Colleen) worked with as she was completing a clinical experience in a hospital in the community where she lived. Kara (a pseudonym) was in her fourth year and close to graduating, and had been evaluated as an excellent nurse throughout her studies. However, on this final clinical placement, she ran into serious trouble for two reasons. First, she was assigned to care for members of her particular ethnic community, and some of the patients and families from that community treated her very disrespectfully. They rudely ordered her about and made demands that she could not meet. For example, one woman repeatedly dropped tissues and asked Kara to pick them up. Kara explained that many in the community do not regard nurses very highly, and that some do not approve of her family. Second, when Kara tried to negotiate a different patient assignment, the nurses in charge were unwilling to change because Kara spoke the language of her ethnic community, making such an assignment 'easier' for the rest of the staff. Kara was not only in a relatively less-powerful position in relation to some patients and families, but was also disadvantaged by her position as a student, and as a minority person in relation to the majority of English-speaking-only staff. Athough this example illustrates that nurses are diverse and varied in terms of their own power, knowledge, and privilege, it also illustrates that we need to consider our privileges not only in relation to patients/families, but also in relation to colleagues and to the contexts within which we live and work.

Throughout this chapter you might feel the double-edged sword of naming difference as you move back and forth between allegiances with people in the stories we offer. As writers, we have felt torn about highlighting particular differences. In order to be able to contextualize issues of culture and name the dehumanizing and stigmatizing treatment of difference, we have at times felt it necessary to use examples that highlight particular differences. At the same time bringing attention to those differences can create the danger of stereotyping and essentializing. For example, in telling the story of Kara, we were tempted not to share the fact that Kara is from a community of people who have emigrated from a non-English-speaking country. To do so invites generalizations and the tendency to 'essentialize culture' and/or dismissal of the adversity she faced as 'merely cultural', yet not to do so makes the adversity less understandable! Thus, we want to emphasize that highlighting difference is a relational process that must always be critically considered and contextually decided.

Explicit Naming of Stigma and Discrimination

Important differences arise when families are in stigmatizing situations or experience stigmatizing health problems. Poverty, drug and alcohol abuse, violence, mental illness, incarceration, homelessness, and HIV/AIDS are some of the more common health challenges that lead to families' experiences of stigma. As the story of Barbara's family suggests, social stigma shapes power dynamics. Given the liberal ideology on which Western health care is based (remember Chapter 1), individuals and families are often held responsible and blamed for their health problems. For example, people who are poor are often treated as though they are poor willfully or through lack of personal initiative, without looking at how a person's life chances are determined by circumstances of birth, geography, and opportunity. People with drug and alcohol abuse are also often treated as though they chose addiction, without taking into account the relationship between addiction and histories of mental illness, child abuse and other forms of severe trauma, poverty, and so on (Bensley, Van Eenwyk, & Simmons, 2000; Clark & Foy, 2000; Craib et al., 2003; Estebaneza et al., 2000; Heffernan et al., 2000; Jasinski, Williams, & Siegel, 2000; Miller, 1999; Mullings, Marquart, & Brewer, 2000; Nair, Schuler, Black, Kettinger, & Harrington, 2003; Parillo, Freeman, Collier, & Young, 2001).

The dynamics of stigma can shape nursing practice. Studies have shown that certain groups of people, such as women, people from ethnic minorities, people who are poor, people who have substance use problems, and/or other stigmatizing health problems, are more likely to experience labeling, stereotyping, and social judgments in health care. When nurses and others care for people who differ from the dominate group in terms of race, class, religion, age, income, or sexual orientation, there is a greater risk of labeling, stereotyping, and social judgments (Carveth, 1995; Corley & Goren, 1998; Grief & Elliott, 1994; Johnson & Webb, 1995; Kelly & May, 1982; Liaschenko, 1995; Stevens, 1992, 1994).

The use of labels, stereotypes, and social judgments in nursing practice affects the quality of patient and family care and is inconsistent with the professional ethical obligations of nurses (Corley & Goren, 1998; Pauly & Varcoe, in review). We believe that as nurses one of our central moral imperatives is to explicitly name and counter such discrimination. However, it is critical to do so without overlooking the power and agency of those experiencing discrimination. As with working across any difference, developing a critical consciousness of one's own power, knowledge, privilege, and biases is the starting point. Developing understanding of stigma and contextual knowledge of the social determinants of stigmatizing situations provides you with a basis for developing alternatives to explanations that blame people for aspects of their health for which they cannot be held responsible. Connecting across stigma occurs within powerful contexts where many forms of stigma are taken for granted. Therefore, once again identifying and enlisting supportive colleagues and resources is crucial to resisting succumbing to norms of practice that are barriers to health-promoting practice.

In Chapter 7 we described recognizing and naming inequities and recognizing and naming structural conditions that compromise health and health promotion as integral to emancipatory practice. In working to connect across difference, these strategies are used to recognize and name discrimination based on difference. So, for example, in Barbara's situation, the relationship between mental illness and poverty (Belle & Doucet, 2003; Chow, Jaffee, & Snowden, 2003; Patel & Kleinman, 2003; Perese & Perese, 2003; Spencer, 2003; Weitoft, Hjern, Haglund, & Rosén, 2003) and discrimination based on mental illness and poverty should be named and taken into account in deciding how to proceed in nursing practice.

Importantly, the language we use to refer to others can be a powerful form of discrimination and can sustain structural inequities. Seemingly innocuous words such as 'they', 'them', and 'those people' can alert us to exclusionary othering. Saying '*they* don't understand parenting the way we do' not only creates a them through exclusionary othering. The speaker also creates an us and invites the listener to side against the other. Generalizations should alert you to stereotyping, the arch enemy of connecting across difference. Paying attention to generalizations assists in identifying and naming discrimination and biases held by yourself and others.

Language about others often obscures power. For example, talking about a person as 'a schizophrenic' rather than as 'a person with schizophrenia' seems a subtle difference. But by using the former, the speaker uses his or her power as a labeler to reduce the person to a problem or disease. Sartorius (2002), a psychiatrist, argues that the 'most obvious source of stigmatization [of people with mental illnesses] is careless use

---

BOX 9.3.	**Manifesting Racism**

How is Racism Commonly Manifest in Everyday Health Care?

- Using racial categories (e.g., 'East Indian', 'Chinese')
- Associating stigmatizing conditions with arbitrary racial or ethnic categories
- Stereotyping
- Using terms such as 'different' and 'other' to imply a dominant norm (e.g. 'I am interested in learning to care for people from a different culture')

How is Racism Manifest in Structures and Delivery of Services?

- Lack of access to appropriate programs and services
- Ethnocentric values in services
- Devaluing the skills and credentials of minority practitioners
- Inadequate funding for ethnoracial community-based agencies
- Lack of minority representation in agency oversight and management
- Monocultural (one dominant culture) models of service delivery

(Adapted from Henry, Tator, Mattis, & Rees, 2000)

---

of diagnostic labels', and urges critical consciousness regarding the power of diagnoses (p. 1471). A more obvious form of othering is language that racializes individuals or groups. Recall from Chapter 2 that 'racialization' refers to the social process by which people are labeled according to particular physical characteristics or arbitrary ethnic or racial categories and then dealt with in accordance with beliefs related to those labels. When people are racialized according to physical characteristics (labeled Chinese, African Americans, East Indian, and so on) and stereotyped according to this racialization, the stage is set for thinking of those being labeled as other, and for exclusionary and discriminatory practices to follow or to be accepted and tolerated. Even language that is intended to name discrimination can be problematic. Browne, Smye, and Varcoe (in press) point out that applying labels such as 'marginalized' and 'disadvantaged' to describe the complexities and diversity of certain peoples' lives risks characterizing them only as victims or as lacking agency or resiliency. Thus identifying and naming discrimination and stigma should take into account the complex dynamics of power without reducing certain groups of people to their experiences of discrimination.

Discrimination is more than just semantics. Racism and other forms of discrimination are built into the everyday practices of health care and very structures of health care delivery. Box 9.3 outlines some of the more common ways that racism, for example, can be seen in the practices, structures, and delivery of health care.

An Example: Teaching Stigma

Several years ago I (Colleen) was asked to consult about a series of case examples that had been developed by a professional organization to guide the teaching of nurses. The cases had been constructed (made up) by a variety of experienced clinical nurses and nurse educators. I was asked to review the cases to see if they covered the required skills for graduate nurses, but my concern with the shocking level of built-in discrimination stopped me from my task. What first struck me was that culture was mentioned primarily where the people in the cases were racialized. For example, in one series, 3 of 18 cases were racialized and culture was considered in all 3; of the remaining 15, culture was only mentioned in 2. Second, racialized people were routinely associated with stigmatizing health issues. For example, in the case involving sexual, emotional, and chemical abuse, the people were identified as 'South Asian', the case involving 'Native' children dealt with lice, the 'Vietnamese' family was associated with child abuse. In the case involving a family of 'immigrants' child malnourishment was the issue and child neglect was explored in a family identified as 'Chinese'. In one series of cases, 8 of 67 cases were racialized, and of these 8, 5 were associated with stigmatizing issues. Of the 59 cases that were not racialized, only 4 were associated with stigmatizing issues, such as abuse, neglect, drug use, or fetal alcohol syndrome. In these cases, racialized people also were associated routinely with 'deficiencies'—for example, a 'Vietnamese' woman was described as being on welfare, an 'East Asian' woman's 'cognitive ability' was in question, and a 'South Asian' woman's commitment to breastfeeding needed to be assessed—associations that were not apparent in the cases that were not racialized.

What disturbed me most was the fact that these cases were being published for widespread use in teaching and evaluating nurses. Along with teaching nurses what was expected in terms of assessment skills, knowledge, interventions, and so on, these cases were subtly building associations between certain groups of people and negative and stigmatizing health issues and 'deficits', entrenching and institutionalizing discrimination.

Explicit naming of discrimination requires being able to *see* discrimination. Try It Out 9.4 asks you to explicitly name both the language of discrimination and the structural practices of discrimination. Such naming is the first step in taking action and can open the way for active reflection on generalizations and bias.

Active Reflection on Generalizations and Biases

Once discrimination is recognized and named, it can be held up for scrutiny and challenge. Active reflection moves beyond naming discrimination and encompasses actions for interrupting discrimination including

---

TRY IT OUT 9.4. **Who are "They"?**

1. *Identify* who is likely to be 'othered' in an exclusionary manner in your community or your clinical area. Think about who might be referred to with phrases such as 'they are our worst families to deal with' or 'they are our biggest problem families'.
2. *List*
   - ways in which this group of people might be labelled,
   - discriminatory ways in which this group of people might be talked about,
   - structures and delivery practices that might limit health care access for this group (review Box 9-3 for ideas here).

> **TRY IT OUT 9.5.** **Safety in Context**
>
> 1. *Share* with at least one other person the discriminatory practices, structures, and delivery practices that you identified in Try It Out 9-4. Compare your analysis with the other person's.
> 2. *Review* the ideas of cultural safety in Box 9-2. Compare your thoughts about the discriminatory practices with the ideas of cultural safety. What direction does this comparison offer?
> 3. *Brainstorm* together the ways that discriminatory practices might be countered.
> 4. *Anticipate* what the risk associated with each action might be.
> 5. *Identify* your limitations in affecting change in relation to the structure and delivery practices.

questioning generalizations and biases and offering alternative perspectives.

In Chapter 6, we identified the skill of interrupting contextual constraints as fundamental to relational practice. In seeking to connect across difference, interrupting contextual constraints becomes the skill of interrupting discrimination. Interrupting begins with naming and proceeds to actions such as countering with questions and alternative perspectives. In the example of the stigmatizing cases, I (Colleen) outlined my concerns in a manner similar to what I wrote earlier, phoned the person who had invited me to do the review and expressed my concern (naming). Then prepared a more detailed analysis of the problem with recommendations regarding how to fix and avoid the problem (countering with alternative perspectives). Taking action was made easier for me in this case because I had been invited to review the cases (although for a different purpose) and because of my privileged position as a professor, my job and work relationships were not at risk in doing so. For many practicing nurses, countering discrimination involves considerably more risk. Try It Out 9.5 invites you to think about the forms of discrimination most relevant to your practice and to anticipate what the risks might be in trying to counter discriminatory practices. As you review the structural forms of discrimination, it will be clear that collective effort and political action are required to address structural forms of discrimination. Despite these limitations, however, at a minimum you can respond in a meaningful manner to a particular patient's and families' claims of discrimination.

Attending to Patient's and Families' Claims of Discrimination

Possible responses to claims of discrimination include:

- ignoring the claim,
- denying the validity of the claim or minimizing the claim,
- acknowledging the claim and taking action based on that acknowledgment.

To ignore or deny claims of discrimination is contrary to the notion of following the lead of families. Regardless of whether *you* would experience a situation or act as discriminatory, the important thing in following the lead of family is whether *they* experienced an act or situation as discriminatory. For example, if you think back to Chris' visit with Barbara, Chris could choose various ways to respond to Adele's contention that their relative poverty made Barbara more vulnerable to being 'locked up'. Chris could dismiss Adele's concerns, argue with Adele and defend the mental health system, or Chris could 'follow the lead' and explore Adele's experience in response to that claim (whether or not Chris agrees).

It is important to emphasize that acknowledging the claim does not mean validating that discrimination 'really' did occur. Rather, what is acknowledged is the person's/families' experience of feeling disadvantaged or discriminated against. At the same time we want to highlight that what is experienced by one family as discrimination may not be experienced in that way by another family. Peggy McIntosh (1988) points out that because she is a white person in the United States and does not face discrimination daily she does not find herself questioning whether there are racial overtones in any negative situation she experiences. However, a black woman in similar experiences might raise such questions as a result of the racialized discrimination that has been part of her everyday experience in life. So experiences of discrimination over a lifetime may lead a person to be alert to and anticipate discrimination, and a person with such experience might be less likely to explain negative experiences in other ways.

Acknowledging discrimination can be the most powerful support you can offer. In the same way that you do not have to fix other problems families encounter, you do not have to fix discriminatory experiences. However, in line with other emancipatory actions, you can take steps to intervene at the level of organizations through coalitions to reduce structural inequities and counter discrimination. Use of these strategies is perhaps easiest to imagine in the situations where difference is foregrounded and explicitly named. Now we invite you to shift your thinking to differences that may not be as obvious.

● Crossing Differences in Healing Modalities

> 66 *[I]f you asked an elder about [mammography] they might say that it would be a test of fire. Of the elements of fire, water, earth and air, that having a mammogram or having radiation might be aligning yourself with the fire spirit to try to make yourself, to try to learn something. . . . On the other side I would say that you're poisoning yourself. You are poisoning. I mean even a tooth x-ray. The radiation. Yeah the radiation is definitely harming you. There is no way around that. (Canales & Geller, 2004, p. 847)* 99

Different healing modalities represent a difference that is a common challenge in Western health care and one that is often conflated with ethnic difference under a narrow understanding of culture. Nurses working within a Western health care system, dominated by biomedicine, are likely to encounter differences between the treatment and healing modalities being offered within the health care system and what is wanted by families. Nurses can often find themselves in the position of negotiating between treatments and practices offered by the formal health care system and a wide range of other health practices. Such practices are variously referred to as 'complementary' practices, 'alternative' practices, 'traditional practices', 'cultural practices', and so on.

What distinguishes these practices is the degree to which they have been accepted and supported by the dominant system and culture. Various nonbiomedical practices enjoy a wide range of acceptance by those practicing within the dominant system. This acceptance shifts continuously and varies from context to context. For example, in health care settings in areas that serve a predominantly Christian population, the importance of certain forms of prayer to healing might be well recognized and tolerated. In that same community, other forms of prayer might be less accepted. To take another example, in some contexts widespread practice (coupled with recent Western scientific validation) has encouraged increasing acceptance of acupuncture as a healing modality.

Keeping in mind that knowledge is ever-evolving, and that today's facts may be tomorrow's fallacies, it is not enough to dismiss nonbiomedical practices as unsubstantiated or lacking in scientific 'proof'. Indeed, many pharmaceuticals and treatments considered routine in Western health care are actively being researched since science has not yet shown their effectiveness. This suggests that in considering nonbiomedical health and healing practices it is important to keep an open mind and to continuously pursue the best information available.

It is also not useful to think of some practices as 'cultural' practices and others as not cultural. This is because in essence *biomedicine is a culture* that has and continues to profoundly shape norms and practices within health care (Coward & Hartrick, 2000). However, because biomedicine is part of dominant Western culture, it is often not recognized as such. Just as through dominance white skin is used in Western countries as an implicit norm to compare and 'other' people, biomedicine is the norm used to compare and 'other' healing modalities. This position within the dominant culture at least partly explains widespread acceptance of biomedical practices with or without evidence of effectiveness and sometimes in the face of evidence of grave side effects. Take, for example, breast implants, a clearly Western 'cultural phenomenon'. In working toward relational practice it is more helpful to understand that acceptance of any treatment or healing practice is influenced by both the cultural beliefs of those advocating the practice and the families receiving or using them.

Finally, a 'recipe' approach to understanding various beliefs about health and healing is inadequate to following the lead of particular families. Although people from particular groups may share certain beliefs and practices, there is great variability among families and within families themselves. For example, although Americans might share certain values and beliefs, not all Americans subscribe to chiropractic treatment, and within any family, members may have different beliefs about any given treatment or practice. As the quote at the start of this section suggests, similar beliefs can be used to either support or dispute a given practice.

An Example: Moving Toward or Away From Mammography

American Indian women studied by Canales and Geller (2004) decided whether to participate in routine mammography screening from their position of living between two cultures, the dominant Western culture and a more traditional, native culture. Specific factors that influenced their decisions included the degree to which the women connected to their 'nativeness', the ways they went about caring for themselves and others, their trust or mistrust of the health care system, and their ability to finance health care. While connecting to their 'nativeness' gave the women more options for healing practices (such as being more in tune with their bodies, following cleansing practices), they interpreted traditional beliefs variously as supporting or not supporting mammography. Other aspects of their experiences were as important in their decisions—for example, as most were poor, whether they could afford a mammogram was a key consideration. Their experiences of racism or of acceptance with the health care system either deterred or encouraged them to have a mammogram. And finally, the importance of family (the need to be healthy for their children, the need to model health practices for other family members) was interconnected to these other factors in their decision making.

Crossing different healing modalities, a nurse can choose to defend one practice over another—he or she can align with the dominant system and promote those practices. Alternatively (following the lead of family), the nurse can try to understand what is health promoting to particular people and families. So, for example, for some women the potential benefits of having a mammogram might be outweighed by the distress of having to endure 'ridicule' and 'being made fun of' due to racism while undergoing the procedure (Canales & Geller, 2004, p. 852). Rather than trying to change women's screening practices (letting be) such understanding (pattern recognition) provides different direction for nursing practice. For example, the women that Canales and Geller interviewed identified trust with health care providers as key, and said that 'if the mammography machine was located in the local clinic and staffed by the personnel they were already connecting to personally, the decision to have a mammogram would not be difficult: they would have one on a routine basis' (p. 853).

> 66 *And when I get an examination, it doesn't matter if it's a Pap smear or if they're doing an annual breast exam or whatever it is. I'm completely comfortable with them. I so totally trust them.* 99

● Crossing Power Differences *Within* Families: From Taking Sides to Building Bridges

Although we have been arguing in this book that nurses ought to follow the lead of family, at the same time it is not helpful to valorize families or see them as faultless victims. Just as there are power differences between families and health care providers, among health care providers, and so on, power differences among family members give rise to challenges. Child abuse and neglect and violence toward women and elders are the more extreme ways that power differences within families manifest. However, less-obvious power differences manifest daily in practice, with nurses commonly feeling like they are caught in between family members (Varcoe et al., 2003). In such situations, nurses often attempt to either be neutral, which leaves the power dynamics of any given situation unchallenged, or to side with one or the other member. However, a relational approach suggests that following the lead of family means looking for the join, seeking common ground, and facilitating change by focusing on the capacity of all involved.

An Example: An Unwanted Transfusion

Woods (1999) describes a situation in which a young child wished to defy his parents wishes and refuse life-sustaining treatment—in this case blood transfusions. Woods described how the nurse negotiated between her own values and those of a little boy to whom she was providing care. Rather than assuming a neutral stance, the nurse took a stand with the little boy against the wishes of his father and others to continue treatment for malignancy. Rather than reducing the challenge to 'to continue or not continue treatment', Woods shows the relational and contextual complexity of the situation. As Woods describes the situation, the nurse took into account the nurse-patient relationship, but aligned with the child, not the whole family.

Let's consider how this situation might be approached from the relational perspective of connecting across difference that we are proposing in this book. For example, as I think about how I (Gweneth) might approach this situation from a relational understanding of family and of nursing practice and attempt to connect across the differences within the family, my first conscious act would be to 'not take sides'. Rather, the focus of my attention would be the relational interdependence and inter-relatedness of all family members. For example, regardless of who makes the decision or what the decision is, it will have a profound impact on each member and the family as a whole. Therefore, although the question of who gets to decide and what will be decided is part of the overall picture, in the foreground of my attention is looking for the join so that the family members might connect across their differences. The overriding question that would guide *my* nursing inquiry is how might this family connect across their differences and experience some common ground from which to make a decision with which they can all live (and perhaps die). Therefore, in approaching the family I would look for the common ground that joins them. This 'looking for common ground within the family' would be facilitated by the processes outlined in Chapter 7 including:

- entering into relation within the whole family,
- following their leads,
- listening to and for what is significant and meaningful to the different family members,
- collaboratively developing knowledge and recognizing patterns (for example, how are they all experiencing and responding to fear, what are they each hoping for and how might those desires be joined),
- naming capacity and adversity (what capacities do they each have and do they share as a family, how can those and other capacities be tapped and support them to be in this adversity and connect across their different views, and so on).

It is important to emphasize that in focusing on the relational connection I am not ignoring the individual rights to autonomy and choice. Rather, I bring my understanding of autonomy as a relational process as described by the domain theorists in psychology and by feminist ethicists (Reed, 2001; Sherwin, 1998). That is, the exercise of autonomy (for example, a child making an autonomous decision and the nurse supporting the right to autonomy) involves a relational process that is shaped through self/other/context. From this perspective, the same processes that support connection will support each person's conscious and intentional autonomous decision making.

These goals of connecting across difference and the relational processes that support those goals can be extended to other situations of power difference among family members. For example, in examining how the dynamics of child custody and access are used as a tool to continue woman abuse after women leave abusive partners, I (Colleen) concluded that approaches in which the 'rights' of children are pitted against the 'rights' of fathers or mothers will never be effective in ensuring the safety of children or their mothers. Rather, a relational understanding is required to take into account the safety of all. Rather than merely requiring the involvement of fathers (which increasingly courts in Western countries tend to do), policies should demand *safe* involvement; ways of fostering safe relationships between abusive partners and their children are required (Varcoe & Irwin, 2004). Thus, the focus of relational practice, although mindful of power differences and not absolving people of responsibility, focuses on relationships and bridge building.

● Crossing Power Differences Between Families, Systems, and Practitioners

Tremendous challenges arise as families bump up against taken-for-granted ideas, policies, and practices within systems that are based on the values of biomedicine, liberal individualism, and the free-market economy that we outlined in Chapter 1. Intensifying the differences that arise between families and systems are the multitude of contrasting values that arise as different health care practitioners come together to provide 'multidisciplinary care'. Within these multidisciplinary situations nurses, who are the ones at the bedside around the clock, or in the home or clinic on a regular basis, often experience being caught in between families, the powerful systemic forces, and the often contradictory values of different health care providers (Varcoe et al., 2003). The following story was shared with me (Colleen) by a palliative care nurse, Val Olynyk.

An Example: Beyond Futility

A few years ago, I looked after 52 year-old woman 'Anna' (a fictitious name), who was being 'medically' treated for lymphoma. She remained on our unit several months and I was often assigned to care for her. As testimony to our long relationship, I admitted Anna when she was first hospitalized in late August and I brought her body to the morgue when she died that November. Anna desperately wanted to live. She was pursuing aggressive chemotherapy. Her condition nonetheless declined, and over time she experienced the devastating side effects of chemotherapy. It was difficult, however, to determine her prognosis from physicians' notes in the chart. Notes written by the general practitioner documented changes in medications, observed shifts in blood work and critical lab values. Mostly, however, 'physicians' notes' consisted merely of simple qualitative statements like 'improved', or 'spirits good today'. By contrast, the oncologist's notes were lengthy, but almost entirely illegible.

Anna would often ask questions. It was difficult, however, to support her emotionally and with information. Her appearance and the severity of her symptoms suggested she was dying, which contradicted the hope she maintained. Nonetheless, aggressive chemotherapy continued. Side effects she experienced included bone marrow suppression, fatigue, mucocytis, nausea, and diarrhea, while increased pain accompanied her advancing disease. Treatment for the side effects of her chemotherapy included reverse isolation as protocol for neutropenia. She also had a central venous line inserted for parenteral nutrition and intravenous antibiotics (because she was unable to eat and had a raging infection).

One Saturday morning, an on-call physician visiting Anna said to her, 'Why are you doing this to yourself? Can't you see you are dying?' Anna was dumbfounded and distraught by his statement. When he left, she asked me, 'Am I really dying?' The oncologist had assured her otherwise, she stated. Then she said without waiting for an answer, 'Who am I to believe?' That evening, the oncologist visited and discontinued all treatments. Anna died two days later. To this day, I do not know why treatment was discontinued at that particular juncture and not another. After Anna died, her husband and sister remarked that because Anna was elementally a very a social person, she had agonized with the reverse isolation. Both stated they wished there had been more consultation and felt that Anna would have abandoned treatment sooner in favour of quality of remaining life, had she realized the ultimate futility (in terms of cure) of the treatment she was receiving. Anna's story exemplifies the varying objectives that exist among disciplines and even within them, case in point being the differing medical objectives found in oncology and palliative care. In those early years of my practice, I was unaware of the limited curative effects of chemotherapy. It is difficult to say how Anna understood or interpreted what the oncologist said to her. The oncologist's mandate is to treat until the treatment offers no further therapeutic effect. There is, however, a big difference between therapy and cure. Anna had proceeded believing she would be cured.

This example provides an excellent illustration of the complexities of differences within health care. In this story you can see the different values of the patient and her family and various health care providers, and the different values inherent in a cure and treatment-oriented model versus a care-oriented model. Val, who has continued to struggle with Anna's story, fully believes that the 'more consultation' for which Anna's family wished could have bridged the differences and allowed both Val and the other health care providers to follow the lead of family toward a much healthier end of life and death for Anna and her family. Once again, naming difference and explicitly seeking to connect across those differences can lead toward more ethical and health-promoting practice.

● Caring For Ourselves and Each Other As We Connect Across Difference

As we have highlighted throughout our discussion there is no 'right' way to connect across difference. Because working across difference and

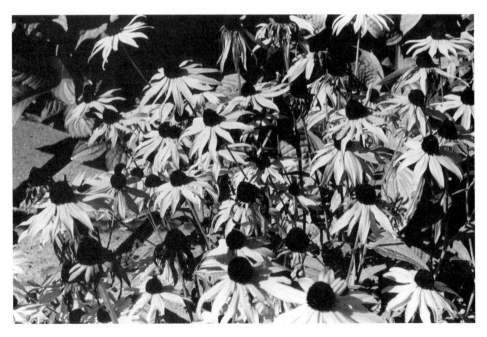

Diversity. (Photograph by Gayle Allison.)

toward an ethic of social justice often involves going against prevailing norms and institutional practices the road is at times daunting. Thus, nurses who seek to practice relationally and connect across difference require courage—courage to confront injustice, to confront their own biases and the biases of other health practitioners, and to challenge the systems within which they work. At the same time connecting across difference requires reaching out to colleagues. A single nurse alone cannot be as effective as a collective of nurses working together.

Our research into nursing ethics has revealed how integral collegial support is to 'good' nursing practice. The nurses we have spoken with have told us that 'taking the wrath' (from colleagues or managers), for example, is often part and parcel of being able to do good. Therefore, as they confront normative practices a central challenge for them is to try and stay intact personally. Many have highlighted the importance of having colleagues who are there for them—to listen, understand, and support them as they take up the moral imperative to do good. Unfortunately there are times when nurses do not experience the support of colleagues—times when their colleagues are in fact the ones giving the wrath. As we conclude we invite you to consider what you (as the particular person you are) might need to support you when you are challenged by the ethics of difference and also how you might more intentionally reach out and support your nursing colleagues as you work to connect across difference. To get you started on this, This Week In Practice suggests a systematic look at othering in your current practice context.

THIS WEEK IN PRACTICE

Investigating Othering

This week in practice we invite you to take up a miniresearch project. Whatever the practice setting in which you are currently working, undertake an examination of how differences are categorized, stereotyped, and/or stigmatized. If you are not currently in practice, conduct similar investigations by reading the paper or watching the television. Begin by looking at written records and documents (e.g., patient charts) to see the various ways in which people/families have been labelled and categorized (e.g., according to culture, economics, family stereotypes, and so forth). Next, listen to the dialogue in the practice setting—how is 'othering' inclusionary and/or how is it dehumanizing? For example, are there particular healing modalities that are assumed to be OK and others that are not? Seek out the resources that the agency may have created and/or uses to address differences of culture and critically consider them in light of the ideas within this chapter. Do they reflect a recipe approach or are they consistent with cultural safety? Finally, take the opportunity to observe yourself in action. How do you locate problems? Do you locate them in people/families, in yourself, and/or in the context? How do you find yourself automatically categorizing people, what generalizations do you make? Finally, take one opportunity to draw on the chapter ideas and relationally connect across difference.

CHAPTER HIGHLIGHTS

1. What ideas have been used to address culture in your education or practice in nursing to this point?
2. As you think about the hard spots in nursing, do you think there is a relationship between what you see as challenging and your choices about where to practice?
3. What do you anticipate the challenges would be in enacting cultural safety in your practice?

REFERENCES

Allen, D. G. (1999). Knowledge, politics, culture, and gender: A discourse perspective. *Canadian Journal of Nursing Research, 30*(4), 227–234.

Anderson, J., Perry, J., Blue, C., Browne, A. J., Henderson, A., Khan, K. B., Reimer-Kirkham, S., Lynom, J., Semeniuk, P., & Smye, V. (2003). 'Rewriting' cultural safety within the postcolonial and postnational feminist project: Toward new epistemologies of healing. *Advances in Nursing Science, 26*(3), 196–214.

Australian Nursing Journal. (2002). Nurses bear the brunt of emergency delays. *Australian Nursing Journal, 9*(9), 13.

Belle, D., & Doucet, J. (2003). Poverty, inequality, and discrimination as sources of depression among U.S. women. *Psychology of Women Quarterly, 27*(2), 101–114.

Bensley, L. S., Van Eenwyk, J., & Simmons, K. W. (2000). Self-reported childhood sexual and physical abuse and adult HIV-risk behaviors and heavy drinking. *American Journal of Preventive Medicine, 18*(2), 151–158.

Bergum, V. 1994). Knowledge for ethical care. *Nursing Ethics: An International Journal for Health Care Professionals, 1*(2), 72–79.

Bhabha, H. (1994). *The location of culture.* London: Routledge.

Bishop, A. H., & Scudder, J. R. (1990). *The practical, moral and personal sense of nursing: A phenomenological philosophy of practice.* Albany: State University of New York Press.

Browne, A. J., & Fiske, J. (2001). First nations women's encounters with mainstream health care services. *Western Journal of Nursing Research, 23*(2), 126–147.

Browne, A., Smye, V., & Varcoe, C. (in press). Postcolonial theoretical perspectives and women's health. In M. Morrow, O. Hankivsky, & C. Varcoe (Eds.), *Women's health in Canada: Critical theory, policy, and practice.* Toronto: University of Toronto Press.

Canales, M. K. (2000). Othering: Toward an understanding of difference. *Advances in Nursing Science, 22*(4), 16–31.

Canales, M. K., & Geller, B. M. (2004). Moving in between mammography: Screening decisions of American Indian women in Vermont. *Qualitative Health Research, 14*(6), 836–858.

Carveth, J. A. (1995). Perceived patient deviance and avoidance by nurses. *Nursing Research, 44*(3), 173–178.

Chow, J. C.-C., Jaffee, K., & Snowden, L. (2003). Racial/ethnic disparities in the use of mental health services in poverty areas. *American Journal of Public Health, 93*(5), 792–798.

Clark, A. H., & Foy, D. W. (2000). Trauma exposure and alcohol use in battered women. *Violence Against Women, 6*(1), 37–48.

Collins, P. H. (1990). *Black feminist thought: Knowledge, consciousness, and the politics of empowerment.* New York: Routledge.

Collins, P. H. (1993). Toward a new vision: Race, class and gender as categories of analysis and connection. *Race, sex & class, 1*(1), 23–45.

Corley, M. C., & Goren, S. (1998). The dark side of nursing: Impact of stigmatizing responses on patients. *Scholarly Inquiry in Nursing Practice, 12*(2), 99–118.

Coward, H., & Hartrick, G. (2000). Perspectives of health and cultural pluralism: Ethics in medical education. *Clinical and Investigative Medicine, 23*(4), 261–265.

Craib, K., Spittal, P. M., Wood, E., Laliberte, N., Hogg, R. S., Li, K., Health, K., Tyndall, M. W., O'Shaugnessey, M. V., & Schechter, M. T. (2003). Risk factors for elevated HIV incidence among Aboriginal injection drug users in Vancouver. *Canadian Medical Association Journal, 168*(1), 19–24.

Culley, L. (1996). A critique of multiculturalism in health care: The challenge for nurse education. *Journal of Advanced Nursing, 23*, 564–570.

Dunn, R. (2003). Reduced access block causes shorter emergency department waiting times: An historical control observational study. *Emergency Medicine, 15*(3), 232–239.

Estebaneza, P. E., Russella, N. K., Aguilara, M. D., Bélandb, F., Zunzuneguib, M. V., & The Study Group on Risk Behaviour in Female Injecting Drug Users. (2000). Women, drugs and HIV/AIDS: Results of a multicentre European study. *International Journal of Epidemiology, 29*, 734–743.

Friere, P. (1994). *Pedagogy of hope.* New York: Continuum.

Fry, S. (1989). Toward a theory of nursing ethics. *Advances in Nursing Science, 11*(4), 9–22.

Gadow, S. (1990). Existential advocacy. In T. Pence & J. Cantral (Eds.), *Ethics in nursing: An anthology.* (pp. 41–51). New York: National League for Nursing.

Gray, P., & Thomas, D. (2002). *Whose cultures count when it comes to cultural competence?* Paper presented at the Critical and Feminist Perspectives in Nursing Conference, Portland, Maine.

Greaves, L., Varcoe, C., Poole, N., Morrow, M., Johnson, J., Pederson, A., & Irwin, L. (2002). *A motherhood issue: Discourses on mothering under duress.* Ottawa: Status of Women Canada.

Grief, C. L., & Elliott, R. (1994). Emergency nurses' moral evaluation of patients. *Journal of Emergency Nursing, 20*, 275–279.

Hartrick Doane, G. (2002). In the spirit of creativity: The learning and teaching of ethics in nursing. *Journal of Advanced Nursing, 39*(6), 521–528.

Heffernan, K., Cloitre, M., Tardiff, K., Marzuk, P., Portera, L., & Leon, A. (2000). Childhood trauma as a correlate of lifetime opiate use in psychiatric patients. *Addictive Behaviors, 25*(5), 797–803.

Henry, F., Tator, C., Mattis, W., & Rees, T. (2000). Racism and human-service delivery. In *The colour of democracy: Racism in Canadian society* (pp. 207–227). Toronto, ON: Hartcourt Brace.

Jasinski, J. L., Williams, L. M., & Siegel, J. (2000). Childhood physical and sexual abuse as risk factors for heavy drinking among African-American women: A prospective study. *Child Abuse & Neglect, 24*, 1061–1071.

Johnson, M., & Webb, C. (1995). The power of social judgement: Struggle and negotiation in the nursing process. *Nurse Education Today, 15*, 83–89.

Kelly, M. P., & May, D. (1982). Good and bad patients: A review of the literature and a theoretical critique. *Journal of Advanced Nursing, 7*, 147–156.

Liaschenko, J. (1993). Can justice coexist with the supremacy of personal values in nursing practice? *Western Journal of Nursing Research, 21*(1), 35–50.

Liaschenko, J. (1995). Ethics in the work of acting for patients. *Advances in Nursing Science, 18*(2), 1–12.

Lipley, N. (2002). Patient experience helps define trolley waits 'tighter'. *Emergency Nurse, 10*(8), 3–6.

Little Bear, L. (2000). Jagged worldviews colliding. In M. Battiste (Ed.), *Reclaiming indigenous voice and vision* (pp. 77–85). Vancouver: UBC Press.

Lugones, M. C. (1987). Playfulness, 'world'-traveling and loving perception. *Hypatia, 2*(2), 3–19.

Lugones, M. C., & Spelman, E. V. (1983). Have we got a theory for you! Feminist theory, cultural imperialism and the demand for 'the woman's voice'. *Women's Studies International Forum, 6*(6), 573–581.

McIntosh, P. (1988). *White privilege: Unpacking the invisible knapsack.* Wellesley, MA: Wellesley Centre for Research on Women.

Miller, M. (1999). A model to explain the relationship between sexual abuse and HIV risk among women. *AIDS Care, 11*(1), 3–20.

Moosa-Mitha, M. (2004). Antiracist pedagogy. Oral conversation, February, 2004, Victoria, BC.

Mullings, J. L., Marquart, J. W., & Brewer, V. E. (2000). Assessing the relationship between child sexual abuse and marginal living conditions on HIV/AIDS-related risk behavior among women prisoners. *Child Abuse & Neglect, 24*, 667–688.

Nair, P., Schuler, M. E., Black, M. M., Kettinger, L., & Harrington, D. (2003). Cumulative environmental risk in substance abusing women: Early intervention, parenting stress, child abuse potential and child development. *Child Abuse & Neglect, 27*(9), 997–1018.

Nye, A. (2000). "It's not philosophy". In U. Narayan & S. Harding (Eds.), *Decentering the center: Philosophy for a multicultural, postcolonial and feminist world* (pp. 101–109). Indianapolis: Hypatia, Indianna Press.

Papps, E., & Ramsden, I. (1996). Cultural safety in nursing: The New Zealand experience. *International Journal for Quality in Health Care, 8*(5), 491–497.

Parillo, K., Freeman, R. C., Collier, K., & Young, P. (2001). Association between early sexual abuse and adult HIV-risky sexual behaviors among community-recruited women. *Child Abuse & Neglect, 25*, 335–346.

Patel, V., & Kleinman, A. (2003). Poverty and common mental disorders in developing countries. *Bulletin of the World Health Organization, 81*(8), 609–616.

Paterson, J. (2003). Bureaucracy drove actress to overdose death, family says. *Times Colonist,* Victoria, BC, November 13, p. 1.

Pauly, B. (2001). *Weaving a tapestry of nursing ethics: Philosophical grounding and future directions.* Unpublished manuscript. University of Victoria.

Pauly, B., & Varcoe, C. (in review). Negotiating difference in everyday ethical practice.

Perese, E. F., & Perese, K. (2003). Health problems of women with severe mental illness. *Journal of the American Academy of Nurse Practitioners, 15*(5), 212–220.

Polaschek, N. R. (1998). Cultural safety: A new concept in nursing people of different ethnicities. *Journal of Advanced Nursing, 27,* 452–457.

Razack, S. (1998). What is to be gained by looking white people in the eye? Race in sexual violence cases. In S. Razack (Ed.), *Looking white people in the eye:Gender, race and culture in courtrooms and classrooms* (pp. 56–87). Toronto: University of Toronto Press.

Reed, D. C. (2001). *Some observations about how moral psychologists have construed autonomy.* Paper presented at the 27th Annual Conference of the Association for Moral Education: Moving Toward Excellence, Vancouver, BC.

Reimer Kirkham, S., Smye, V., Tang, S., Anderson, J., Blue, C., Browne, A., Coles, R., Dyck, I., Henderson, A., Cynam, J. M., Perry, J., Semeniuk, P., & Shapera, L. (2002). Rethinking cultural safety while waiting to do fieldwork: Methodological implications for nursing research. *Research in Nursing and Health, 25,* 222–232.

Rogers, C. (1961). *On becoming a person.* Boston: Houghton Mifflin Company.

Sartorius, N. (2002). Iatrogenic stigma of mental illness. *British Medical Journal, 324*(7352), 1470–1471.

Sherwin, S. (1998). A relational approach to autonomy in health care. In S. Sherwin (Ed.), *The politics of women's health: Exploring agency and autonomy* (pp. 19–47). Philadelphia: Temple University Press.

Simmington, J. (2004). Ethics for an evolving spirituality. In J. Storch, P. Rodney, & R. Starzomski (Eds.), *Toward a moral horizon. Nursing ethics for leadership and practice* (pp. 465–484). Toronto: Pearson Prentice Hall.

Smye, V., & Browne, A. J. (2002). Cultural safety and the analysis of health policy affecting aboriginal people. *Nurse Researcher, 9*(3), 42–56.

Spencer, N. (2003). Social, economic, and political determinants of child health. *Pediatrics, 112*(3), 704–707.

Spooner, M. H. (2002). Long waits in NHS casualty departments. *Canadian Medical Association Journal, 167*(3), 292–295.

Stephenson, P. (1999). Expanding notions of culture for cross-cultural ethics in health and medicine. In H. Coward & P. Ratanakul (Eds.), *A cross-cultural dialogue on health care ethics* (pp. 68–91). Waterloo, ON: Wilfried Laurier University Press.

Stevens, P. E. (1992). Who gets care? Access to health care as an arena for nursing action. *Scholarly Inquiry in Nursing Practice, 6*(3), 185–200.

Stevens, P. E. (1994). Lesbians' health related experiences of care and noncare. *Western Journal of Nursing Research, 16,* 639–659.

Swendson, C., & Windsor, C. (1996). Rethinking cultural sensitivity. *Nursing Inquiry, 3,* 3–12.

Varcoe, C., Doane, G., Pauly, B., Rodney, P., Storch, J. L., Mahoney, K., et al. (2003). Ethical practice in nursing—Working the in-betweens. *Journal of Advanced Nursing, 45*(3), 1–10.

Varcoe, C., & Irwin, L. (2004). 'If I killed you, I'd get the kids': Women's survival and protection work with child custody and access in the context of woman abuse. *Qualitative Sociology, 27*(1), 77–99.

Watson, J. (1988). *Nursing: Human science and human care.* New York: National League for Nursing.

Weitoft, G. R., Hjern, A., Haglund, B., & Rosén, M. (2003). Mortality, severe morbidity, and injury in children living with single parents in Sweden: A population-based study. *Lancet, 361*(9354), 289–296.

Wilbur, K. (1985). *No boundary: Eastern and Western approaches to personal growth.* Boston: Shambala.

Wood, P. J., & Schwass, M. (1993). Cultural safety: A framework for changing attitudes. *New Praxis in New Zealand, 8*(1), 4–15.

Woods, M. (1999). A nursing ethic: The moral voice of experienced nurses. *Nursing Ethics, 6*(5), 423–433.

Yeo, M. (1989). Integration of nursing theory and nursing ethics. *Advances in Nursing Science, 11*(3), 33–42.

10 Inquiry in Family Nursing

OVERVIEW

In this final chapter we focus on the integral link between family nursing *as* inquiry and inquiry *in* family nursing. We illuminate how the knowledge, skills, and processes that serve as the foundation for relational family nursing practice also serve as the foundation for you as a nurse to competently draw on other peoples' research to inform your practice and/or to participate in more formal research projects.

● Research As Everyday Practice

Throughout this book we have sought to offer a picture of family nursing in which little is fixed or given. We have invited you to develop the capacity to be open, aware, and intentional as you engage and 'inquire with' families. Overall we have emphasized that nursing is a process of inquiry that involves constant questioning, adjustment, and responsiveness. Everything that we have discussed in reference to family nursing *as* inquiry is also relevant when thinking about inquiry *in* family nursing. Basically, when you approach family nursing as a process of inquiry you automatically engage in a form of research. The very nature of the process leads you to pose questions and inquire into those questions to develop the knowledge you need for practice. Therefore, any practicing nurse potentially is doing research.

Overall the relational approach to knowledge, and the skills and processes we have delineated within that approach, offers a strong foundation for reading and integrating other people's research and/or participating in more formal research projects of your own or with others. For example, as you engage as an inquiring nurse with a family who has a member who is experiencing depression, it is likely that you will identify areas where you need to 'find out more'. You may need to learn more about depression and about current treatment options. To engage with the family in an informed way you might also turn to existing research to learn more about families' experiences of living with depression and the contextual aspects that might shape those experiences. Similarly, as described in Chapter 8, your work will require an ethical inquiry including an examination of the ethical tensions and competing obligations that are arising for you as a nurse and for the family and individual members who are living with this health challenge. Ideologically it might be important to inquire into what is shaping the family's view and your own view of depression. For example, in research that a colleague Rita Schreiber and I (Gweneth) carried out with adults living with depression we found that people were drawn to the dominant biomedical explanatory model of 'depression as a biochemical condition' to diminish the stigma that accompanied both their experience of living with depression and other people's (including family members') responses to the diagnosis of depression (Schreiber & Hartrick, 2002). Taking up this explanatory model profoundly shaped the way people approached treatment and healing including who they sought out during their illness and what healing modalities they engaged in.

In addition to intentionally enlisting family knowledge and/or other people's research to inform your practice, you may also find yourself developing research questions of your own. For example, Rita and I formed our research question and undertook our inquiry into people's understanding of depression as a result of our experiences as practitioners. We had both found that many people/families with whom we worked did not connect previous life experiences that had been deeply traumatic with their subsequent depression. Interestingly, to us as practicing nurses there often seemed to be a link. We became curious about this difference in perspective and wanted to better understand how people made sense of their depressive illness in order to more effectively and responsively 'connect across that difference'. In a way you could say we 'followed the lead of the person/family' through a more formal process of research. Through this research we came to understand the profound impact of stigma on people living with depression. This understanding sensitized us to the potential connection between stigma and explanatory models and ultimately led us to pay closer attention and more intentionally inquire into the ideology shaping people's experiences and their health and healing choices as they lived with depression.

● Role of the Practicing Nurse in Research

Whether you are enlisting the research of others to inform your nursing practice or carrying out your own formal research projects, research is part of every nursing moment. And, research is a way of being/doing and a form of learning that is accessible to all practicing nurses. Overall, it is our intent to demystify the research process—to challenge the notion that research is something that academic researchers do to seeing all nurses, regardless of their role or position, as researchers. We believe strongly that practicing nurses have the potential to identify and carry out research that can 'make a difference' in people's lives. Being inside the experience or situation is the most authentic way of coming to understand, explore, and articulate both family's health and healing and the art and science of nursing. As nurses who are practicing relationally, you are automatically 'inside the experience'. This location offers a view and understanding from which to identify domains where knowledge is lacking, identify questions that need to be asked, and explicate what it is that needs further research.

An Example: Naming the 'Everyday'

Following a workshop on health-promoting relational practice I (Gweneth) conducted with public health nurses in the Northern Region of British Columbia, a group of the nurses invited me to collaborate with them on a research project to examine the 'working relationships' between families in the north who lived in rural and often isolated areas and the public health nurses in that region. The nurses wanted to know how the relationships between themselves and families were working and/or *if* they were 'working'. Through their practice experiences they had come to believe that it was these relationships that determined how families accessed public health programs and resources and also the efficacy of those programs. They wanted to simultaneously document the importance of those working relationships, find out if the families saw it in similar ways, and also learn more about how they might enhance their relational practice. Together the nurses, some other researchers, and myself met to think through how we might best go about the research. What was striking about the conversations we had as part of this research conceptualization process was the way in which the practicing nurses were able to articulate the subtle and complex aspects of their relational practice. As we struggled to articulate the 'research phenomena' it was the public health nurses who were able to give voice to those phenomena. Often they did so by telling a story of an experience they had had that pointed to what it was we were trying to articulate. They 'knew' it but had not necessarily put their knowing into words before. When I brought this to the attention of the group and commented on how valuable their knowledge and articulation was, the public health nurses responded with surprise saying 'it's just everyday stuff'. They had not explicitly seen how very important that everyday knowledge was to conducting research that could potentially advance public health nursing practice as well as family health.

It is this naming of 'everyday stuff' that is vital to advancing nursing knowledge. And the research process creates the opportunity and means for making this familiar everyday stuff unfamiliar. Research allows observation of oneself and one's experience in such a way that the taken-for-granteds begin to be seen more clearly and more fully. At the same time the aspects that are positive and/or problematic have a chance to be named (Bray, Lee, Smith, & Yorks, 2000). A good example of this is a project in which we are currently involved. As we described in Chapter 9, as part of a team of researchers we are collaborating with nurses on two hospital units (a medical oncology and an emergency unit) to research their ethical practice. We have designed the research as a participatory action form of research. The intent is not only to document the personal and contextual elements that shape ethical practice but also to affect change to enhance the nurses' ability to 'do good' in practice. As the nurses have begun examining their everyday practice more thoughtfully through the research process, they have gained insight into the relational nature of their work—how their individual practice is shaped not only by themselves but by everything else in their relational world. They have begun to see the subtle and at times not so subtle ways that systemic structures and policies constrain the choices they make. Gadamer (1993) describes that 'insight . . . always involves an escape from something that had deceived us and held us captive' (p. 356). In working with the nurses we are witnessing this escape. That is, as the nurses further their insight into the complex, relational nature of their ethical practice they have begun to think creatively of how they might more effectively work within the system of constraints and perhaps even effect change. For example, in the emergency unit, there are serious problems with the volume of patients for which the nurses are expected to care—the unit was designed and staffed to handle 28,000 visits per year, whereas over 68,000 visits actually occur. Together we (emergency nurse researchers and academic researchers) have come to see that framing problems as 'communication problems' or as 'organizational development problems' distracts our attention from the resource issues and nurse/patient ratios that prevent nurses from even carrying out routine checks as required in their clinical standards. This insight has led us to develop an action plan in which, rather than being the center of attention, issues such as 'communication' are understood to be symptomatic of the larger issue of being able to provide quality patient/family care and safe nursing practice. As carriers of creative thought the nurses are living their potential as 'authors of action' (McDermott, 1973, p. 54). This project is a wonderful example of how practicing nurses have the potential and capacity to play a role in moving toward change not only in their immediate place of practice but also at the policy, systemic, and theoretical levels.

● Entering Into Inquiry Through Everyday Practice

As one begins to approach everyday practice through an inquiry lens and see oneself increasingly as a researcher, the multitude of entry points for more focused research become evident. Research questions may arise through aspects related to family health and healing as you 'follow the family's lead', including the personal and contextual elements that shape families' experiences and resources. Similarly, you may enter into a more focused inquiry process to affect your own experience and practice as a nurse and/or the treatment protocols or policies that are shaping your practice. Following up on our discussion in Chapter 3 regarding the inter-connectedness of self/other/context, it is possible that as a nurse you may be sparked to undertake a research project to examine the interface of contextual elements, family health and your own practice as a nurse.

Often research in everyday practice is sparked through nurses' own self-knowing. As we described in Chapter 5, our bodies offer us a site where multiple forms of knowing come together. By listening to our bodily sensing—to the knowing that is coming together as we work with people/families—we are not only better able to identify issues that need to be addressed in practice, but also able to identify research questions that need to be asked. For example, when you feel a deep sense of discomfort at something you are experiencing in your practice, that discomfort is a signal that inquiry is needed. Although it may not necessarily require a formal research project, as we described in Chapter 5, listening to our bodily sensing (for example, to discomfort) is the first step toward knowledge development. As you inquire into your discomfort you simultaneously have the opportunity to gain insight into the aspects that may be troubling you and also explore and illuminate the situation or issues more fully. Such an inquiry process provides the means to both rethink practice and identify whether more formal research is required. For example I (Gweneth) had always felt a strong discomfort with the label 'high-risk families' and with the screening tools that many agencies use 'on' families to screen for risk assessment. Although I knew that, according to existing research, families who meet indicators specified by the assessment tools are statistically linked to greater health risks, my bodily knowing informed me that somehow the practice of assessing and labeling families in such a way was not conducive to relationally responsive practice. As I inquired into my discomfort and examined this practice empirically, contextually, ethically, and ideologically (remember Chapter 8) I was able not only to articulate the issues and problems of such practice, but also to raise important questions concerning the efficacy of such practice. In particular I was able to question the limitations of such practice. As it became clear to me that (for all of the reasons we described in Chapter 7) the screening tools presented a partial and reduced view of any family, I was able to identify what knowledge the tools failed to offer that was vital to assessing and intervening with families effectively. In a similar way I (Colleen) experienced discomfort regarding screening when I first encountered the CAGE alcohol screening (as described in Chapter 7). Prior to that, I had accepted literature that advocated such screening and literature that advocated screening for woman abuse as well. However, my dismay at the way the CAGE questionnaire was implemented in practice led me to raise concerns regarding the literature and to extend those concerns to woman abuse screening. As we came together to write this book we found ourselves compelled to raise this 'practice issue' and explicitly articulate our concerns about such screening and assessment tools. At the same time, we are in the process of thinking through how we might address our concerns about screening practices through more formal research.

● Transferable Skills for Reading and Using Other People's Research

As we have mentioned earlier, the knowledge, processes, and skills that support relational practice are transferable to the research process. Just as they can help you pay attention to the philosophical, theoretical, and practical congruence of your everyday nursing work they can support your 'research work' by:

- providing direction for reading other people's research and using it to inform your practice,
- carrying out formal research projects of your own.

The relational approach to knowledge and the lenses, skills, and processes we have presented to support relational nursing practice also provide an excellent foundation for the *how* and *what* of reading, interpreting, and using other people's research. For example, the relational approach to knowledge we described in Chapter 1 reminds us that any knowledge is partial, that research is not read in order to learn the 'truth' but rather to help us be as responsive and health promoting as possible. This relational, pragmatic approach directs us to take up any research as a 'confident unconfident' (Flanagan, 1996) to always ask the questions: 'How will this knowledge enhance my responsiveness to people/families?' 'How is this knowledge limited?' and 'What more do I need to learn/know to enhance my responsiveness?' At the same time, the relational approach to 'knowing' reminds us that everything we know and experience is relationally derived. That is, people's experiences and our knowing of those experiences is affected by everything else in their/our relational world. This understanding highlights that any knowledge must be considered contextually. So, for example, the latest research on the efficacy of certain treatments for depression must be considered within the experience and context of the particular people with whom we are working, as well as the other 'knowing' that families and we, as nurses, bring to the situation.

Using the Theoretical Lenses to Read Other People's Research

The hermeneutic phenomenological, critical, and spiritual lenses we present in Chapter 2 offer a way of both illuminating what we know and what we need to know more about. Subsequently these lenses can offer direction for 'what' and 'how' to read research in order to become a more informed and responsive practitioner. For example, if you are working with new mothers, the fact that as of 2003 only one randomized trial has evaluated the pharmacological treatment of postpartum depression (Hendrick, 2003) means that all other research regarding various drugs will have unknown applicability to the women with whom you may be working. Considering this research through the hermeneutic phenomenological and critical lenses (that we described in Chapter 2) sparks important questions such as:

- With what sorts of people and within what contexts have various treatments been studied?
- What is the availability of treatment to various groups of people and how might this availability (and the way it has subsequently shaped who has and/or has not participated in the research) shape the research findings?
- Are there different treatments for different groups of people based on social determinants of health?
- What are the implications of the research for this particular woman with whom I am working?

In addition to providing an excellent foundation for *what* and *how* to read research, a relational approach to knowledge highlights the ever-changing nature of knowledge—how what we know today is limited and temporary. Subsequently, the relational approach directs us to continually question existing knowledge and seek out new knowledge. Once again the hermeneutic, critical, and spiritual lenses provide ways of approaching this knowledge development process. Together the lenses help us 'see through' the taken-for-granteds that might be shaping us and help us identify ambiguities and complexities within our knowing and within the lives of the people with whom we are working. In this way they illuminate not only *what* we know and what we might need to know more about but also *how* to go about interpreting, scrutinizing, and using the knowledge available to us. For example, Crystal, Sambamoorthi, Walkup, & Akincigil (2003) analyzed an extensive data base in the United States and found that people aged 75 and over, people who were of 'Hispanic and other' ethnicity, and those without supplemental insurance were significantly less likely to receive treatment for depression, and when they did get treatment it was in the form of drugs, as they were less likely to receive psychotherapy. By thinking about this research through our hermeneutic and critical lenses all sorts of other questions arise for us. We find ourselves wondering why it is that those who are more advanced in years and of other (read nondominant) ethnic groups are less likely to receive treatment for their depression. What is it like for people without supplemental insurance to live with and heal their depression without treatment? And, once again what implications does this research have for the particular people with whom we are working and for the action we as nurses might take?

Using the Skills and Processes to Read Other People's Research

Just as the lenses can be valuable as we read research, the skills and processes that we outlined in Chapter 7 offer particular ways to read, interpret, and use existing research. These skills and processes are transferable to and support the intentional and rigorous integration of existing research. We briefly describe the relevance of these skills and processes to reading research and then offer an example to illustrate.

Entering Into Relation

Understanding a family requires that we enter into relation with that family in a conscious and intentional manner. Similarly, reading and interpreting research requires *entering into relation* with existing research and knowledge. This entering into relation requires that we *get in sync* with the researchers who have conducted the research to *walk alongside* their thinking and approach to research. As one stops to listen, look, and hear what has inspired the researchers, what the research is all about, and what it has to offer we are more able to determine the knowledge that is relevant to our own practice and understanding. For example, nurses working with new mothers might be particularly interested in an article that reports research by two health visitors and a community mental health nurse in the United Kingdom (Davies, Howells, & Jenkins, 2003) who wanted to improve the early detection and treatment of postnatal depression. Reading that these nurses were concerned about the lack of both recognition and treatment of postnatal depression might mirror your own nursing concerns. In contrast, a study to see if it is feasible to have patients with congestive heart failure and major depression participate in clinical trials (Lesperance et al., 2003) may be of less interest to a nurse working with new mothers. However, this study might be of interest to a nurse working with families with a history of cardiac disease. Getting in sync with research means figuring out where you are 'at' in relation to the body of research that can best inform your practice and seeking out and keeping up with new knowledge as it evolves.

Being in Collaborative Relation

Similar to relational nursing practice, any engagement with existing research can be enhanced by *being in collaborative relation.* Approaching any research in the spirit of collaboration leads you to look for the knowing the research results offer, the knowing you as a reader bring, and how those two forms of knowledge might be brought together. Rather than focusing merely on the knowledge gleaned from the research, being in collaborative relation directs attention to the interface between the knowing gleaned from the research and your knowing as a nurse. For example, in our earlier discussion of Crystal and colleagues' (2003) research into who receives treatment for depression, we engaged in collaborative relation interfacing their findings with our own critical and hermeneutic perspectives to raise other pertinent questions related to the research and to our practice.

Inquiring Into the Family Health and Healing Experience

The interpretation and enlistment of other people's research can also be enhanced by *inquiring into families' health and healing experiences.* By keeping families at the center of your mind as you read, you will be automatically sparked to read relationally—to question the assumptions the researchers are making about families and consider how researchers are or are not bringing a contextual understanding of families and of health and healing to the research process. Similarly, as with the example of Crystal and colleagues' research, by keeping families at the center, other questions about existing practice and knowledge can be raised.

Following the Lead of Families

By *following the lead of families* as you look to existing research to inform your practice you are better able to illuminate what, within the large body of existing research, is meaningful and significant to the particular people/families with whom you are working and to your own particular knowledge development process. For example, in Rose Steele's (2002) research (which we described in Chapter 7), families caring for children with life-threatening neurodegenerative illnesses were desperate to find basic information about their children's conditions. At the same time, following the lead of families can help you scrutinize the research against family experience. Our example of the way we evaluated the research about screening tools was facilitated by our 'following the lead of families'. By scrutinizing the research and the use of research for the development of screening tools against the experience of families, we have been able to challenge existing knowledge and begin to consider other possibilities for practice.

Listening to and for

The process of *listening to and for* is also central to reading and interpreting research. As we read existing research and engage in a process of listening to and for certain things, we are able to read more intentionally and critically. This approach to reading helps us relate new knowledge to our existing knowledge and consciously integrate that knowledge to evolve our own theories and theoretical practice. Similar to our relational work with families, the hermeneutic phenomenology, critical, and spiritual lenses sensitize us to look and listen more thoughtfully as we read an article or listen to a presentation. In Chapter 3, we invited you to develop knowledge about families and about the contexts in which they are living. As you proceed in developing your knowledge, try purposefully donning the 'lenses' as you read and learn about various studies.

Self-Observation

An important aspect of reading, scrutinizing, and taking up the knowledge that is offered by existing research is reflexivity. As we mentioned earlier, our bodies offer a site where our knowing comes together. Therefore, by listening to ourselves and to our bodily knowing we are able to access knowing that we may not yet have put into words. Just as in relational practice with families, the process of *self-observation* helps us tune into that knowing. For example, as we read a research article or listen to a research presentation we pay attention to what makes us sit up in excitement, what leaves us feeling confused and questioning our knowing, what leaves us feeling concerned, and so forth. As we listen we reflexively inquire into our response to tap the knowing to which it is alerting us.

Letting Be

Also helpful for reading and using other people's research is the process of *letting be.* As one reads research or listens to a research presentation and intentionally lets the knowledge 'be' (for example, by reflecting on the knowledge that is being presented and letting it percolate within you) the possibility for learning and change is potentiated. In his classic book *The Courage to Create*, Rollo May (1975) describes that it is during the states of nonaction and nonwork that most creative products come to the surface. He explains that although the 'work' of creativity may happen when we are focused and intent on the project, the outcome of our creative work most often emerges when we are not working—when we have created enough space within ourselves to let the product or breakthrough emerge. This means that although we may read and work at developing knowledge, it is often when we take the time to 'let be' that we have the 'ah has' and/or are able to see how what we have been reading is integrally linked to our practice. According to May (1975) these breakthroughs often happen as we walk home at the end of the day or even while we are in the shower. In this way the process of letting be can facilitate knowledge development. Try going for a 10-minute walk (or wheel, if you are in a chair or prefer a bike) next time you are 'stuck' on an assignment, paper, or problem you are studying.

Collaborative Knowledge Development

The process of *collaborative knowledge development* also supports our interpretation and use of existing research. Collaborative knowledge development provides a way of bringing multiple forms of existing research together to develop wider patterns of knowledge both within nursing and interdisciplinarily. For example, as a nurse who is also a psychologist I (Gweneth) have found that as I have brought the knowledge from research in these two disciplines together 'collaboratively' my ability to know and respond to people/families has expanded greatly. For example, by bringing psychological research in identity together with women's experiences of mothering during a research project I was able to more fully articulate women's experiences while actively engaged in motherhood (Hartrick, 1996, 1998). Similarly, the psychological research in identity more recently helped me articulate the processes of nurses' moral identity during an ethics research project (Hartrick Doane, 2002). To take another example, I (Colleen) have found my work with economists and political scientists

---

TRY IT OUT 10.1.   **Whose Knowledge?**

1. *Identify* any practice area in which you are interested. This could be a setting (e.g., community), a practice area (e.g., mental health), or a particular age group or health issue.
2. *List* the range of disciplines and types of knowledge that could inform nursing practice in an important way.
3. *Compare* your list to the usual sources of knowledge that inform that area.
4. *Talk* to someone practicing in a knowledge-based manner in the area you choose (for example, an experienced nurse, a clinical leader or manager), ask what he or she thinks are the important forms and sources of research for his or her practice, and have a conversation about it.

---

helped me better understand nursing. Understanding how health care economists do evaluations helped me to critique and offer alternatives to the way nursing is evaluated and its potential impact on families (Rodney & Varcoe, 2001). Though as nurses your primary sources of formal research may be nursing, you will undoubtedly find that other disciplines and various specialties within nursing will be important to your practice. Try It Out 10.1 suggests enumerating the range of knowledges and disciplines that potentially could inform any practice area.

Pattern Recognition

Paying attention and recognizing patterns is an integral part of reading research and expanding one's knowledgeable practice. As you read in the spirit of collaborative knowledge development you automatically begin linking what you are reading or hearing with other knowledge you bring to the situation. For example, during the ethics research project I (Gweneth) mentioned earlier, as I listened carefully to the nurses discuss their experience of practicing ethically, I was struck by how their descriptions exemplified the identity process articulated in the psychological literature I had read. In *recognizing the pattern* within the data I began to wonder if identity construction was central to the nurses' experience of ethical practice. This led me to go back and more intentionally read the psychological research about moral identity development and consider it in light of the 'knowing' in the nursing data. The psychological literature served as a resource to help me more fully articulate the construction of nurses' moral identity. So, for example, by conducting a secondary analysis of the data I was able to look beyond the surface of the nurses' descriptions to examine how systemic and organizational structures that were limiting nurses' practice were shaping their identity as moral agents—and how their ability to identify themselves as moral agents was being chipped away as a result of health care reform (Doane Hartrick, 2002). As you read the next research article you pick up, look for the relationship between what you are reading and what you know from practice and your other experiences. How does what you read inform those experiences and vice versa?

Naming and Supporting Capacity

The value of existing research can be more clearly considered by purposefully *naming and supporting the capacity* and adversity within the research. That is, as a reader it can be helpful to ask yourself in what ways this research might enhance your capacity for responsive practice. Similarly, it is important to ask in what ways the research might constrain that capacity. For example, the study about postnatal depression by Davies and colleagues (2003) describes offering the women 'listening visits', which might be an idea to incorporate within your practice. On the other hand, the study relied on the use of a depression scale, which might influence you to practice from more of an expert 'knower' stance than you would like. Considering research in view of the adversity within families' health and healing experiences can also shed light on what the research contributes, what it doesn't, and how you might go about developing the knowing that might enable you to better attend to family adversity. If, for example, you work with families who do not have permanent homes (for example, migrant farm workers), the study examining treatment that involves a series of four home visits over a year may not offer much useful direction for your practice.

Emancipatory Action

As you read existing research to inform your practice, the process of *emancipatory action* can shape how you take up existing research and the reasons for doing so. For example, tuning into the emancipatory potential of any research can help us identify how any particular research is promoting and/or perpetuating inequities and limiting existing views and practices. Similarly, with this emancipatory action in mind, as we read research we can ask ourselves how the research might support alternate discourses that could be more health promoting and/or how we might connect with researchers who share the ethic of social justice and relational practice. So, for example, the research we cited earlier that showed that people over 75 years of age and of 'Hispanic or other' ethnicity were less likely to receive treatment for depression might lead you to be more alert to depression in the elderly or to share with your colleagues how certain groups are systematically disadvantaged. To take another example, Averitt's (2003) research into the experience of homelessness for women with preschool children not only challenges the discourse of 'homelessness as a choice' but also makes a compelling call for nurses practicing in inner-city hospitals, in public health, and/or in the community to more fully understand and respond to the plight of women faced with homelessness. As researchers we have found that many of our most important collegial relationships have arisen either as we ourselves have followed up research that resonates with us and have contacted the researchers or when others have read our work and have contacted us. Through such connections we have the opportunity to 'join' around common concerns.

An Example: Reacting to What 'Is Known'

The importance of carefully, intentionally, and critically engaging with and scrutinizing existing research was brought home to us during a recent discussion we had in our ethics research team. One of our team members had attended a nursing conference the week before our meeting. During the conference one of the keynote speakers (a non-nurse) had presented her research about children with a particular 'disorder' and family 'dysfunction'. Our colleague described how throughout the presentation the researcher kept using the phrase 'we now know' in a way that implied that the research offered not only a complete picture of how the disorder arises (as opposed to a partial picture) but also that it was a 'certain' and 'true' picture—that there was a truth and the research she was presenting was it! Not only was the way she presented the results problematic, but the content of her presentation was highly concerning. Our colleague described that she was so upset at the content of the presentation she was 'literally shaking with anger' as she listened to the presenter make broad generalizations about how particular behaviours in children were indicative of a particular type of family pathology and how nurses could take a half-day workshop to learn how to assess for those behaviours to diagnose such pathology in families, in less than 3 minutes. As our colleague reported the researcher's claims about what was now known all of us on our research team were left aghast! Not only were the generalizations the researcher had made incredulous, it seemed to us that there was no way that the claims the researcher was making could be substantiated or 'proven' by the research that had been undertaken. What was perhaps most distressing as we listened to her story was our colleague's description of how the nurses in the audience had responded to the presentation. Not only had they enjoyed the presentation and taken up what the researcher had presented as a researched and reliable 'truth', many nurses from the audience lined up following the talk to learn more about how they might participate in the workshop that could teach them how to use this knowledge to diagnose family dysfunction in their practice!

Unfortunately this story is not unusual. We have often heard presentations and read research reports that have what we consider to be harmful potential. For this reason, we believe that some of the most important skills you require as a practicing nurse are those that allow you to not only critically scrutinize research but thoughtfully consider how any particular research might potentiate and/or diminish family well-being. For example, had the nurses in the audience brought these relational skills and processes to the research presentation, they might have 'entered into relation' with the research in quite a different way. They might have 'stopped, looked, and listened' to how this researcher was taking up an expert stance of 'knower of truth' and questioned the way the research was being presented as a proven fact. Similarly, they might have engaged in more of a collaborative relation with the research. Rather than focus on the content of the research and take it up as a truth, they might have focused on how this research interfaced with what they already knew of families. If they had 'inquired into family health and healing experiences' and 'followed the lead of families' they may have been compelled to question the pathologizing that the research was supporting and also the decontextualized way the knowledge was being used. In 'listening to and for' using the lens from Chapter 2 they may have been able to identify inconsistencies and limitations of the research. Paying attention to their own response and reflexively considering that response may have enabled them to articulate more subtle aspects of their knowing. For example, as our colleague experienced herself 'shaking

> **TRY IT OUT 10.2.** **Reading Other People's Research**
>
> Choose a research article that is of interest to you and has the potential to inform your current practice. Review the earlier section in this chapter on Using Skills and Processes to Read Other People's Research—and review these processes in preparation for reading the article. To help you review the skills and processes you might also review Box 7.1 (in Chapter 7). Now, as you read the article enlist the help of the processes. For example, as you begin reading pay attention to how you are 'entering into relation' with the article. Are you getting 'in sync' by 'stopping to look, listen, and hear' what the article is saying or are you distracted by other things in your life-world? As you read, try 'inquiring into what is meaningful and significant' to the researchers who conducted the research and to yourself as a practicing nurse. Similarly, look for how the researchers are 'following the lead of people/families' both in the research questions that are guiding the research and how they have conducted the research. What theoretical and experiential knowledge informs the research? How have they 'collaboratively developed knowledge' by drawing on other existing research, family knowledge, and so forth? Carry on 'using the processes' to guide your reading and knowledge development. Once you have finished reading, have a discussion with two classmates or colleagues about your experience and consider how the relational processes effected each of you in your reading and knowledge development. What did you experience that was similar and/or different?

with anger' during the presentation she was able to name specific things that were problematic and more clearly see where the research was lacking and how it was also potentially harmful. If there had been a chance for the nurses to 'let be' and reflect on it and also for 'collaborative knowledge development' by considering the research in light of other existing knowledge and in light of their experience with families they may have been able to recognize patterns of both capacity and adversity within the research and within how the researcher was proposing the research findings might be used in practice. In particular, they might have been able to question the simplistic picture of diagnosing and treating 'pathology' that was being proposed. Finally, had the nurses in the audience looked at what the researcher was proposing through an emancipatory action lens, the incredibly harmful potential of the research and the proposed use of the research would have likely become evident and the opportunity to interrupt such harmful potential would have been created.

In summary, the skills and processes you have studied throughout this book in relation to family will support your inquiry processes as you integrate research about families and family nursing. Try It Out 10.2 suggests that you choose a research article and try out the relational processes in the way we have suggested transferring the skills to integrate research with your practice.

● Undertaking Research Projects

The knowledge, processes, and skills that we have described to support relational family nursing practice throughout the book also provide a strong foundation for carrying out more formal research projects. Using the theoretical lenses, paying attention to the connection between theory and practice, engaging in reflexive practice, drawing on the relational skills and processes, and considering how to connect across difference are all integral to conducting rigorous research.

Using the Theoretical Lenses When Undertaking Research Projects

Each of the theoretical lenses we described in Chapter 2 and have used throughout this book form the basis of important research approaches in family nursing. The hermeneutic phenomenological lens has been used to guide research regarding the families' lived experiences of health and illness and the meanings of those experiences within the context of families' lives. The critical lenses have been used to examine the context of families' lives: feminist lenses have turned attention to gender inequity as it intersects with other inequities in families' lives, poststructural lenses have turned attention toward discourses that shape those lives and experiences, and postcolonial lenses have been used to guide research toward culturally safe and decolonizing research practice. We have used examples of such research throughout this book, and undoubtedly when you read research you will be able to recognize these lenses in action. As you study further, also note what such lenses *might* offer you as a reader when they are not being used by the authors of research.

Paying Attention to the Connection Between Theory and Practice

Our description in the first four chapters about the importance of understanding the connection between the theories you hold and how you enact your practice is also relevant to conducting formal research. Just as the beliefs, values, and theories that you hold as a nurse determine what you take note of when assessing and intervening with families, a researcher's beliefs, values, and theories also determine how he or she goes about 'doing' research. The research questions that you ask, the research method you choose to collect data, how you analyze and interpret the data, and the conclusions you reach are all shaped by the values, beliefs, and theories you hold as a researcher. Rigorous research involves explicating (as much as possible) the 'biases' and knowing that you bring as a researcher and the limitations that are created through those biases. For example, recognizing that each researcher's philosophical and theoretical location affects the research process, in presenting the findings of qualitative research it is common for researchers to articulate an auditable decision-making trail so that people reading the research are able to judge the viability of the research method and the researcher's conclusions for themselves.

Approaching Research as Reflexive Practice

As the understanding that researchers can profoundly affect the research process has grown, within the research world there has been greater and greater emphasis on developing ways to attend to this researcher effect. Similar to the way we have emphasized the importance of conscious and intentional practice in each moment of nursing, the research world is recognizing the importance of conscious and intentional research practice. For example, in describing action inquiry research Torbert (1991) contends that 'consciousness in the midst of action . . . is . . . both the ultimate aim and the primary research instrument' (p. 221). Torbert contends that widened attention to 'primary data . . . in the midst of perception and action' (p. 41) is central to research. And, the skill of reflexivity that we described in Chapter 5 is the skill that gives rise to this consciousness-in-the-midst of action.

It is fair to say that during the last decade reflexivity has 'exploded in academic consciousness' (Finlay & Gough, 2003). As Finlay (2003) describes, in the world of qualitative research reflexivity has become a given and is seen as a central ingredient of any research process. Reflexivity supports researchers to examine the impact of their own position and presence on the research process, opens up a more radical consciousness between the researcher, participants, and the phenomenon being studied, and helps researchers evaluate the research process, method, and outcomes (Finlay, 2003). The skill of reflexivity we described in Chapter 5 to support your everyday nursing practice can also support you to do research. Both relational nursing practice and rigorous research are supported by the nurse/researcher's ability for:

- self-observation,
- critical scrutiny of the knowing that arises both personally and contextually,
- conscious participation.

The reflexive skill of paying attention to the thoughts and emotions and bodily responses you are having at any moment to the contextual elements and relationships that are shaping your responses and reflexively considering those responses and contextual elements in order to more consciously and intentionally choose how to act and respond is not only transferable to the research process but is central to carrying out rigorous research (Doane, 2003).

Enlisting Relational Skills and Processes to Support Rigorous Research

Just as the skill of reflexivity is transferable, the other relational skills and processes we articulated in Chapters 6 and 7 are also transferable. For example, throughout the past couple of decades the nature of relationships in research has shifted in ways comparable to the responsive relationships we have described in Chapter 6. Within some realms of formal research there has been a shift from I-It relationships where people are labelled 'subjects' and treated as objects to be studied and known, to I-Thou relationships where people are 'participants' and more actively involved in developing knowledge and collaborating with researchers. Similarly, the researcher's position has moved from 'researcher as expert knower' to more of a participant in the collaborative process of knowledge development. Within the research process there has been a move away from doing research to and on people and a move toward doing research with people.

For example, in some research designs such as collaborative inquiry (Bray et al., 2000; Reason & Torbert, 2001) and participatory action research (Heron, 1997; Kemmis & McTaggart, 2000; Maguire, 1987) participants play an active role in all phases of the research process including the research design, participant selection, data collection, data analysis, and so forth. In this way the power relations between researchers and participants have shifted in ways comparable to those between families and nurses. That is, there has been a move from the expert researcher wielding the power and making the decisions to shared power relations. Similar to how the practice of nursing has moved beyond a sterile and detached procedure that is method bound, research has become more fluid and relationally determined. Similar to relational nursing practice, rather than using a pre-determined method, many studies, particularly qualitative ones, proceed in such a way that decisions about how best to proceed are reflexively made along the way (Denzin & Lincoln, 2000). For example, in our participatory research with nurses on their practice environments and ethical practice, we are collaboratively making decisions regarding how to proceed. One such decision has been in response to escalating staff turnover. The emergency nurses have decided to conduct a survey to find out what staff are staying and what keeps them, and who is leaving and why. In addition, both the emergency nurses and the medical oncology nurses have decided to conduct a survey measuring the ethical climate of their units.

Another commonality between relational nursing practice and current research approaches is the growing understanding that research is potentially more than a data-collection process. Just as assessment cannot be separated from intervention in practice, it is becoming evident that undertaking and participating in a research project often results in change even if one does not directly set out to create change. For example, recently in my research on the relationship between the risk of HIV and violence against women, I (Colleen) conducted a focus group in which a community nurse participated. This nurse was dismayed that she had not previously thought of the connection between coerced sex and the risk of HIV. A few weeks later, her community health unit joined in World AIDS Day activities, action that was sparked by the 'changed understanding' that had resulted from her participation in the focus group.

Finally, just as we have highlighted that as a person/nurse you are never '*not* involved'—that by virtue of being human you bring your concerns, values, and beliefs with you to any nursing moment—this understanding has also permeated the world of research. As we described earlier, most researchers today recognize the importance of their person in research relationships and the necessity of critically scrutinizing how they are shaping those relationships and ultimately effecting the research and the research 'findings'.

Doing Research to Connect Across Difference

The knowledge and processes that support connecting across difference also support the doing of formal research. Differences and the hard spots are often the areas that require inquiry. Identifying differences offers the potential not only to connect, but also to raise questions about what is known, what is not known, and where inquiry might be fruitful. At a minimum, identifying differences points to the need for inquiry about the differences themselves—what are the differences you are encountering? What factors influence and shape these differences? Where is the common ground? Overall a critical awareness of difference helps you to identify and work with biases and taken-for-granted assumptions. For example, in my (Colleen) research regarding the relationship between the risk of HIV and violence against women, initially some people in the community thought that a key difference was ethnicity—that the central difference of concern was that Aboriginal women were more vulnerable to both violence and HIV than non-Aboriginal women. However, when the heightened risk due to rural geography and the risks associated with poverty were considered, it became clear that all of these differences intersected. The key difference on which we focused became gender—women were at heightened risk of HIV due to violence, and their risk was compounded by rural isolation, poverty, and racism. Thus we focused the study on all women in the community, seeking women with a range of experiences, from a range of income levels and ethnicities. Awareness of difference can also guide how research is conducted—who needs to be involved, who will be supportive, and what the resources might be. Again, in the HIV and violence study, awareness of the particular differences in the experiences of Aboriginal women (and a postcolonial lens) led us to ensure that an Aboriginal researcher was a key leader on the research team, that participation was negotiated with elders, and that focus groups were held in a variety of rural communities.

● The Art of Inquiry in Family Nursing Research

As we have described earlier, basically everything we have discussed in this book is about doing and using research. By its very nature the approach we propose for family nursing practice is an inquiry process. Overall, the approach highlights the importance of practicing nurses taking a more active and central role in research. And, as we have just discussed, the knowledge, processes, and skills we have offered throughout the book are transferable to formal research projects. To involve oneself in research—to take up inquiry *in* family nursing involves:

- taking an active stance,
- raising questions,
- identifying the issues,
- working the context,
- enlisting support,
- moving forward.

We will explicate these processes by sharing an example of how one nurse moved from family nursing *as* inquiry to undertaking inquiry *in* family nursing.

An Example: Researching Practice With an Eye to Prevention

During a recent trip to New Zealand I (Gweneth) met Mary Cleland who is an experienced district nurse (Home and Community Care Nurse) employed by the Waikato District Health Board. Mary has worked in the same community for 24 years and so has been involved in the care of families over many of their life course events and health changes. She has a wealth of practice knowledge and deeply understands the effects of ill health on the lives of people and those who care for them—their families and whanau (the term for extended family used by New Zealand indigenous Maori people who make up a high proportion of Mary's patients). I met Mary when she arrived for a research meeting with Trish Wright, a faculty member and research coordinator at Waikato Institute of Technology where I was visiting. In hearing about their research project I asked Mary and Trish if I might include their research story in this book because it offered a wonderful example of 'the art of inquiry in nursing' and highlighted how research is a part of and supports the everyday practice of nurses. Mary shares her story below in her own words.

Children who have had rheumatic fever are often referred to me (Mary) in order to be given their monthly intramuscular injections of penicillin. These children require injections for a period of between 10 and 20 years. The injections are renowned for being particularly painful at the time of injection and for the 24 hours or more following the injection. Because of the pain, some children opt out of their treatment, which places them in danger of a recurrence of rheumatic fever and subsequent heart valve damage and even death. In the past, when nurses were able to reconstitute penicillin themselves, it was possible to add xylocaine to the compound, which considerably reduced the pain experienced by children. Now, bicillin, the product of choice, comes in a premixed cartridge that means that the addition of local unaesthetic is precluded.

I also had cared for people who had recurrences of rheumatic fever and were in terminal stages of the illness and people who had cardiac surgery to repair valve damage from rheumatic fever and who were required to take warfarin for life with all that that means for their health. Thus, I began to ponder the implications for the children I was caring for—what would it mean if these children who were currently receiving bicillin injections chose to opt out of treatment? It became evident that somehow we needed to find a way to lessen the pain of the injections so children would get the treatment they needed to prevent further problems. I tried using topical creams, that for a variety of reasons (cost, access, time, and accuracy of application) became too difficult to use in practice for all patients. One day while meeting with a rheumatic fever resource nurse I noticed some cans of spray and asked what they were for. The nurse told me that they were ethyl chloride spray which they were going to be trying to address the bicillin injection pain. Returning to my rural area of practice I insisted that we also try the ethyl chloride. I contacted pharmacists to try and find out the best way of applying the spray so that it would have the best effect. However, I wasn't sure how to go about evaluating the efficacy of the ethyl chloride—how to go about this in a planned way that would provide reliable and acceptable evidence for continued and more widespread use. I decided to create a form asking patients who were used to having the injection without any anesthetic to comment on how they found the injection with the spray on a graded 1–10 scale. Patients commented in a surprised manner that the pain after the injection was 1.

At the same time I was studying for my degree in nursing. I had my registration through hospital training. I started the research paper and throughout that course kept in mind the trial I was undertaking. As part of my coursework I undertook liter-ature searches around ethyl chloride and rheumatic fever and found ways to improve my application technique. I also found evidence that ethyl chloride did help with pain relief in other procedures but no direct evidence related to the use of ethyl chloride and injections for rheumatic fever. During the ethics course in the degree program I began to think deeply about the importance of consultation with Maori people and formal ethical approval. At the same time I developed increasing aware-ness of what has now become evidence-based practice—that is practice where what is done by nurses has some justification in the literature.

Once my degree was completed, because of the apparent success of ethyl chloride in helping people maintain their injection program, I decided to apply my time to pursuing this research rather than undertaking further study toward a mas-ter's program. I approached my managers and they directed me to work with a clin-ical resource nurse with regional rather than local responsibility. This provided the means for the research to be undertaken in a fresh way with people who had not experienced the difference with ethyl chloride administered by nurses and who did not have the commitment to its utility that I had come to have.

Together, the resource nurse and I began to think about the research and find out about what the process required. At this time there was no nursing research support in the institution on which we could draw for help and guidance. We accessed the ethics form and had a copy of one that had been completed for a previous study. Consulta-tion with Maori proved a stumbling block because an introduction by someone is required to begin. A colleague suggested that I make contact with Trish with whom I had previously worked in practice. Together we were able to establish a formal process to undertake the research collaboratively between the two institutions (the Institute of Technology and the Health Board). The research is now nearing completion.

Taking An Active Stance

In talking with Mary and Trish about their research it became evident to me (Gweneth) that it was Mary's long-standing clinical practice with the same families over many years that provided the impetus for this research. In particular it was her reflective and inquiring way of being that supported her sensitivity to both the physical and social concerns that accompany a chronic illness such as rheumatic fever and the severe impact of those concerns on people/families. Mary's story offers a wonderful example of 'taking an active stance'. Having seen the long-term effects of opting out of treatment and knowing that because of the painful injections children might potentially do so, Mary was not content to accept painful injections as 'just the way things are'. Taking an active stance, Mary decided to do something about the situation and work to effect a change that might not only make treatment more palatable but also prevent future difficulties for the children she cared for.

Raising Questions

An important aspect to highlight in Mary's story is how she looked beyond the surface of the nursing task of injecting antibiotics to see what was meaningful and significant to children and their families. By 'following the lead' of the children, she was compelled to raise questions—to inquire empirically, contextually, ethically, and ideologically into how children come to be in this situation, how the health care context was shaping their health and healing experience, and how she might better respond in a care-full way that did not perpetuate further disadvantage. Although Mary could have proceeded by ignoring the complexity of the situation (for example, just assume that pain on injection was the way it is and carry on giving the injections) her deep sense of inquiry and persistence in making her own practice as good as it could possibly be created the impetus to take up a formal research project that could potentially effect nursing practice more generally (for example, more effective protocols for injections). Integral to this was her ability to research existing empirical knowledge and also raise questions about its limitations. At the same time, by expanding her nursing inquiry to question the efficacy of the treatment contextually, ethically and ideologically, she was able to identify what needed to be more formally researched—what it was that she and other nurses required to enhance the responsiveness of their practice. Her willingness to actively take up the research challenge and raise these questions served to not only enhance her own practice but created the potential to inform nursing practice more generally.

Identifying the Issues

In raising the questions Mary simultaneously was able to identify the issues within the situation. These issues provided not only direction for the research but also the justification and importance of carrying out such research both empirically and ethically. One of the issues Mary identified was the physical pain with which children had to cope in order to receive the medication. However, this physical pain was not the only 'issue' that was central to this research. 'Looking over the shoulders' of the children she cared for, Mary was able to see that contextually, these children had already been disadvantaged and compromised in their access to health care by not having received treatment for the streptococcal infections that were the precursor to rheumatic fever. This contextual understanding raised questions of ethics—what knowledge was necessary for Mary as an ethical nurse to practice relationally and be able to respond in a socially just way? How could she ensure that the children were not further disadvantaged? At the same time, Mary identified and challenged the ideological issue of 'painful injections as the only option'. The way the lives of the adults with whom she worked had been affected by reoccurrences helped Mary identify the importance of challenging such an ideology. The severe impact of the pain required moving beyond existing empirical knowledge and the ideological assumptions that were currently underpinning practice.

Working the Context

Central to this research process was working the context. In many ways it was Mary's understanding of the contextual elements that led her to the conclusion that something had to be done to create more adequate treatment. Similar to the questions of adequacy we posed in Chapter 1,

Mary's contextual understanding of both the historical aspects that had led to children developing rheumatic fever and the current lives of the adults who had opted out of treatment raised questions of treatment adequacy. It became clear to Mary that the current treatment was not adequate for either treatment or prevention for children with rheumatic fever. In addition to this understanding of the children's context, Mary brought an understanding of how to work the health care context to effect more responsive care. Her inquiring way of practicing led her to discover the ethyl chloride in the rheumatic fever resource nurse's office and to transfer that approach to her rural practice setting. However, understanding the value of evidence-based practice that dominates the health care world, Mary recognized the importance of conducting more formal research in order to support her practice and to effect practice on a larger scale. Mary also worked the educational context to her advantage. She made her academic studies work *for* her by using her coursework to enhance her knowledge in ways that could help her more knowledgeably respond to the children for whom she cared.

Enlisting Support

In order to make the research happen Mary recognized that she needed to enlist support. Although she brought her strong knowledge of children, rheumatic fever, and current treatment options to the research she realized that she needed the support of people who were more knowledgeable about research methodology and also in working with Maori to undertake research in culturally safe ways. She began by turning to her nurse managers as a resource to help her know how to move forward. Her discussions with them pointed her in the direction of the regional clinical resource nurse. What is important to highlight is the reflexive process in which she was engaged throughout the research project. She continually asked herself what she knew, what she didn't know and how she might gain the knowledge and/or support she needed to carry out the research project and ultimately be more responsive to the children and families she nursed. This is an important aspect of rigorous research—that if one engages in a reflexive way, the questions that need to be asked and the knowledge and resources that need to be accessed to carry out research in a sound way, will become readily apparent. And, it highlights how any research process involves collaboration. No one nurse may have the knowledge, expertise or even time to develop and undertake a research project. However, this is not a problem. Rather, it is an opportunity to connect with other colleagues to draw on and share knowledge and expertise.

Moving Forward

As Mary took an active stance, raised questions, identified the issues, worked the context, and enlisted support she was able to move forward in her research project. By the time that I (Gweneth) met Mary she had moved from being frustrated at the limitations of existing practices to effecting change in her workplace, to being at the point of almost completing formal research that could further inform her practice and the practice of other nurses working with children with rheumatic fever. As I listened to the description of her research journey I was struck by the synergy of relational nursing practice and research in nursing. As can be seen in the description earlier, when nursing is approached *as* a process of inquiry the integral role of research and the need for further research becomes evident. At the same time approaching nursing *as* inquiry supports nurses' ability to conduct relevant and important inquiry *in* nursing. Finally, Mary's story exemplifies the potential impact of a practicing nurse 'moving forward' in research—how such action might positively effect people/families, other nurses, nursing knowledge, and health care practice more generally.

● Bringing the Voice of Practice to Family Nursing Knowledge

From Mary's story the value of bringing the voice of practicing nurses to family nursing knowledge becomes evident. The story also highlights the continual and lifelong journey of developing the knowledge to be a responsive nurse in practice. We have found that as we have entered into nursing as inquiry the quest for knowing and learning has taken on an energy and excitement of its own. Experiencing and witnessing the value of researching what it is we know and the value of inquiry in everyday practice has fundamentally shaped how we think of ourselves as nurses. In particular we find that the role distinctions of practicing nurse and/or academic researcher hold less meaning. In many ways we have approached our work in similar ways regardless of which role we have been in. For example, both of us began our nursing lives and spent many years in practice positions prior to taking up our current academic positions. Our experience as practitioners has profoundly shaped our research work. Similarly, it has been our experience in practice that has led us to seek out more formal study at the graduate level and develop our capacity as researchers. At the same time, our research endeavors serve to continually evolve our way of practicing nursing.

We are not alone in this blending of practice and research. We continuously meet nurses in practice who feel compelled to take up more formal processes of research to inform and enhance their everyday practice and who want to engage in more formal study at university in order to enhance their inquiring nursing practice. Mary's story offers a wonderful example of this. Although Mary undertook a leadership role in formal research, there are many ways to enact this blending of practice and research. For example in our current participatory action research into ethical practice, the nurses have arranged themselves according to how much they are able and want to be involved in the research. They have self-selected into those who are centrally involved and very active in undertaking the research to those who are only kept informed of our progress.

As well as meeting nurses in direct practice who are engaged in formal research projects, we have met many academics whose research is

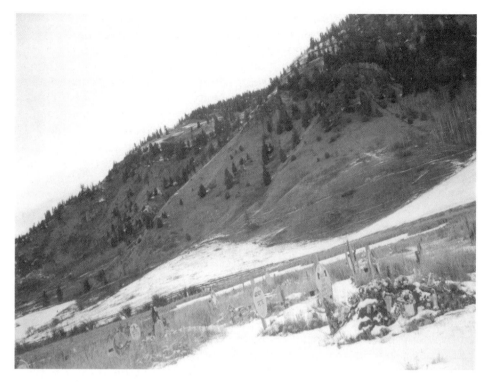

Bereaved. (Photograph by Maria Walther.)

integrally connected to and arises out of their practice. These academic nurses are called by the kinds of research that speak to them about their practices. The following story is of one such academic nurse. Nancy Moules is a nursing professor at the University of Calgary in Canada who became interested in the human experience of loss and grief as a result of her work with parents whose children had died. The bereaved parents and other people experiencing profound losses in their lives with whom she worked as a practicing nurse showed her how the ideas and theories we hold as a culture, society, and a profession about grief are not necessarily the most useful ones in assisting people who are grieving. As Nancy describes, her experiences in practice highlighted how generally accepted and sanctioned beliefs, such as the belief that grief is a time limited experience that ends in resolution and recovery or that grief is a task of saying goodbye to the lost person, defy the experiences of those suffering in loss. Thus, as an academic who teaches 'theory' at the undergraduate and graduate level, Nancy was compelled to bring not only the voice of practice to inform loss and grief theory but also the voices of families.

 An Example: Walking Backward with the Bereaved

In working with families who are grieving I (Nancy) have found that those who have lost a loved one continue to experience aspects of grief throughout their lifetime, though these aspects do change over time and they become comforting and connecting rather than only painful. Similarly, rather than saying goodbye to the lost other, people continue to stay in relationship with, and connected to, the person who has died, in a changed relationship that, in spite of physical absence, holds new possibilities and dimensions. The juxtaposition of these experiences of grief against discourses that offer a normalized contrary expectation serves to create more suffering in the life of one who has lost, at times even inviting the person into a self critique of dysfunction, failure, or pathology.

Having observed this paradox in my clinical work, I, along with a group of student research assistants at the undergraduate and graduate level, decided to undertake some research that explored the beliefs about grief held by bereaved parents—including beliefs that are helpful and those that seem to create more suffering. We also wanted to look at the practices of nurses and other helping professionals that are received as healing practices by the families who are bereaved.

This research is now in process and we are finding that our understanding of grief is being expanded substantially. We are beginning to view grief with a useful metaphor of grief as an uninvited houseguest. This houseguest arrives without invitation and remains in such a way that it touches all aspects of one's life, family, relationships, and health. If room is not made for this uninvited houseguest, it has a tendency to take over the house, claiming the bathroom as one tries to get ready for work, sneaking into children's rooms and affecting their lives, sneaking into the bedrooms of partners. Metaphorically, invited or not, grief sneaks in and becomes a part of the family and household. The more efforts are made to keep it out, the more it makes its presence known. If, however, room is made for this houseguest, its presence becomes expected at times, its comings and goings are not surprises, its intrusions not unanticipated. In time, its presence even becomes welcomed as something familiar. This visitor, welcome or not, does come and go over time and it changes in appearance, but its very absence and presence serves to sustain a mutable, evolving, sometimes intermittent, but lifelong, relationship with the loss. Grief has intensive, and sometimes unrelenting, elements of suffering and pain, but it also has attributes of comfort, connection, and celebration. Grief is the experience of keeping in relationship with the lost person, who although physically absent, is still profoundly a member of the family. Death does not mean the end of a relationship, but a change in the relationship, with new depths and possibilities.

As we have conducted the research and begun to articulate this fuller understanding of grief in people's everyday lives we have continually asked ourselves: 'How then can nurses be helpful to the bereaved?' Although the research around this question is not completed, we are beginning to understand that nurses can play a role in challenging culturally accepted, yet experientially contradicted discourses or beliefs. Finding ways to help normalize what one actually feels in loss—a continued, yet changing, experience of grief and a continued and binding relationship with the lost person and being willing to enter into conversations of remembrance and stories of loss and connection could support the grieving person. We have come to see the importance of nurses and other professionals in contact with bereaved people recognizing, inviting, and even challenging beliefs that are not particularly helpful to or consistent with experiences of grief.

As I have conducted the research I have been reminded of China's ancient Mountain and Sea scripture that records the exploits of an itinerant immortal who could walk backward faster than the eye could see. Walking backward in China has been popular ever since and it is not unusual to observe a person (most often an older person) walking backward. The movement exercises muscles that are not used in ordinary walking, especially in the back, waist, thighs, knees, and lower legs. Some people believe walking backward is akin to a karmic reverse allowing you to correct mistakes and sins of the past. This idea of walking backward seems to be a fit in the movement associated with grief. This art of grieving requires the use of different muscles than we are used to using in our lives and grief appears as perversely different from what is expected as does an old man walking backward. Walking backward allows the strengthening of part of ourselves that we were not aware of or did not have to use. It allows one the ability to look to the past and recall what was, and yet continue to move along. Walking backward is not a permanent state or gait, nor does the research suggest that the bereaved should not ever look ahead and walk in more typical fashion, but perhaps grief requires this occasional and periodic walk backwards. In thinking of this scripture in light of our research findings I have begun to wonder if perhaps the work of nurses and other health professionals is to learn how to best walk backward at times with bereaved clients, while keeping a careful watch for bumps on the road.

● Moving Forward Together

Together Mary and Nancy's research projects illuminate that whether one's role is as a nurse in direct care or as an academic researcher the integral link between family nursing *as* inquiry and inquiry *in* family nursing is at the center of our work. If, as members of a professional practice discipline, we are to move forward in our desire to promote the health and healing of people/families in knowledgeable and responsive ways, we must bring the knowledge, skills, and abilities of practicing nurses and academic researchers together. It is through this collaborative knowledge development process that the spark to ignite and sustain research at both the formal and informal levels might be generated. And it is through this collaborative process that we might all be more able to do good in our work with people/families. Try the exercise in This Week In Practice to help you consider the link between research and your own everyday practice.

THIS WEEK IN PRACTICE

Research Possibilities

As you go about your work in practice this week pay attention to any questions or knowing that arise. For example, you might find yourself curious about something related to the people/families you are caring for, something in the way practice or treatment is given or something about the way in which people/practice/context interfaces. Or you might find yourself feeling a sense of discomfort about something. As you pay attention, consider how the questions that arise might inform your knowledge. Explore them in light of a possible research project. If you were to take up an active stance, what questions and concerns would provide the impetus for the research? How would this research be important to promoting knowledge of family health, nursing, and/or health care practices? What issues can you identify? How does the context come into play? What within the context might you need to address/explore? Who might you enlist for support? For example, reflexively consider the knowledge and skills you bring to the research. Then ask yourself what other resources you would need to be able to carry out the research? Are they ones you can access or would you need to enlist the skill and knowledge of others? To help you with this reflexive process, try talking your research project through with a classmate and have them ask questions that come to mind for them. This can help further your own more in-depth thinking about the project and also about the skills, knowledge, and resources that would be necessary to carry out the research. Finally, consider how you might move forward. What might get in the way? How might you work around that? What might you learn through such a research project and how might it ultimately contribute to others? Does working through a practice issue in this way help you identify the researcher that is already living within you?

CHAPTER HIGHLIGHTS

1. As you read, what were you able to identify about your ideas about yourself as a 'researcher'?
2. How does the understanding of research offered in this chapter compare to your understanding of research from other sources (other courses, previous experience, and ideas?)
3. What is one way you will be able to bring inquiry *in* family nursing into your practice?

REFERENCES

Averitt, S. (2003). "Homelessness is not a choice!" The plight of homeless women with pre-school children living in temporary shelters. *Journal of Family Nursing, 9*(1), 79–100.

Bray, J., Lee, J., Smith, L., & Yorks, L. (2000). *Collaborative inquiry in practice. Action, reflection, and meaning making.* Thousand Oaks, CA: Sage.

Crystal, S., Sambamoorthi, U., Walkup, J. T., & Akincigil, A. (2003). Diagnosis and treatment of depression in the elderly medicare population: Predictors, disparities, and trends. *Journal of the American Geriatrics Society, 51*(12), 1718–1729.

Davies, B. R., Howells, S., & Jenkins, M. (2003). Early detection and treatment of postnatal depression in primary care. *Journal of Advanced Nursing, 44*(3), 248–256.

Denzin, N. K., & Lincoln, Y. S. (2000). *Handbook of qualitative research.* Thousand Oaks, CA: Sage.

Doane, G. (2003). Reflexivity as presence: A journey of self-inquiry. In L. Finlay & B. Gough (Eds.), *Reflexivity. A practical guide for researchers in health and social sciences* (pp. 93–102). Oxford: Blackwell.

Doane Hartrick, G. (2002). Am I still ethical? The socially mediated process of nurses' moreal identity. *Nursing Ethics, 9*(6), 623–635.

Finlay, L. (2003). The reflexive journey: Mapping multiple routes. In L. Finlay & B. Gough (Eds.), *Reflexivity. A practical guide for researchers in health and social sciences* (pp. 3–20). Oxford: Blackwell.

Finlay, L., & Gough, B. (2003). Prologue. In L. Finlay & B. Gough (Eds.), *Reflexivity. A practical guide for researchers in health and social sciences* (pp. ix–xi). Oxford: Blackwell.

Flanagan, O. (1996). *Self expression. Mind, morals and the meaning of life.* New York: Oxford University Press.

Gadamer, H. G. (1993). *Truth and method* (J. Weinsheimer & D. G. Marshall, Trans.) (2nd rev. ed.). New York: Continuum.

Hartrick, G. (1996). The experience of self for women who are mothers: Implications for the unfolding of health. *Journal of Nolistic Nursing, 14*(4), 316–331.

Hartrick, G. (1998). Women who are mothers: The experience of defining self. *Health Care for Women International, 18,* 263–277.

Hendrick, V. (2003). Treatment of postnatal depression. *British Medical Journal, 327*(7422), 1003.

Heron, J. (1997). A participatory inquiry paradigm. *Qualitative Inquiry, 3*(3), 274–294.

Kemmis, S., & McTaggart, R. (2000). Participatory action research. In N. K. Denzin & Y. S. Lincoln (Eds.), *Handbook of qualitative research* (2nd ed., pp. 567–605). Thousand Oaks, CA: Sage.

Lesperance, F., Frasure-Smith, N., Laliberte, M.-A., White, M., Lafointaine, S., Calderone, A., Taljie, M., & Rouleau, J. L. (2003). An open-label study of Nefazodone treatment of major depression in patients with congestive heart failure. *Canadian Journal of Psychiatry, 48*(10), 695–701.

Maguire, P. (1987). *Doing participatory research: A feminist approach.* Amherst: Center for International Education, School of Education, University of Massachusetts.

May, R. (1975). *The courage to create.* New York: Norton.

McDermott, J. (Ed.). (1973). *The philosophy of John Dewey: Vol. 1, The structure of experience, Vol. 2, The lived experience.* New York: Putman.

Reason, P., & Torbert, W. (2001). Toward a transformational science: A further look at the scientific merits of action research. *Concepts and Transformations, 6*(1), 1–37.

Rodney, P. A., & Varcoe, C. (2001). Toward ethical inquiry in the economic evaluation of nursing practice. *Canadian Journal of Nursing Research, 33*(1), 35–57.

Schreiber, R., & Hartrick, G. (2002). Keeping it together: How women use the biomedical explanatory model to manage the stigma of depression. *Health Care for Women International, 23*(2), 91–105.

Steele, R. G. (2002). Experiences of families in which a child has a prolonged terminal illness: Modifying factors. *International Journal of Palliative Care, 8*(9), 418–434.

Torbert, W. R. (1991). *The power of balance.* Newbury Park, CA: Sage.

Conclusion

Based on previous writing that I (Gweneth) have done in the area of family nursing, I have received invitations to speak and work with different groups of students, practicing nurses, and nurse educators. During these times I am often asked if what I am presenting is written anywhere. The reason that many of the nurses ask for something in writing is because although what I have said affirms their own knowing of families and of nursing practice the contexts they work in do not necessarily support such practice. One such experience was during a conversation with a group of nurses in New Zealand. As I described a relational view of nursing to a group of public health nurses one nurse declared, 'I have been waiting 25 years to hear someone say what you just did.' This nurse went on to describe how very early on in her career she had come to see and join families similar to the way I suggested; however, she never really spoke about it with anyone because the policies and practice guidelines that focused on service delivery and problem resolution did not condone such practice. Her story echoed what I had heard from many nurses over the years—that approaching their practice relationally 'works' (in terms of promoting family health and capacity) yet is not necessarily valued or supported in practice guidelines, policy and/or procedures. As a result of these experiences, I decided that it was time to write about relational practice in a way that articulates how it is not only theoretically sound but how it is also more adequate and ethical than many of the currently sanctioned approaches.

At the time of my decision I was working on a research project with Colleen in the area of nursing ethics. Through our passionate and challenging conversations it became clear to me that (because of our similarities and differences) together we might offer a picture of family nursing that could more adequately respond to the diversity of people/families and the complexity of nursing today. One thing I did not fully appreciate was how writing this book would expand my own knowing of family nursing and enable me to bring another level of form to my thinking. And, being able to share that creative process with Colleen has been wonderful—we have supported, inspired, and challenged each other and through it all somehow it has not really felt like 'work'.

When Gweneth first invited me to write this book with her, I (Colleen) thought that she had either misunderstood what my interests and commitments were, had seriously overestimated my abilities, or both! 'No way', I said. 'I don't do that stuff—I do violence, substance abuse, racism'. Here I both betrayed my narrow understanding of 'family nursing' and revealed how my forays into the family nursing literature had left me cold. What I had read of family nursing had not resonated with either my personal experience of family, nor with how I had come to practice as a nurse with families. Now, thanks to Gweneth, I have had an opportunity to try to bring my experience, practice, and theory more closely together, learning continuously in the process.

My (Colleen) research and writing in areas such as women's health, violence, racism, and the culture of health care often seems to be of interest only to those nurses who have particular interests in those areas. Yet as I believe that all nurses need to have understanding in these areas, I weave such ideas into my work with all nurses and students with whom I work. And, I realized that women's health, violence, racism, and experiences of health and health care are lived by and within family. Thus in this book I have had the opportunity to bring these substantive concerns into thinking about family nursing.

The process in which we have engaged together mirrors the process we hope you will pursue in using this book. We brought our ideas together and they became something more than either of us could have done separately, and in the process each of us has been changed. In this book we describe what it is 'we set our hearts on' as nurses. In offering an approach to family nursing as a relational inquiry, we have attempted to highlight the complex, interconnected nature of health and healing and of family nursing practice. In so doing, we have emphasized the significance of sociocontextual structures and illustrated how people/families can only be understood in relation to their social, historical, political, and economic circumstances. Overall we have invited you to join us in examining what it is you 'know' about family, to expand your knowledge by looking through different lenses, and to reflexively consider how you live knowledge in your everyday practice.

From the stories we have told and the literature we have cited throughout this book it is evident that there have been many who have contributed to the knowing and knowledge we have presented. In essence the process of writing this book has served as an opportunity for us to bring our own previous work and understandings forward, collaboratively explore the knowledge others have offered, and ultimately re-search and articulate new possibilities for family nursing practice. As we reach the end of our writing, we find the process has brought us full circle to begin again. As we have said throughout, knowledge is at best partial, always provisional, and forever in the process of developing. Thus, we anticipate that we will learn much more as we carry on in our work and as we engage with you, our readers, with your ideas, critiques, and suggestions.

As we stated at the beginning of this book, we view nursing practice as a way of being as much as a particular form of action. We believe that it is the *way* a nurse works with people/families; what the nurse sees, thinks, and takes note of when assessing families; and *how* he or she goes about engaging with knowledge and promoting health that makes practice relational. Relational practice involves a deeply embodied process of thoughtful knowing-in-action. Therefore, our overall intent has been to foster a more critically conscious way of being that is evidenced in respectful, compassionate, equitable, and socially just nursing actions. We hope that what we presented offered you 'food for thought' and that it also supported the development of your own capacity as a knowledgeable, relational practitioner. In closing, we wish you well as you continue to expand your knowledge and understanding of family and family nursing and we hope that you continue to imagine new possibilities as you carry on in your practice.

Gweneth and Colleen

INDEX

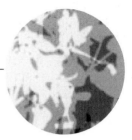